T0306108

Single Embryo Transfer

Single Embryo Transfer

Edited by

J. Gerris
Ghent University, Belgium

G. D. Adamson
Fertility Physicians of Northern California, USA

P. De Sutter
Ghent University, Belgium

C. Racowsky
Brigham & Women's Hospital, Harvard Medical School, USA

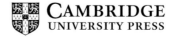
CAMBRIDGE
UNIVERSITY PRESS

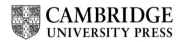

CAMBRIDGE
UNIVERSITY PRESS

Shaftesbury Road, Cambridge CB2 8EA, United Kingdom

One Liberty Plaza, 20th Floor, New York, NY 10006, USA

477 Williamstown Road, Port Melbourne, VIC 3207, Australia

314–321, 3rd Floor, Plot 3, Splendor Forum, Jasola District Centre, New Delhi – 110025, India

103 Penang Road, #05–06/07, Visioncrest Commercial, Singapore 238467

Cambridge University Press is part of Cambridge University Press & Assessment, a department of the University of Cambridge.

We share the University's mission to contribute to society through the pursuit of education, learning and research at the highest international levels of excellence.

www.cambridge.org
Information on this title: www.cambridge.org/9780521888349

First published 2009
First paperback edition 2012

A catalogue record for this publication is available from the British Library

Library of Congress Cataloging-in-Publication data
Single embryo transfer / edited by J. Gerris . . . [et al.].
    p. ; cm.
Includes bibliographical references and index.
ISBN 978-0-521-88834-9 (hardback)
1. Fertilization in vitro, Human.   2. Human embryo – Transplantation.
I. Gerris, Jan.
[DNLM: 1. Embryo Transfer – methods.   2. Pregnancy Complications.
3. Pregnancy, Multiple. WQ 208 S617   2009]
RG135.S57   2009
618.1´780599 – dc22   2008030870

ISBN   978-0-521-88834-9   Hardback
ISBN   978-1-107-41152-4   Paperback

Contents

Section 3: Controversies

Color plate section is between pages 150 and
   151.

Contributors

G. David Adamson MD
Fertility Physicians of Northern California, Palo Alto, CA, USA

Christina Bergh MD PhD
Department of Obstetrics & Gynecology, Sahlgrenska University Hospital, Göteborg, Sweden

Siladitya Bhattacharya MD PhD
Department of Obstetrics & Gynaecology, Aberdeen Maternity Hospital, Aberdeen, UK

Didi D. M. Braat MD PhD
Department of Obstetrics & Gynecology, Radboud University Nijmegen Medical Center, Nijmegen, The Netherlands

John Collins MD
Department of Obstetrics & Gynecology, McMaster University, Hamilton, Ontario, Canada

Sharon N. Covington MSW
Shady Grove Fertility Reproductive Science Center, Rockville, MD, USA

Alan H. DeCherney MD
Reproductive Biology & Medicine Branch, National Institute of Child Health & Human Development, NIH, Bethesda, MD, USA

Petra De Sutter MD PhD
Center for Reproductive Medicine, Ghent University, Ghent, Belgium

Hasan M. El-Fakahany MD
Department of Obstetrics, Gynecology & Reproductive
Sciences, Yale University School of Medicine, New
Haven, CT, USA

Ofer Fainaru MD PhD
Center for Reproductive Medicine, Brigham &
Women's Hospital, Boston, MA, USA

Reginald Finger MD MPH
Southeastern Center for Fertility & Reproductive
Surgery, Knoxville, TN, USA

Jan Gerris MD PhD
Center for Reproductive Medicine, Ghent University,
Ghent, Belgium

Mark D. Hornstein MD
Center for Reproductive Medicine, Brigham &
Women's Hospital, Boston, MA, USA

Robert P. S. Jansen MD
Sydney IVF, Sydney, Australia

Per-Olof Karlström MD PhD
Center of Reproduction Academish Hospital,
Uppsala, Sweden

Jeffrey A. Keenan MD
Southeastern Center for Fertility & Reproductive
Surgery, Knoxville, TN, USA

Jan A. M. Kremer MD PhD
Department of Obstetrics & Gynecology, Radboud
University Nijmegen Medical Center, Nijmegen,
The Netherlands

Eric D. Levens MD
Reproductive Biology & Medicine Branch, National
Institute of Child Health & Human Development, NIH,
Bethesda, MD, USA

Anne Loft MD
The Fertility Clinic, Copenhagen University Hospital,
Copenhagen, Denmark

Steven J. McArthur BSc
Sydney IVF, Sydney, Australia

Janetti Marotta PhD
Fertility Physicians of Northern California, Palo Alto,
CA, USA

Marius Meintjes MD PhD
Presbyterian Hospital ARTS Program, Dallas, TX, USA

John M. Norian MD
Reproductive Biology & Medicine Branch, National
Institute of Child Health & Human Development, NIH,
Bethesda, MD, USA

Guido Pennings MD PhD
Center for Environmental Philosophy & Bioethics,
Department of Philosophy, University of Ghent,
Ghent, Belgium

Anja Pinborg MD DMSci
The Fertility Clinic, Copenhagen University Hospital,
Copenhagen, Denmark

Karen J. Purcell MD PhD
Fertility Physicians of Northern California, Palo Alto,
CA, USA

Catherine Racowsky PhD
Department of Obstetrics, Gynecology & Reproductive
Biology, Brigham & Women's Hospital, Harvard
Medical School, Boston, MA, USA

Denny Sakkas PhD
Department of Obstetrics, Gynecology & Reproductive
Sciences, Yale University School of Medicine, New
Haven, CT, USA

Lynette Scott PhD
The Fertility Centers of New England, Reading,
MA, USA

Emre U. Seli MD
Department of Obstetrics, Gynecology & Reproductive
Sciences, Yale University School of Medicine, New
Haven, CT, USA

Christine C. Skiadas MD
Department of Obstetrics, Gynecology & Reproductive
Biology, Brigham & Women's Hospital, Harvard
Medical School, Boston, MA, USA

Viveca Söderström-Anttila MD PhD
The Väestöliitto Fertility Clinic, Helsinki, Finland

Ann Thurin-Kjellberg MD PhD
Department of Obstetrics & Gynecology, Sahlgrenska
University Hospital, Göteborg, Sweden

Aila Tiitinen MD PhD
Department of Obstetrics & Gynecology, Helsinki
University Central Hospital, Helsinki, Finland

Jonathan Van Blerkom PhD
Department of Molecular, Cellular & Developmental
Biology, University of Colorado, Boulder, CO, USA;
Colorado Reproductive Endocrinology, Rose Medical
Center, Denver, CO, USA

Aafke P.A. van Montfoort PhD
IVF Laboratory, Department of Obstetrics &
Gynecology, Academic Hospital of Maastricht,
Maastricht, The Netherlands

Arno M. van Peperstraten MD
Department of Obstetrics & Gynecology, Radboud
University Nijmegen Medical Center, Nijmegen, The
Netherlands

André Van Steirteghem MD PhD
Center for Reproductive Medicine, Vrije Universiteit
Brussel, Brussels, Belgium

Willem Verpoest MD
Center for Reproductive Medicine, Vrije Universiteit
Brussel, Brussels, Belgium

Ulla-Britt Wennerholm MD PhD
Perinatal Center, Department of Obstetrics &
Gynecology, Sahlgrenska University Hospital East,
Göteborg, Sweden

Foreword

In 1980 in the United States, that is before in vitro fertilization (IVF) or the widespread use of ovulatory drugs, some 1.8% of all births were multiple – mostly twins. By the mid first decade of the twenty-first century, this figure has doubled and many of the births have been of triplets or more. Other nations have had a similar experience.

This is no trivial matter.

Fortunately, most neonate twins and triplets are normal, but multiples have problems – even twins – and these problems can be serious, such as mental retardation.

Many reproductive endocrinologists and other users of ovulatory drugs are really not focused on the plight of multiples for the simple reason that in this age of specialization they do not participate in the obstetrical or pediatric care of their successful patients.

In this twenty-first century, it is truly time that those called upon to overcome infertility strive to produce not a baby, but a normal healthy baby.

If these observations have merit, every reproductive endocrinologist or other user of ovulatory drugs would benefit his or her patients by reading the first chapter of *Single Embryo Transfer*. This chapter by Wennerholm titled, "The risks associated with multiple pregnancies" spells out the reasons to do everything possible to avoid multiples.

For those who use ovulatory drugs, one of the things possible is elective single embryo transfer (eSET) by those who use IVF and have a patient to which it can be applied. *Single Embryo Transfer* is a comprehensive and authoritative resource to consider and to apply the option of eSET.

Before further consideration of eSET as a solution to the problem of multiples, an overall view of the cause of multiples might be in order.

Multiples can occur naturally or by ovulation induction or ovulation enhancement (OI/OE) or by IVF. Using 2003 data of the United States Bureau of Vital Statistics [1], it was shown that for all twins 60% were natural, 8% were caused by IVF and 32% by OI/OE. For triplets, 20% were natural, 14% were caused by IVF and 66% were caused by OI/OE.

Ovulation induction/ovulation enhancement is far more responsible for multiples and their problems than IVF. These data point to the proposition that many patients now treated by OI/OE might well be good candidates for IVF if they qualified for eSET.

It is significant that some of the physiological principles of eSET so well covered in this book also are fundamental to IVF in general. Thus, these chapters are well worth the attention of all who use IVF in any form.

We might mention a few. We still struggle to identify the egg, sperm, or embryo which has pregnancy potential. To be updated on this elusive goal will be rewarding. Thus, a reading of Chapter 2 by Van Blerkom titled, "An overview of determinants of oocyte and embryo developmental competence: specificity, accuracy and applicability in clinical IVF" will be extremely rewarding as will be a reading of Chapter 8, "Sequential embryo selection for single embryo transfer" by Lynette Scott.

Oddly enough, not all IVF programs have the capability of cryopreservation. In this twenty-first century, such a capability is essential. The rationale and options for cryopreservation as practiced in Europe and America are set out in Chapters 9A and 9B, specifically, 9A by Tiitinen titled, "Cryo-augmentation after single embryo transfer: the European experience," and Chapter 9B by Meintjes titled, "Cryo-augmentation after single embryo transfer: the American experience."

These few examples and others show that *Single Embryo Transfer* deals with topics which should be mastered by all of those who practice IVF in any form.

Those who pioneered IVF share a heavy responsibility for its unintended complications and for their elimination.

The use of eSET when applicable would be a giant step to a better reproductive world. *Single Embryo Transfer* admirably points the way.

Howard W. Jones, Jr., MD
Professor Emeritus
Department of Obstetrics and Gynecology
Eastern Virginia Medical School
Norfolk, Virginia
Professor Emeritus
Department of Gynecology and Obstetrics
Johns Hopkins University School of Medicine
Baltimore, Maryland

REFERENCE

1. H W. Jones, The iatrogenic multiple births: a 2003 checkup. *Fertil. Steril.*, **87** (2007), 453–455.

Preface

The idea to transfer just one embryo in a treatment cycle of in vitro fertilization (IVF) or intracytoplasmic sperm injection (ICSI) was launched 10 years ago [1] and applied in a first series of patients with medical contraindications for multiple pregnancies [2]. These included women with diabetes mellitus, congenital anomalies of the uterus, isthmic insufficiency or with a history of early loss of (multiple) pregnancy.

Ten years later, SET (single embryo transfer) has acquired a certain place in the practice of IVF/ICSI. This place is by no means uncontroversial. Intended to be a reasonable answer to the very high proportion of multiple pregnancies [3, 4], it has been advocated vividly by some clinicians [5] and antagonized by others [6].

During the last few years, numerous articles have appeared that have addressed varying aspects of SET: patient selection, embryo selection, health-economic aspects, the definition of what counts as a success and what as a complication, the complication itself, counseling, patient's autonomy, impediments to SET, arguments in favor or against SET. It seems that the possibility of SET has provided a new and invigorating perspective to IVF. Single embryo transfer has allowed us to study the relationship between the morphology of individual embryos and their implantation potential, the true incidence of monozygotic twinning and, to some extent, the black box of early pregnancy. Single embryo transfer illustrates that "good clinical practice" for some consists of transferring just one embryo in over 80% of their patients, whereas others transfer three or more embryos in first attempts. These contrasts suggest that although under certain circumstances the application of SET can be considered, the process of finding an appropriate place for SET is far from concluded. Single embryo transfer has led some clinicians to consider less aggressive stimulation schemes on the basis of the assumption that less eggs are needed because less embryos are needed and cryopreservation does not work too well anyway. All of this remains open to debate. Some have tried to give natural cycle IVF or minimally modified natural cycle IVF a place in the spectrum of possibilities. Single embryo transfer has introduced the notion of patient-friendly IVF or minimally invasive IVF. Some are delving deep into the embryo to single out the 100%-implanter by studying chromosomes and metabolism. All in all, the introduction of SET has spurred reflection over the whole range of aspects related to IVF treatment.

The goals of this book are several. It is not our goal to convince or to criticize, but to make aware. We defend the value of a neutral view based on data for all to see and use to the perceived benefit of their patients. What SET is, should be or cannot be depends in a very large measure on societal factors for which practicing physicians cannot be held responsible. So, whether SET is applied in up to 80% of an IVF population, as is the case in some Scandinavian countries, or given no place at all, is not problematic *in se*. More problematic is the fact that complications of multiple pregnancies are minimized or the fact that prevention of triplets is considered a goal worth achieving whereas decreasing the huge incidence of twin pregnancies is not. There is an impact in this debate of semantics. What *is* a complication? What is a risk? For some, a twin pregnancy *is* a complication, for others it *may but not necessarily entail* complications, for others a human twin pregnancy has the status of normal reproductive activity given the possibilities of perinatal medicine *anno* 2008.

Nevertheless, it is generally accepted that multiple pregnancies constitute the most frequent and serious (cause of) complications of IVF/ICSI. Both higher-order multiple and twin pregnancies do

entail, in a different degree of frequency and of severity, a number of sequels that affect the children, the mother, the parents, the families and society as a whole.

It is also recognized that limiting the number of embryos to transfer is the only effective method to decrease the incidence of multiple pregnancies. However, due to the societal circumstances in which IVF/ICSI is performed, limitations on the number of embryos to transfer and more specifically the introduction of SET has been met with more enthusiasm in some countries than others. Whereas in some countries, laws regulate the number of embryos to transfer, in others, different mechanisms have been employed to decrease the twinning rate. In others still, the debate is just beginning or there is even an anti-SET attitude.

In order to safeguard its potential value and at the same time acknowledge its limitations, we think that the time is ripe to assess the possibilities and limitations of SET.

On a couple of things there seems to be increasing agreement.

First, SET works. Countries where it is implemented on a large scale, have seen their multiple pregnancy rates drop dramatically without the much feared decrease in their own pre-SET pregnancy rate as a consequence of the introduction of SET. This is, e.g., the case in Sweden, Finland and Belgium. In contrast, the overall pregnancy rate in countries where SET is difficult to introduce, e.g. the United States of America, is significantly higher, but at the price of a much higher rate of multiple pregnancies. We should try to find an equilibrium between results and complications, which is acceptable *in that particular society*.

Second, SET has spurred embryologists to search for more effective methods of embryo selection. Because morphological criteria are and will probably remain for some time to come the cornerstone of embryo selection, there has been a great effort to optimize the use of traditional morphological criteria and to validate new criteria [7]. Other, non-invasive, methods of embryo assessment, derived from their metabolic activity, are the focus of research. Invasive techniques, such as aneuploidy screening, have also been proposed [8]. Much of this is the consequence of the increased need to select the high implantation potential or top quality embryo.

Third, SET seems to do more than just decrease the number of twin births, thereby increasing the obstetrical and neonatal outcome of the average child after IVF/ICSI. Singletons born after SET perform as well as naturally conceived singletons; and singletons after SET perform better than singletons after double embryo transfer [9, 10]. The allegedly decreased outcome of singletons after IVF/ICSI on the basis of meta-analysis of IVF/ICSI comprising all transfers (from one to many embryos) in all cycles (first until high rank trials) in all patients (young and old) reflects an average that does not exist, since both good prognosis patients (the ones that used to end up with twins in first cycles after two-embryo or three-embryo transfer) and bad prognosis patients (the ones that ended up with singletons after transfer of many embryos in high rank trials) were included in this analysis [11]. On the other hand, it has to be admitted that this meta-analysis is based on very large numbers of pregnancies and children, whereas the data on SET children have considered much smaller numbers.

Fourth, SET is a prism through which the light of assisted reproductive technology (ART) breaks into new perspectives. Patient counseling has become very important. Cryopreservation has been upgraded from a solution for an ethical problem (what to do with supernumerary embryos?) to a goal in itself (how to optimally use one oocyte harvest?) [12]. Oocyte harvest (what is achieved with the total number of eggs retrieved in a single oocyte pick-up, replaced in both the fresh and subsequent thaw cycles), and certainly not an individual embryo transfer, has become the clinical, financial and philosophical unit of thinking in IVF/ICSI. Even the definition itself of what success is, has been the topic of an international debate.

Many of these effects of SET are still under discussion, as is SET itself. Each country, each region, each center has to find out for itself whether and how to introduce SET. Financial constraints (patients having to pay for ART but not for neonatal costs), league-tables (mixing up soccer with medicine) and other imperative conditions make it much harder for some centers to adopt SET than for others. For that reason, the editors of this book explicitly aim at giving a free voice to different convictions and tendencies which are present in different parts of the world. There is no better and worse, just difference. From those differences, we can all learn. Conditions in which we work may change more quickly than we can imagine.

Generally speaking, the will to optimize IVF/ICSI outcome and the readiness to accept the birth of a healthy singleton as the ideal outcome are present.

We hope that bringing together expert opinions, often from pioneers and opinion leaders in the world, on varying aspects of SET, from the clinical to the embryological, from the patient perspective to the insurer's perspective, may help the open-minded reader to see for her- or himself what best use can be made of SET in her or his particular practice. All should strive towards an ideal start for tomorrow's children.

For SET to work, four elements are critically important: (1) creating awareness among all practitioners, patients and other stakeholders of reproductive medicine; (2) creating a continuous marketing effort of SET; (3) creating agreement and adjustment among clinical embryologists regarding embryo criteria for selection prior to transfer or/and cryopreservation; and (4) increasing access to treatment by creating funding or financing of ART which keeps a balance between social justice and a reasonable remuneration of all practitioners. These principles are meant to be applicable worldwide, not only in the richer parts of the world but in third-world settings as well.

This book can be of interest to all involved directly or indirectly in IVF and ICSI: physicians (reproductive endocrinologists, pediatricians, gynecologists, urologists, general practitioners, etc.) patients, embryologists, nurses and midwives, counseling and mental health specialists, administrative personnel, insurers, politicians and technocrats, civil servants of governments concerned about reproduction as a public health issue, ethicists and philosophers, and medical journalists. Single embryo transfer is a sign of maturation of IVF/ICSI and all who speak out on it must take their responsibilities. This holds for all countries, whatever their actual position, since it is likely that SET will slowly be implemented until it has attained a level of universal judiciousness that can be shared by the large majority of those involved.

REFERENCES

1. T. Coetsier and M. Dhont, Avoiding multiple pregnancies in in-vitro fertilization: who's afraid of single embryo transfer? *Hum. Reprod.*, **13** (1998), 2663–2664.

2. S. Vilska, A. Tiitinen, C. Hydén-Granskog and O. Hovatta, Elective transfer of one embryo results in an acceptable pregnancy rate and eliminates the risk of multiple birth. *Hum. Reprod.*, **14** (1999), 2392–2395.

3. J. Gerris, Single embryo transfer and IVF/ICSI outcome: a balanced appraisal. *Hum. Reprod. Update*, **11** (2005), 105–121.

4. C. Bergh, Single embryo transfer: a mini-review. *Hum. Reprod.*, **20** (2005), 323–327.

5. J. A. Land and J. L. H. Evers, What is the most relevant standard of success in assisted reproduction? Defining outcome in ART: a Gordian knot of safety, efficacy and quality. *Hum. Reprod.*, **19** (2004), 1046–1048.

6. N. Gleicher and D. Barad, The relative myth of elective single embryo transfer. *Hum. Reprod.*, **21** (2006), 1337–1344.

7. J. Holte, L. Berglund, K. Milton *et al.*, Construction of an evidence-based integrated morphology cleavage score for implantation potential of embryos scored and transferred on day 2 after oocyte retrieval. *Hum. Reprod.*, **22** (2007), 548–557.

8. C. Staessen, P. Platteau, E. Van Assche *et al.*, Comparison of blastocyst transfer with or without preimplantation genetic diagnosis for aneuploidy screening in couples with advanced maternal age: a prospective randomized controlled trial. *Hum. Reprod.*, **19** (2004), 2849–2858.

9. P. De Sutter, J. Bontinck, V. Schutyser *et al.*, First trimester bleeding and pregnancy outcome after assisted reproduction. *Hum. Reprod.*, **21** (2006), 1907–1911.

10. P. De Sutter, I. Delbaere, J. Gerris *et al.*, Birth weight of singletons in ART is higher after single than after double embryo transfer. *Hum. Reprod.*, **21** (2006), 2633–2637.

11. F. M. Helmerhorst, D. A. Perquin, D. Donker and M. J. Keirse, Perinatal outcome of singleton and twins after assisted conception: a systematic review of controlled studies. *BMJ*, **328** (2004), 261.

12. A. Tiitinen, M. Halttunen, P. Härkki, P. Vuoristo and C. Hyden-Granskog, Elective embryo transfer: the value of cryopreservation. *Hum. Reprod.*, **16** (2001), 1140–1144.

SECTION 1

Preliminaries

The risks associated with multiple pregnancies

Ulla-Britt Wennerholm

Introduction

The incidence of multiple pregnancies has increased dramatically during the past three decades primarily owing to the expanded use of infertility therapies and higher childbearing ages.

Women who become pregnant later have an increased risk of dizygotic twins, up to 37 years of age. Older maternal age accounts for 25–30% of the rise in multiple birth rates since 1970. Infertility treatment includes the use of ovulation-inducing drugs and assisted reproductive technology (ART). Births resulting from infertility treatment account for around 1–3% of all singleton live births, 30–50% of twin births and more than 75% of higher-order multiple births [1].

Multiple pregnancies are associated with considerable medical risks for the mother and offspring as well as excess obstetric and neonatal costs. It is increasingly thought that the high frequency of multiple births after ART is not acceptable, and strategies to reduce this frequency are being developed. However, patients and physicians all sometimes seem to underestimate the negative consequences of multiple pregnancy. This review therefore addresses the complications of multiple pregnancies, focusing on twin pregnancies, which constitute the vast majority (95–98%) of multiple pregnancies.

The PubMed and Cochrane databases were searched for relevant articles published in English before September 2007.

Trends in multiple births

In many countries, multiple birth rates began to decline in the 1950s, reaching a low point in the 1970s. Since then there has been a continuous increase in the frequency of twin pregnancy rates and twin birth rates in many countries in Western Europe and North America (Figure 1.1).

In most countries, rates of triplets and higher-order multiple births fluctuated around a relatively constant level until the mid 1970s. This was followed by a steep rise, after which there has been decline since 2000. In 11 European countries in 2000, multiple birth rates ranged from 11.7 to 19.0 per 1000 for twins and from 0.16 to 0.62 per 1000 for triplets and higher-order multiple births [2]. The latest report from the USA from 2004 showed that the twin birth rate was 32.2 per 1000, another record high. In contrast, the rate of triplet and higher-order multiple births showed a downward trend, the rate being 1.77 per 1000 [3].

Infertility treatment has played a major role in the increase in multiple pregnancies. The contribution of ART to multiple pregnancies is better known than that of ovulation stimulation without in vitro

Single Embryo Transfer, ed. J. Gerris, G. D. Adamson, P. De Sutter and C. Racowsky. Published by Cambridge University Press.
© Cambridge University Press 2009.

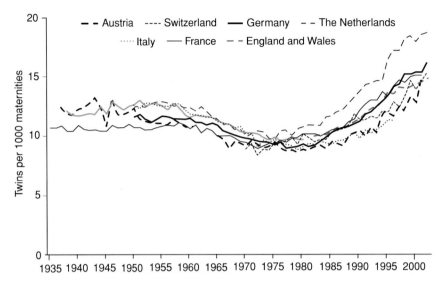

Figure 1.1 Twin births in selected European countries. Adapted from [52], with permission.

Table 1.1 Approximate risk of multiple birth after infertility treatment

	Multiple of population frequency[a]	
Infertility treatment	Twins	Triplets
Clomiphene citrate	12	200
Gonadotropins	20	500
IVF/ICSI cycles	30	500

[a] Population frequency is 1% for twins and 1 per 10 000 for triplets; ICSI, intracytoplasmic sperm injection. Adapted from Collins (49).

fertilization (IVF), because several countries have established national registries for ART outcomes. Table 1.1 presents the approximate risks of twins and triplets, relative to population frequency, after infertility treatment.

Recent reports from ART registries show a decline in multiple birth rates after ART. Data from the latest report from the European Society of Human Reproduction and Embryology (ESHRE) on ART results in Europe showed a multiple birth rate of 23.1% in 2003 (22% twins and 1.1% triplets) as compared with 24.5% in 2002 [4]. However, data from the USA showed that, in 2004, 51% of infants born after ART were still multiple birth babies (45% twins and 6% triplets) [5]. A dramatic decrease in the multiple birth rate after ART has occurred in a few European countries during recent years after the introduction of single embryo transfer. For example, in Sweden the multiple birth rate was 5.7% in 2004 as compared with 35% in 1991 and in addition delivery rates were maintained at around 26% [6].

Zygosity and chorionicity

There are two major types of twin pregnancies: dizygotic and monozygotic twin pregnancies. Dizygotic twins result from the fertilization of two separate eggs. They have two functionally separate placentas (dichorionic) although these may fuse to resemble one single placenta macroscopically at birth. A thick membrane consisting of two layers of chorion and two layers of amnion separates the cavities. Monozygotic twin pregnancies arise from the fertilization of a single egg. If the split occurs within 3 days of conception the result will be a monozygotic dichorionic twin pregnancy with two placentas (which may also fuse as mentioned above). Later splitting, between days 4 and 8, will result in a monozygotic monochorionic twin pregnancy with a single placenta and two amniotic cavities with a thin dividing membrane consisting of two layers of amnion. Splitting after day 8 will result in a monochorionic monoamniotic twin pregnancy with a single amniotic cavity and a single placenta. Conjoined twinning occurs rarely, in about 1: 50 000 pregnancies. It is caused by failure of complete separation of the embryo around the 15th to 17th day after conception.

The incidence of dizygotic twinning in the population is affected by many factors such as race, heredity, maternal age and ovulation induction with or without IVF. The rates vary from 3 to 40 per 1000 pregnancies. The rate of monozygotic twinning in the general population is thought to be fairly stable around the world and over time, 3 to 4 per 1000. In whites, about 30% of twin pregnancies are monozygotic and about 70% are dizygotic, about one third of the monozygotic twins are dichorionic and two thirds are monochorionic. Approximately 1 per 100 of monozygotic twins are monoamniotic.

The proportions of monozygotic and dizygotic twins are very different in spontaneously conceived twins as compared with iatrogenic twins; 95% of iatrogenic twins are dizygotic.

Zygosity and chorionicity are important variables for outcomes in multiple pregnancies. Perinatal mortality and morbidity are elevated in monozygotic and particularly in monochorionic twins. Monochorionic twins have a fivefold increase in fetal/perinatal loss, a tenfold increase in antenatally acquired cerebral lesion and almost twice the incidence of intrauterine growth restriction. The key to management of multiple pregnancies is accurate determination of chorionicity, which is best performed in the first trimester where accuracy rates approach 100% [7, 8].

Maternal morbidity and mortality

Multiple pregnancies are associated with a range of well-documented risks to the health of the mother. Multiple pregnancy increases the risk of maternal mortality as compared with singleton pregnancies, especially in developing countries. A mortality rate of 14.9 per 100 000 pregnancies was reported for multiple pregnancies in Europe in 1994, as compared with 5.2 per 100 000 for singleton pregnancies. In France, the corresponding figures were 10.2 per 100 000 and 4.4 per 100 000 [9]. In contrast, maternal mortality rates of 77 per 100 000 were associated with multiple pregnancies in Latin America between 1985 and 1997, as compared with 43 for singleton pregnancies [10]. Maternal deaths were caused by eclampsia, excessive blood loss and pulmonary edema following administration of parenteral beta-mimetics as tocolytics. Since maternal deaths are rare in the developed world, other measures of pregnancy outcome have been suggested such as "near misses" or severe obstetric morbidity (severe pre-eclampsia including eclampsia and HELLP [hemolysis elevated liver enzymes and low platelets] syndrome, severe hemorrhage, severe sepsis, uterine rupture). In a case–control study comprising 50 000 pregnant women, over 1 out of every 100 women suffered from severe obstetric morbidity [11]. Two thirds of these cases were related to obstetric hemorrhage and one third to severe pre-eclampsia. Multiple pregnancy was found to be an independent risk factor (adjusted odds ratio (OR) = 2.21, 95% confidence intervals (CI) = 1.24–3.96) for such a life-threatening event. In a retrospective Canadian cohort study the incidence of maternal complications in 165 188 singleton pregnancies and 44 674 multiple pregnancies were compared [12]. Multiple pregnancies were associated with significant increases in cardiac morbidity (myocardial infarction, pulmonary edema and heart failure), hemorrhage, pre-eclampsia, amniotic fluid embolism, gestational diabetes, and the need for obstetric interventions, hysterectomy and blood transfusion. A recent population-based report by Luke and Brown confirmed that higher plurality and higher maternal age were associated with increased risk of many pregnancy complications, e.g. diabetes, hypertension and excessive bleeding [13]. Multiple pregnancy is an independent risk factor and has a 2.3 OR for the woman (or mother) to be admitted to an intensive care unit [14].

Hypertensive disorders of pregnancy

Hypertension with or without proteinuria is one of the main maternal complications associated with multiple pregnancy. As compared with singleton pregnancies women with twin gestations have higher rates of hypertensive disorders; the OR in twins as compared with singleton pregnancies varies from 1.8 to 3.4 according to one review [15]. Pregnancy-induced hypertension and pre-eclampsia are both more common in women carrying twins. For example, in a secondary analysis of a large prospective multicenter trial of women with twin ($n = 684$) and singleton ($n = 2946$) pregnancies, designed to investigate the efficacy of low dose aspirin for the prevention of pre-eclampsia, rates of gestational hypertension and pre-eclampsia were twice as high in twin as compared with singleton pregnancies (13% vs. 5–6% for both) [16]. In addition, early severe pre-eclampsia and HELLP syndrome were seen more frequently with twin pregnancies. Moreover, women with twin pregnancies and hypertensive complications had higher rates of adverse neonatal outcomes than those with singleton pregnancies.

In triplet pregnancies the incidence of pre-eclampsia is between 24% and 60%, and it may be as high as 90% in quadruplet pregnancies [17].

A sixfold relative risk (RR) of eclampsia in multiple, when compared with singleton, pregnancies was found in a survey in the UK (28.1/10 000 vs. 4.7/10 000 pregnancies, respectively) [18].

No intervention (e.g., low dose aspirin) has shown to prevent or reduce the incidence of hypertensive complications in multiple pregnancies.

Obstetric hemorrhage

Severe obstetric hemorrhage contributes to severe maternal morbidity and is the third most common cause of direct maternal death in the UK. It was found that severe hemorrhage was 2.3-fold more common in multiple pregnancies [11]. The high incidence of uterine atony and dystocia, both contributing to postpartum hemorrhage and an increased rate of operative deliveries, are important reasons. Placental abruption and placenta previa are seen slightly more often in multiple pregnancies and may cause bleeding. Iron and folate deficiency are more often seen in multiple pregnancies and the incidence of anemia is doubled in twin pregnancies.

Obstetric intervention

Maternal morbidity is also related to mode of delivery, particularly emergency Cesarean section. Cesarean section is associated with more complications than vaginal deliveries, e.g. infections, hemorrhage and thrombo-embolic disease. A much higher frequency of Cesarean section is seen in multiple pregnancies as compared with singleton pregnancies, mainly attributable to malpresentations. Cesarean section in multiple pregnancies has been shown to be associated with an additional risk of endometritis and abdominal wound infections, as compared with Cesarean section in singleton pregnancies according to a Finnish study [19].

Prophylactic cervical cerclage has been used to prevent preterm birth in multiple pregnancies. A meta-analysis from two randomized controlled trials showed no benefit, and the routine use of cerclage cannot be recommended [20].

Emergent peripartum hysterectomy, defined as a hysterectomy performed at the time of delivery or in the immediate postpartum period, has been shown to be more common in multiple pregnancies than in singletons [21].

Maternal complications in triplet, quadruplet and higher-order multiple pregnancies

Maternal morbidity is related to the number of fetuses. A recent population-based study showed that the risks of maternal morbidity and obstetric complications (e.g., pregnancy-associated hypertension and eclampsia, anemia, diabetes mellitus, abruptio placentae, premature rupture of the membranes and Cesarean delivery were increased in triplet pregnancies ($n = 5491$), quadruplet pregnancies and higher-order multiple pregnancies

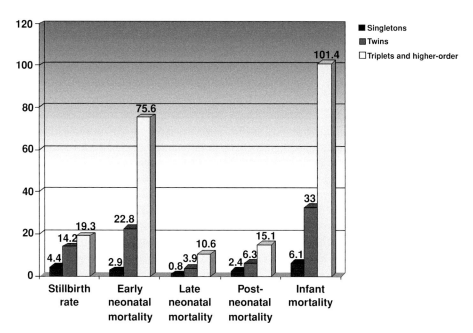

Figure 1.2 Mortality and multiplicity of birth in England and Wales 1991. Adapted from Doyle [53]. Stillbirth rate: late fetal deaths/1000 total births; Early neonatal mortality: deaths in first 6 days/1000 live births; Late neonatal mortality: deaths 7–27 days/1000 live births; Post-neonatal mortality: deaths 28 days to 1 year/1000 live births; Infant mortality: deaths < 1 year/1000 live births.

($n = 423$) as compared with twin pregnancies ($n = 152\,238$), even after adjustment for the main confounding factors. A dose–response relationship was observed for pregnancy-associated hypertension, diabetes mellitus and abruptio placenta with higher ORs in women with quadruplet and higher-order multiple gestations than in women with triplet pregnancies [22].

Fetal and neonatal outcome

Mortality

Early fetal loss in the form of "vanishing twin" is a rather common occurrence following ART. In a review, the rates of "vanishing twin" were 33% and 56%, respectively when two or three gestational sacs were detected initially. When two or three embryos were initially detected, the rates were 28.5% and 51.5%, respectively [23].

All mortality rates (stillbirths, early neonatal, late neonatal and infant mortality) are higher in multiple pregnancies as compared with singletons and the rates increase with the number of fetuses. Differences in mortality rates from a population-based registry in England and Wales, are shown in Figure 1.2. The figure shows that multiple births contribute greatly to overall mortality rates, despite their relative rarity. In England and Wales, multiple births represented 2.5% of all births and 8% of stillbirths, 19% of all neonatal deaths and 7% of all post-neonatal deaths in 1991. Disparity related to multiplicity was greatest when it came to neonatal deaths, the rate for twins being 7 times higher and the rate for triplets and higher-order multiple births more than 20 times higher than the singleton rate.

Recent data from the USA show that the infant mortality rate in 2000 was 6.1 per 1000 live births for singleton pregnancies and 31.1 per 1000 for multiple pregnancies [24]. As in the UK, this rate increased with the number of fetuses, from 28.9 per 1000 live births for twins, to 63.2 per 1000 for triplets and 95.5 per 1000 for quadruplets. Although multiple births account for only 3% of births, they account for 14% of infant deaths in the USA.

A large population-based cohort study of more than 1 000 000 births in Australia and the USA, of which more than 20 000 were twins, found that twins had an approximately fivefold increase in the risk of fetal death and a sevenfold increase in the risk of neonatal death as compared with singletons. However, the risk varied between twin pregnancies, with second-born twins, twins from the same-sex or growth-discordant pairs and twins whose co-twin died in utero having an increased risk of death [25]. No significant difference was seen in gestational age-specific mortality rate between gestational week 23 and 35 when singletons, twins and triplets were compared [26].

Gestational age and birth weight

Preterm delivery (before 37 completed weeks) and low birth weight (< 2500 g) are the main factors accounting for the excess in neonatal morbidity seen in the infants from multiple births. On average, multiple birth infants are born much earlier and are smaller than singletons. A generally accepted clinical rule for multifetal pregnancies is that gestational age at delivery is about 3 weeks less for every additional fetus. As in singletons, the causes of preterm birth can be divided into three groups: spontaneous preterm labor; preterm premature rupture of the membranes (PPROM); and indicated preterm delivery on maternal or fetal indications. One study comprising 434 sets of twins found that spontaneous labor accounted for 54%, PPROM for 22% and indicated delivery for 23% of the preterm deliveries. (The corresponding figures for preterm singleton deliveries were 44%, 31% and 23%, respectively) [27]. Chorionicity plays an important role: the risk of preterm birth before 32 weeks is almost doubled in monochorionic twins compared with dichorionic twins [28]. Table 1.2 shows the main differences between singletons, twins and triplets and higher-

order multiples in gestational age and birth weight using the latest National Vital Statistics Report for the year 2004 in the USA [3]. In 2004, the average birth weight of twins was nearly 1000 grams lower than that of singletons and the average triplet weighed about 50% less than the average singleton.

There is controversy concerning which fetal growth curve should be used in multiple pregnancies. Fetal growth curves are similar for singletons, twins and triplets up to about 28 weeks of gestation. After this the curve of multiples begins to deviate from that of singletons and at approximately 35 weeks of gestation the curve of triplets begins to deviate from that of twins. Some investigators suggest that plurality-specific birth-weight-by-gestation standards should be used for assessment of fetal growth in multiple births, rather than singleton standards.

In general, twin pregnancies are at tenfold risk of resulting in growth-restricted babies as compared with singletons. The risk is higher in monochorionic pregnancies than in dichorionic pregnancies. One study demonstrated that the chance of having at least one growth-restricted twin was 34% in monochorionic and 23% in dichorionic twin pregnancies. The chance of both twins having growth restriction was fourfold higher in monochorionic pregnancies [3, 28].

Perinatal morbidity and mortality in twin pregnancies is related to intrapair birth weight discordance. The birth weight discordance for twins is calculated by dividing the difference between the weights of the two fetuses by the weight of the largest fetus. Compared with the less than 5% birth weight discordance category, the adjusted OR for stillborn fetuses associated with 20% to 29%, 30% to 39% and > 40% discordance was 1.7, 3.1 and 4.3, respectively, for the smaller twin and 1.8, 3.4 and 2.9, respectively, for the larger twin in same-sex twin pairs and 2.7, 6.2 and 12.8, respectively for the smaller twin in opposite-sex twin pairs [29]. The association of fetal death with birth weight discordance is also seen in triplet pregnancies. A birth weight discordance of 29% or more is associated with a significant risk of fetal death when compared

Table 1.2 Gestational age and birth weight characteristics by plurality: USA 2004

	Singletons	Twins	Triplets	Quadruplets	Quintuplets and higher-order multiples
Number	3 972 558	132 219	6 759	439	86
Percent very preterm	1.6	11.8	35.9	64.9	81.4
Percent preterm	10.8	59.7	93.0	95.9	100.0
Mean gestational age in weeks (standard deviation)	38.7 (2.4)	35.2 (3.6)	32.1 (83.9)	29.7 (4.5)	28.4 (2.7)
Percent very low birth weight	1.1	10.2	33.2	65.1	84.9
Percent low birth weight	6.3	56.6	94.1	98.4	100.0
Mean birth weight in grams (standard deviation)	3 316 (570)	2 333 (634)	1 700 (559)	1 276 (552)	1103 (383)

Very preterm is less than 32 completed weeks of gestation.
Preterm is less than 37 completed weeks of gestation.
Very low birth weight is less than 1500 grams.
Low birth weight is less than 2500 grams.
Source: From [3].

with less than 10% discordance. For the smallest, middle and largest triplets, the adjusted ORs are 10.9, 22.6 and 2.4, respectively.

Neonatal morbidity

The vast majority of excess morbidity in multiple births is attributable to preterm delivery and intrauterine growth restriction. Many multiples require treatment and extended care in neonatal intensive care units (NICUs) [30]. According to one study, 15% of singletons, 48% of twins and 78% of triplets and higher-order multiples were admitted to NICUs. In the study by Gardner and colleagues, twins, who constituted only 2.4% of all neonates, contributed disproportionately to neonatal morbidity, e.g. low Apgar score at 5 minutes (7.9%), intraventricular hemorrhage (IVH) grades 3 and 4 (11.4%), sepsis (7.6%), necrotizing enterocolitis (NEC) (9.9%) and respiratory distress syndrome (13.8%) [27]. In view of the large differences in gestational age at birth between singletons, twins and higher-order multiple births, several investigators have tried to correct for this and other confounding variables. One study with data from a large neonatal database showed that the gestational age-specific

long-term adverse outcome (NEC, IVH grade 3 or 4 or severe degrees of retinopathy of prematurity) was similar for singletons ($n = 36\,931$), twins ($n = 12\,302$) and triplets ($n = 2155$) at all viable premature weeks of gestation (week 23–35) [26]. In an Israeli national population-based study, respiratory distress syndrome was found to be more common among multiples despite higher exposure to antenatal steroids [31].

Fetal abnormalities

An individual fetus in a multiple gestation may be affected by both chromosomal and structural abnormalities. Women pregnant with twins are at greater risk of fetal chromosomal abnormalities than those with singletons. The increased risk of chromosomal abnormalities may be partially attributable to the fact that many mothers of dizygotic twins are of advanced maternal age. In a dizygotic pregnancy, each fetus has its own independent risk of a chromosomal or structural abnormality, so the overall risk of an abnormality increases as the number of fetuses increases. In a dizygotic twin pregnancy the risk of one fetus being aneuploid is approximately twice that in a singleton pregnancy. The risk of a chromosomal abnormality in a monozygotic multiple gestation is similar to the risk in a singleton pregnancy. However, monozygotic gestations are also at increased risk of other complications unique to monochorionic gestations, such as twin-to-twin transfusion syndrome (TTTS), twin reversed arterial perfusion syndrome and conjoined twins.

There are few large population-based studies comparing the prevalence of congenital malformations in twins and higher-order multiple pregnancies with singletons. In a review, Little and Bryan concluded that there is "almost certainly" an excess of malformations in twins as compared with singletons, the RR varying between 0.9 and 1.5 [32]. Monozygotic twins seem to be more affected than dizygotic twins, and the highest figures are found in monoamniotic twins.

All anatomical sites are involved but some specific malformations have been found to occur excessively in twins (e.g., cardiac, neural tube and brain defects and gastrointestinal and anterior abdominal wall defects). A large international registry study ($n = 260\,865$ twins) recently confirmed the higher risk of malformations in twins, as compared with singletons, the RR being 1.2 (95% CI 1.21–1.28). It was not possible to distinguish the RR between dizygotic and monozygotic twins [33].

Genetic counseling and testing is complex and challenging in multiple pregnancies. Options for screening tests are limited and less effective and amniocentesis or chorionic villus sampling may be associated with a higher risk of miscarriage. The ethical dilemmas facing the patient and doctors are complex when there is a diagnosis of a fetus with a non-fatal abnormality in a multiple gestation. Options include expectant management, termination of the entire pregnancy, or selective termination of the abnormal fetus. The procedural complications (e.g., miscarriage and preterm birth) after selective feticide seem to have decreased with greater experience. However, chorionicity should be determined before the procedure, since the technique is different in monochorionic and dichorionic pregnancies.

Special considerations

Twin-to-twin transfusion syndrome

Twin-to-twin transfusion syndrome usually presents in the mid-trimester with gross discordance in amniotic fluid volume, and it complicates one in five of all monochorionic pregnancies. This results from chronic circulatory imbalance between the vascular anastomoses that occur in practically all monochorionic placentae. It is associated with high rates of perinatal mortality from ruptured membranes, hydrops and growth restriction, and significant morbidity from cardiac and neurological sequelae. If untreated, early onset, severe TTTS is associated with perinatal mortality rates of more than 90% and more than 30% of survivors have abnormal neurodevelopment as a result of the combination of a severe antenatal insult and the complications of severe prematurity [34]. Ultrasound may be valuable in the prediction of TTTS. Increased nuchal translucency in weeks 10–14 has been found to be an early sign of TTTS, as has folding of the intertwin membrane in weeks 15–17. Since there is a wide clinical and sonographic variation in the manifestation of the syndrome, use of a specialized staging system of TTTS by Quintero *et al.* was proposed in 1999 [35]. Treatment strategies for this serious condition have remained controversial but two main approaches have been used. Serial aggressive amniodrainage is commonly used, being a relatively simple technique. It involves the repetitive percutaneous removal of 1–2 liters of amniotic fluid. The rationale for this technique is mainly to prevent preterm labor related to hydramnios. However, despite reported survival rates of up to 83%, this therapy has been associated with high perinatal morbidity, especially long-term neurodevelopmental damage, of between 5% and 58%. Fetoscopic selective laser photocoagulation of the vascular anastomoses at the intertwin membrane has been advocated at specialist centers. This treatment has been associated with survival rates of between 55% and 69% and reduced neurologic morbidity of between 5% and 11% in survivors. In a systematic review of observational and randomized controlled studies, laser photocoagulation seemed to be more effective than serial amnioreduction, with less associated perinatal morbidity and mortality [36]. The OR for overall survival ranged from 1.3 to 2.1, and for survival of at least one twin 2.4–2.9 for laser photocoagulation versus amnioreduction. Fetoscopic treatment was also associated with a significant reduction in neurological morbidity (OR 0.15–0.43). However, given the potential benefits of fetoscopic procedures, it is also important to consider the maternal risks. Maternal risks associated with maternal–fetal surgery are pulmonary edema and placental abruption, and anecdotal cases of maternal death have occurred [37].

Monoamniotic twins

Monoamniotic monochorionic twins are a rare but significant event, occurring in about 1% of monozygotic twins. An increased rate of monoamniotic twins has been reported following zona pellucida manipulation and IVF. Diagnosis is most typically by ultrasound, with the inability to distinguish a dividing membrane between the fetuses being the most typical feature. Monoamniotic twin pregnancies are associated with high rates of fetal mortality, cited at between 30% and 70%. In addition to the other complications that can occur in monochorionic pregnancies, monoamniotic twins are at elevated risk of fetal death owing to cord entanglement. Obstetric management protocols are based on several retrospective case series. Large well-controlled studies are needed to provide guidance in the management of monoamniotic twin pregnancies. In a recent report 96 monoamniotic twin sets from 1993 to 2003 were studied [38]. Perinatal death excluding lethal anomalies was 12.6%. Improved neonatal survival and decreased perinatal morbidity were seen among women admitted electively for inpatient fetal monitoring after 24 weeks of gestation, as compared with those who required an indicated admission. Elective admission patients underwent non-stress tests one to three times a day, whereas outpatients were tested one to three times a week.

No fetal deaths occurred in the inpatient group, while a 14.8% (13/88) death rate was noted in the outpatient group.

At many institutions today, elective Cesarean delivery between 32 and 34 weeks of gestation is recommended for women with monoamniotic twins, after administration of corticosteroid for enhancement of fetal lung maturation.

Long-term outcome

Cerebral palsy

There is an increased risk of neurological sequelae in multiple pregnancies, in general, as compared with singletons. Multiple as compared with singleton gestations are at a five- to tenfold increased risk of cerebral palsy. One of the main reasons for the increased risk of cerebral palsy is the higher proportion of multiples born preterm with cerebral impairment from periventricular hemorrhage or leukomalacia. Monochorionic placentation is also associated with an increased risk of cerebral palsy. This is seen in particular in survivors when there is a fetal or early fetal death of the co-twin. Petterson et al. examined the rate of cerebral palsy (excluding post-neonatal causes) in twins and triplets born from 1980 to1989 in Western Australia [39]. Twins have an increased risk and triplets a severely increased risk for cerebral palsy in 1000 survivors, and this is found by several authors. Risk increased further for the surviving twin after a fetal death (96/1000) as compared with twins in pregnancies where both survived (12/1000). Pharoah and Cooke reported on the prevalence of cerebral palsy in births in the UK between 1982 and 1989. Overall, the prevalence of cerebral palsy was 7.3 per 1000 infant survivors in singletons, 12.6 per 1000 twin survivors and 44.8 per 1000 triplet survivors [40] (Figure 1.3).

Pharoah and Adi collected data on all registered twin births in England and Wales between 1993 and 1995, in which one twin was registered as having died in utero [41]. For same-sex twins surviving to infancy, cerebral palsy rates were 106 per 10 000 as

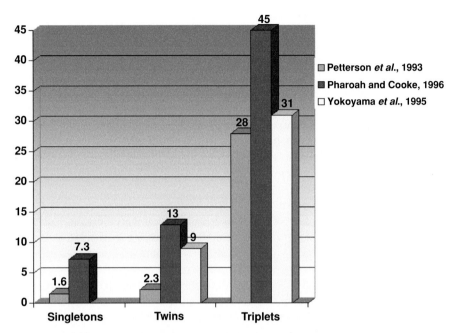

Figure 1.3 Published rates of cerebral palsy per 1000 infant survivors in singletons, twins and triplets. Data from Petterson *et al.* [39], Pharoah and Cooke [40]; Yokoyama *et al.* [54]. Adapted from Wimalasundera *et al.* [55].

compared with 29 per 1000 in the surviving twin in different-sex pair. A meta-analysis of six studies of cerebral palsy in twins and two in triplets showed a 4.5-fold risk for twins and 18.2-fold risk for triplets as compared with singletons [42].

Cognitive development and social development

Many studies have reported that twins have poorer cognitive abilities than singletons although one recent study from the Netherlands twin registry found no evidence of a difference in cognitive ability between singletons and twins in the same family [43]. Another recent cohort study from Aberdeen found that twins had substantially lower IQs in childhood than singletons in the same family. At age 7 years, the mean IQ score of twins was 5.3 points lower and at 9 years 6.0 points lower than in singletons. At least partly, the lower IQ was a consequence

of restricted fetal growth and shorter gestation in twins [44].

ART twins versus spontaneous twins

A more adverse outcome in IVF twins as compared with twins after spontaneous conception might be expected for reasons of maternal characteristics, similar to the situation for IVF singleton pregnancies. However, the higher rates of monozygotic twinning in spontaneous twins as compared with IVF twins (30% vs. 1–5%), may influence outcome, i.e. IVF twins would be expected to have better outcomes than spontaneously conceived twins. However, there are conflicting findings in the case-control and cohort studies in the literature. There are two recently published meta-analyses of perinatal outcomes in IVF twins and the results are summarized in Table 1.3. Overall, the reviews indicate

Table 1.3 Data from two systematic reviews of perinatal outcomes of twins conceived by IVF as compared with twins conceived spontaneously

Outcome	Helmerhorst *et al.*, 2004 [50] Summary relative risk (95% CI)	McDonald *et al.*, 2005 [51] Summary odds ratio (95% CI)
Preterm birth < 37 weeks	1.07 (1.02–1.13)	1.41 (0.96–2.08) 1.57 (1.01–2.44)[a] week 32–36: 1.48 (1.05–2.10)
Very preterm birth < 32–33 weeks	0.95 (0.78–1.15)	1.03 (0.4–2.9)
Low birth weight < 2500 g	1.03 (0.99–1.08)	1.13 (0.85–1.51)
Very low birth weight < 1500 g	0.89 (0.74–1.07)	1.22 (0.50–2.9)
Small for gestational age	1.27 (0.97–1.65)	0.92 (0.62–1.38)
Cesarean section	1.21 (1.11–1.32)	1.33 (1.06–1.67)
NICU admissions	1.05 (1.01–1.09)	2.22 (1.64–3.02)
Perinatal mortality	0.58 (0.44–0.77)	1.40 (0.22–9.11)

[a] Adjusted for parity.

few differences between outcomes in ART twins as compared with twins conceived spontaneously. The significant findings are those related to late preterm birth, admission to NICU and Cesarean delivery, with a slightly more adverse outcome for IVF twins as compared with non-IVF twins.

One study not included in the meta-analyses compared only opposite-sex twins (= only dizygotic twins). They found evidence of more obstetric complications (e.g. placenta previa and antepartum hemorrhage) in IVF twins as compared with non-IVF twins. This may explain the higher preterm delivery rates [45]. A study from the East Flanders prospective twin survey confirmed higher late preterm delivery rates in twins after subfertility treatment, including both IVF/ICSI and ovulation induction, compared with spontaneously conceived twins when controlled for birth year, maternal age, parity, fetal sex, Cesarean section, zygosity and chorionicity (OR 1.6) [46].

A comprehensive Danish systematic review of IVF/ICSI twins concluded that, with few exceptions, IVF twins had similar neonatal outcomes as non-IVF twins [47]. Significantly more IVF/ICSI mothers were on sick leave and with hospitalization during pregnancy than the mothers of spontaneous twins. In vitro fertilization twins had similar

long-term outcome as non-IVF twins, with no differences in the rates of cerebral palsy, chronic disease, surgery, or hospital admissions. Nor were there any differences in growth, motor or cognitive development. This review also included comparisons between IVF twins and IVF singletons. Surprisingly, no differences were seen between IVF singletons and IVF twins in neurological sequelae. One possible explanation for this, according to the author, could be a higher risk of cerebral palsy in IVF singletons than in the general population. However, for most other short- and long-term outcomes, IVF twins had considerably higher risk than IVF singletons. The conclusion was that there should be a general change in the embryo transfer policy towards more elective single embryo transfer.

Conclusions

Women with a multiple pregnancy face greater risks for themselves than women with a singleton pregnancy, and multiple birth babies have much higher rates of perinatal mortality, neonatal morbidity and long-term neurological impairment than singletons. Twins also fare considerably less well than singletons. Adverse perinatal outcomes relate to the high rate of preterm births and intrauterine growth restriction, and these factors are exacerbated for monozygotic and monochorionic twins.

Although the rates of triplets and higher-order multiple births have declined, the high twin birth rates and the larger number of adverse outcomes in twins remain a major concern in relation to ART. Women offered ART should be provided with adequate counseling about the increased risk of twin pregnancy and the potential complications. Primary prevention of multiple pregnancies, including twin pregnancies, after ART is desirable and single embryo transfer, particularly emphasized in Finland and Sweden, has been shown to be an effective means of reducing multiple pregnancies after IVF/ICSI with maintenance of acceptable pregnancy rates [6, 48].

REFERENCES

1. B. C. Fauser, P. Devroey and N. S. Macklon, Multiple birth resulting from ovarian stimulation for subfertility treatment. *Lancet*, **365** (2005), 1807–1816.
2. B. Blondel and M. Kaminski, Trends in the occurrence, determinants, and consequences of multiple births. *Semin. Perinatol.*, **26** (2002), 239–249.
3. J. A. Martin, B. E. Hamilton, P. D. Sutton *et al.*, Births: final data for 2004. *Natl. Vital Stat. Rep.*, **55** (2006), 1–101.
4. A. N. Andersen, V. Goossens, L. Gianaroli *et al.*, Assisted reproductive technology in Europe, 2003. Results generated from European registers by ESHRE. *Hum. Reprod.*, **22** (2007), 1513–1525.
5. C. Wright, J. Chang, G. Jeng, M. Chen and M. Macaluso, Assisted reproductive technology surveillance – United States, 2004. *MMWR Surveill. Summ.*, **56** (2007), 1–22.
6. P. O. Karlström and C. Bergh, Reducing the number of embryos transferred in Sweden-impact on delivery and multiple birth rates. *Hum. Reprod.*, **22** (2007), 2202–2207.
7. N. J. Sebire, R. J. Snijders, K. Hughes, W. Sepulveda and K. H. Nicolaides, The hidden mortality of monochorionic twin pregnancies. *Br. J. Obstet. Gynaecol.*, **104** (1997), 1203–1207.
8. R. Bejar, G. Vigliocco, H. Gramajo *et al.*, Antenatal origin of neurologic damage in newborn infants. II. Multiple gestations. *Am. J. Obstet. Gynecol.*, **162** (1990), 1230–1236.
9. M. V. Senat, P. Y. Ancel, M. H. Bouvier-Colle and G. Bréart, How does multiple pregnancy affect maternal mortality and morbidity? *Clin. Obstet. Gynaecol.*, **41** (1998), 78–83.
10. A. Conde-Agudelo, J. M. Belizan and G. Lindmark, Maternal morbidity and mortality associated with multiple gestations. *Obstet. Gynecol.*, **95** (2000), 899–904.
11. M. Waterstone, S. Bewley and C. Wolfe, Incidence and predictors of severe obstetric morbidity: case-control study. *BMJ*, **332** (2001), 1089–1093.
12. M. C. Walker, K. E. Murphy, S. Pan, Q. Yang and S. W. Wen, Adverse maternal outcomes in multifetal pregnancies. *BJOG*, **111** (2004), 1294–1296.
13. B. Luke and M. B. Brown, Contemporary risks of maternal morbidity and adverse outcomes with increasing maternal age and plurality. *Fertil. Steril.*, **88** (2007), 283–293.
14. M. H. Bouvier-Colle, N. Varnoux, B. Salanave, P. Y. Ancel and G. Bréart, Case-control study of risk factors for obstetric patients' admission to intensive care units. *Eur. J. Obstet. Gynecol. Reprod. Biol.*, **74** (1997), 173–177.
15. J. G. Santema, I. Koppelaar and H. C. Wallenburg, Hypertensive disorders in twin pregnancy. *Eur. J. Obstet. Gynecol. Reprod. Biol.*, **58** (1995), 9–13.
16. B. M. Sibai, J. Hauth, S. Caritis *et al.*, Hypertensive disorders in twin versus singleton gestations. National Institute of Child Health and Human Development Network of Maternal-Fetal Medicine Units. *Am. J. Obstet. Gynecol.*, **182** (2000), 938–942.
17. J. P. Elliott and T. G. Radin, Quadruplet pregnancy: contemporary management and outcome. *Obstet. Gynecol.*, **80** (1992), 421–424.
18. K. A. Douglas and C. W. Redman, Eclampsia in the United Kingdom. *BMJ*, **309** (1994), 1395–1400.
19. S. Suonio and M. Huttunen, Puerperal endometritis after abdominal twin delivery. *Acta Obstet. Gynecol. Scand.*, **73** (1994), 313–315.
20. A. Grant, Cervical cerclage to prolong pregnancy. In I. Chalmers, M. Enkin and M. Keirse, eds., *Effective Care in Pregnancy and Childhood.* (Oxford: Oxford University Press, 1989), pp. 633–645.
21. K. François, J. Ortiz, C. Harris, M. R. Foley and J. P. Elliott, Is peripartum hysterectomy more common in multiple gestations? *Obstet. Gynecol.*, **105** (2005), 1369–1372.
22. S. W. Wen, K. Demissie, Q. Yang and M. C. Walker, Maternal morbidity and obstetric complications in triplet pregnancies and quadruplet and higher-order

multiple pregnancies. *Am. J. Obstet. Gynecol.*, **191** (2004), 254–258.

23. H. J. Landy and L. G. Keith, The vanishing twin: a review. *Hum. Reprod. Update*, **4** (1998), 177–183.

24. R. B. Russell, J. R. Petrini, K. Damus, D. R. Mattison and R. H. Schwarz, The changing epidemiology of multiple births in the United States. *Obstet. Gynecol.*, **101** (2003), 129–135.

25. A. I. Scher, B. Petterson, E. Blair *et al.*, The risk of mortality or cerebral palsy in twins: a collaborative population-based study. *Pediatr. Res.*, **52** (2002), 671–681.

26. T. J. Garite, R. H. Clark, J. P. Elliott and J. A. Thorp, Twins and triplets: the effect of plurality and growth on neonatal outcome compared with singleton infants. *Am. J. Obstet. Gynecol.*, **191** (2004), 700–707.

27. M. O. Gardner, R. L. Goldenberg, S. P. Cliver *et al.*, The origin and outcome of preterm twin pregnancies. *Obstet. Gynecol.*, **85** (1995), 553–557.

28. N. J. Sebire, C. D'Ercole, W. Soares, R. Nayar and K. H. Nicolaides, Intertwin disparity in fetal size in monochorionic and dichorionic pregnancies. *Obstet. Gynecol.*, **91** (1998), 82–85.

29. K. Demissie, C. V. Ananth, J. Martin *et al.*, Fetal and neonatal mortality among twin gestations in the United States: the role of intrapair birth weight discordance. *Obstet. Gynecol.*, **100** (2002), 474–480.

30. T. L. Callahan, J. E. Hall, S. L. Ettner *et al.*, The economic impact of multiple-gestation pregnancies and the contribution of assisted-reproduction techniques to their incidence. *N. Engl. J. Med.*, **331** (1994), 244–249.

31. E. S. Shinwell, I. Blickstein, A. Lusky and B. Reichman, Effect of birth order on neonatal morbidity and mortality among very low birthweight twins: a population based study. *Arch. Dis. Child. Fetal Neonatal Ed.*, **89** (2004), F145–F148.

32. J. Little and E. Bryan, Congenital anomalies in twins. *Semin. Perinatol.*, **10** (1986), 50–64.

33. P. Mastroiacovo, E. E. Castilla, C. Arpino *et al.*, Congenital malformations in twins: an international study. *Am. J. Med. Genet.*, **83** (1999), 117–124.

34. S. P. Walker, S. A. Cole and A. G. Edwards, Twin-to-twin transfusion syndrome: is the future getting brighter? *Aust. N. Z. J. Obstet. Gynaecol.*, **47** (2007), 158–168.

35. R. A. Quintero, W. J. Morales, M. H. Allen *et al.*, Staging of twin-twin transfusion syndrome. *J. Perinatol.*, **19**: 8 Pt. 1 (1999), 550–555.

36. C. Fox, M. D. Kilby and K. S. Khan, Contemporary treatments for twin-twin transfusion syndrome. *Obstet. Gynecol.*, **105** (2005), 1469–1477.

37. K. Golombeck, R. H. Ball, H. Lee *et al.*, Maternal morbidity after maternal-fetal surgery. *Am. J. Obstet. Gynecol.*, **194** (2006), 834–839.

38. K. D. Heyborne, R. P. Porreco, T. J. Garite, K. Phair and D. Abril, Improved perinatal survival of monoamniotic twins with intensive inpatient monitoring. *Am. J. Obstet. Gynecol.*, **192** (2005), 96–101.

39. B. Petterson, N. B. Nelson, L. Watson and F. Stanley, Twins, triplets, and cerebral palsy in births in Western Australia in the 1980s. *BMJ*, **307** (1993), 1239–1243.

40. P. O. Pharoah and T. Cooke, Cerebral palsy and multiple births. *Arch. Dis. Child. Fetal Neonatal Ed.*, **75** (1996), F174–F177.

41. P. O. Pharoah and Y. Adi, Consequences of in-utero death in a twin pregnancy. *Lancet*, **355** (2000), 1597–1602.

42. F. Stanley, E. Blair and E. Alberman, The special case of multiple pregnancy. In *Cerebral Palsies: Epidemiology and Causal Pathways*, Clinics in Developmental Medicine, 151 (London: Mac Keith Press, 2000), pp. 109–123.

43. D. Posthuma, E. J. De Geus, N. Bleichrodt and D. I. Boomsma, Twin-singleton differences in intelligence? *Twin Res.*, **3** (2000), 83–87.

44. G. A. Ronalds, B. L. De Stavola and D. A. Leon, The cognitive cost of being a twin: evidence from comparisons within families in the Aberdeen children of the 1950s cohort study. *BMJ*, **331** (2005), 1306.

45. P. R. Smithers, J. Halliday, L. Hale *et al.*, High frequency of cesarean section, antepartum hemorrhage, placenta previa, and preterm delivery in in-vitro fertilization twin pregnancies. *Fertil. Steril.*, **80** (2003), 666–668.

46. H. Verstraelen, S. Goetgeluk, C. Derom *et al.*, Preterm birth in twins after subfertility treatment: population based cohort study. *BMJ*, **331** (2005), 1173.

47. A. Pinborg, IVF/ICSI twin pregnancies: risks and prevention. *Hum. Reprod. Update*, **11** (2005), 575–593.

48. A. Thurin, J. Hausken, T. Hillensö *et al.*, Elective single-embryo transfer versus double-embryo transfer in in vitro fertilization. *N. Engl. J. Med.*, **351** (2004), 2392–2402.

49. J. Collins, Global epidemiology of multiple birth. wwwrbmonlinecom/Issue/118, 2006.

50. F. M. Helmerhorst, D. A. Perquin, D. Donker and M. J. Keirse, Perinatal outcome of singletons and twins after assisted conception: a systematic review of controlled studies. *BMJ*, **328** (2004), 261.

51. S. McDonald, K. Murphy, J. Beyene and A. Ohlsson, Perinatal outcomes of in vitro fertilization twins: a systematic review and meta-analyses. *Am. J. Obstet. Gynecol.*, **193** (2005), 141–152.

52. A. B. Macfarlane, Demographic trends in Western European countries. In I. Blickstein and L. Keith, eds., *Multiple Pregnancy*, 2nd edn. (London; New York: Taylor and Francis, 2005), pp. 11–21.

53. P. Doyle, The outcome of multiple pregnancy. *Hum. Reprod.*, **11** (2006), 110–117.

54. Y. Yokoyama, T. Shimizu and K. Hayakawa, Prevalence of cerebral palsy in twins, triplets and quadruplets. *Int. J. Epidemiol.*, **24** (1995), 943–948.

55. R. C. Wimalasundera, G. Trew and N. M. Fisk, Reducing the incidence of twins and triplets. *Best Pract. Res. Clin. Obstet. Gynaecol.*, **17** (2003), 309–329.

2

An overview of determinants of oocyte and embryo developmental competence: specificity, accuracy and applicability in clinical IVF

Jonathan Van Blerkom

The need for non-invasive marker of developmental competence

It is a tribute to the success of in vitro fertilization (IVF) as a primary treatment of human infertility that the subject of an entire volume is devoted to the notion that single embryo transfers can and perhaps should become the worldwide standard of practice. The intent of this chapter is to provide a general survey of research that has sought to identify cellular, molecular and developmental (i.e., performance in vitro) characteristics of hyperstimulated ovarian follicles, oocytes and cultured preimplantation stage embryos that may relate to or predict competence and outcome after uterine transfer. The need for predictors of competence is related to the basic clinical strategy of this treatment; namely, induce large numbers of follicles to develop coordinately by managed or "controlled" ovarian hyperstimulation, so that a corresponding number of aspirated oocytes will be meiotically mature (i.e., meiosis arrested at metaphase II, MII), fertilizable and capable of normal development in vitro. Selection for transfer is usually made at a set time after insemination (program-specific protocol) from a cohort of embryos in which those deemed stage- and performance-appropriate are selected for transfer or cryopreservation.

While the first human IVF birth in 1978 was conceived during a "natural cycle" [1] and sporadic reports of positive outcomes with this approach were reported in subsequent years [2, 3], it soon became evident that the efficacy of this process could be significantly increased if more oocytes were available to produce more than a single embryo for transfer. Existing protocols of controlled ovarian hyperstimulation that produced multiple oocytes were rapidly applied to IVF and as new modalities were introduced and successful outcomes reported, there were no apparent reasons to change the paradigm of exogenous management of the menstrual cycle. The origin of the central issue to which this volume is devoted stems from the occurrence of twin and higher-order gestations at frequencies that could be described as reaching "epidemic" proportions in IVF treatments [4].

The practice of replacing multiple embryos after 2 or 3 days of culture was a standard for many IVF programs that began operation in the late 1970s and early 1980s, and was based on a prevailing notion of human reproductive biology; namely, that a high degree of inherent developmental heterogeneity and "embryonic wastage" occurs in our species such that a sizeable percentage of embryos undergo demise during the pre- and early postimplantation stages [5, 6]. Estimates of the frequency of early demise during natural (i.e., unassisted) pregnancy in the 70% range [7, 8] suggested that defects inherent to the oocyte could compromise competence to

Single Embryo Transfer, ed. J. Gerris, G. D. Adamson, P. De Sutter and C. Racowsky. Published by Cambridge University Press.
© Cambridge University Press 2009.

a greater degree than those which may be related to hormonal stimulation protocol or IVF methodology (i.e., iatrogenic). In this regard, it was not surprising that some of the earliest studies of ploidy in mature (MII) human oocytes that would normally be available for IVF after exogenous ovarian stimulation reported frequencies of aneuploidy > 50% [9]. In this context, the combined effects of aneuploidy resulting from non-disjunction, anaphase lag and premature centromeric division during preovulatory meiosis in the oocyte [10–12], and spontaneous chromosomal malsegregation during the early mitotic divisions of the embryo [13], were largely considered natural and unavoidable phenomena in the human, and with respect to outcome after IVF, the most significant determinants of developmental competence.

In addition to underlying chromosomal defects, specific disorders in cellular organization for the MII oocyte [14, 15], termed "cytoplasmic dysmorphisms" by Van Blerkom and Henry [16], were described as competence-associated and commonplace within cohorts obtained for IVF after ovarian hyperstimulation. Certain disorders, such as severe organelle clustering, were correlated with higher frequencies of aneuploidy [16], while others, such as abnormal aggregations of the smooth surfaced endoplasmic reticulum, were shown to have adverse affects on embryo performance in vitro [15] and, in one study, suggested to be associated with the occurrence of genomic imprinting defects in newborns [17].

The use of routine light microscopy to identify specific morphological characteristics that appeared to be competence-associated has been incorporated into most oocyte assessment schemes for human IVF [18, 19]. However, some reports discounted the validity of morphology-based selection of MII oocytes because fertilization could be achieved in some instances by intracytoplasmic sperm injection (ICSI) [20, 21]. However, the utility of these assessment criteria was supported by high frequencies of embryo demise and spontaneous abortion during the pre- and postimplantation stages, respectively, where ICSI was performed

on dysmorphic oocytes [18, 22]. The finding that specific cytoplasmic dysmorphisms occurred repeatedly in multiple cycles of IVF with different protocols of ovarian stimulation suggests that defects in cytoplasmic organization could be a proximal cause of idiopathic infertility in some women, and, similar to chromosomal aneuploidy for the human oocyte, may be both unavoidable and uncorrectable [18]. It was also well known from the field of reproductive genetics that the presence of certain genetic defects does not preclude development to birth, and early studies of triploid embryos that developed in vitro after dispermic penetration showed common instances of morphologically normal development during days 2 and 3 of culture, at which cleavage stage embryos were, and for many programs still are, transferred to the patient [23]. This was among the first suggestions that normal blastomere morphology and organization within the embryo during early development was not a reliable indicator of either chromosomal normality or competence.

Against a presumed high background of pre-existing and seemingly unavoidable nuclear and cytoplasmic defects that likely predisposed oocytes and embryos to developmental failure or early demise, the replacement of multiple embryos was generally considered necessary to bias the treatment cycle to a successful outcome. Sporadic reports of higher-order gestations with normal-appearing oocytes could be viewed as an unexpected and perhaps inevitable consequence of the protocols necessary to achieve a successful outcome, and as further evidence that unique differences in competence between similar-appearing oocytes could not be easily distinguished or detected [24]. Given the inability to reliably predict the competence of each normal-appearing oocyte or stage-appropriate embryo, and the perceived necessity of replacing multiple embryos that most often resulted in singleton or twin pregnancies, there was no imperative to limit the number of embryos transferred and with respect to outcome, it could be argued that such efforts would likely be counterproductive.

The notion that higher-order gestations are an unavoidable complication of clinical IVF was often indirectly supported by the press and popular media in articles that focused on how parents had to adapt their lives to accommodate the needs of their multiple "miracle babies." To this author's recollection, few, if any, of these written articles or television programs emphasized the considerable hazards to the mother and progeny associated with multiple gestations, as well described in this volume. In no small measure, this view was abetted by some prominent IVF practitioners who were shown proudly displaying the quadruplets or quintuplets their program had produced, and by extolling the virtues of advances in perinatal medicine that allowed potentially deleterious complications for mother and offspring to be addressed, seemed to displace criticisms that such outcomes should be considered as failures rather than successes of this enterprise. The frequent portrayals of the long-standing desperation of infertile couples followed by the elation of birth, even when multiples, was commonplace during the proliferation of clinical IVF programs. In what was becoming a highly competitive atmosphere in some countries, such as the United States, displays of this type were often a financial boon for a program and, for some, resulted in statements of outcomes presented as babies born rather than successful pregnancies initiated per cycle. Against a generally positive background for the accomplishments of clinical IVF, it is not surprising that calls for limiting the number of transferred embryos gained little attention or support. In an anecdotal context, during an interview with a producer who was preparing a television program on infertility treatments, I asked why higher-order gestations are commonly presented as an unavoidable "complication" of IVF and why there was little mention that its potential could be reduced by limiting the number of transferred embryos and emphasizing cryopreservation as a viable alternative. The response was informative – "no one wants to read about or see sick babies and distraught parents."

For some patients, the potential for a higher-order gestation was an unacceptable consequence of their attempts to overcome infertility, but rather than go against the conventional wisdom of transferring high numbers of embryos, "selective fetal reduction" was introduced as an effective remedy to address an unwanted outcome. The avoidance of limiting the number of embryos replaced coupled with increasing use of the fetal reduction option persisted through the 1990s, but as the overall rates of success for IVF rose, so did the frequency of multiple births, which along with the use of selective fetal reduction were reaching alarming proportions [4]. What could account for this relatively rapid improvement in outcome in general and, in particular, why had the frequency of multiple births increased in a relatively short period of time such that so-called "take-home baby" rates in the 30% to 40% range were commonplace? Because the basic biology of human sperm, oocytes and early embryos had not undergone a spontaneous improvement in quality, it seems most likely that the following were significant factors:

1. increased experience with embryo culture;
2. newer culture media formulations optimized for the human development, especially to the blastocyst stage;
3. improved catheter designs for atraumatic embryo transfer;
4. ICSI, which effectively extended treatment to severe male factor infertility;
5. increased use of and successful outcomes with embryo cryopreservation;
6. a more precise characterization and use of morphological criteria to detected stage-specific features indicative of normal development.

The use of morphological criteria in oocyte and embryo competence assessment

In addition to the progressive improvements in methodology, IVF programs developed various schemes to predict competence by incorporating oocyte cytoplasmic phenotype and morphological characteristics of embryos during cleavage in their assessments. Confidence in these schemes was largely the result of increased demand for IVF, which enabled oocytes and embryos to be evaluated in numbers sufficient to correlate light microscopic features with outcome, and to detect subtle stage-specific differences in embryo performance that could be related to competence. While the underlying biological influences and causes of different oocyte phenotypes and patterns of early embryo development were largely unknown, for the newly fertilized egg and early cleavage stage embryo, common morphological characteristics that could be readily identified by routine light microscopic examination were suggested to be markers of competence. The occurrence of dispermic penetration was the most obvious development defect owing to the presence of three distinct pronuclei, and during the first decade of clinical IVF, reported frequencies of dispermic penetration for > 20% of the MII oocytes obtained per cycle were common [25]. Thus, the importance of detecting dispermic penetrations was evident relatively early in the evolution of clinical IVF because the performance and behavior of triploid embryos during the cleavage stages was often equivalent to their normally fertilized (i.e., monospermic) siblings [23].

The high frequency of dispermic penetrations reported by IVF programs following the introduction of this treatment for infertility was largely attributed to "defects" that arose in a certain proportion of oocytes as a consequence of the endocrine protocols used to stimulate the growth and development of multiple ovarian follicles. However, while no alterations in specific molecular pathways or cellular conditions that could account for dispermic penetrations were identified, it was generally assumed that the causative agent had such a basis and likely involved a defective or abnormally slow cortical granule reaction that permitted penetration by more than one sperm. The "standard" protocol of conventional IVF in use at this time involved insemination with sperm numbers in the tens-to-hundreds of thousands. Van Blerkom and Henry [25] reported that the probability of dispermic penetration was directly related both to sperm numbers and, more importantly, the proportion of sperm

exhibiting rapid linear (progressive or directed) motion. These authors noted that dispermic penetrations became increasingly infrequent in their program when the number of sperm used for insemination was based on the proportion showing this motility pattern and, in many cases, the presence of 1000 or fewer sperm with this behavior was sufficient to achieve monospermic penetration. The point of raising this issue is that the basis of observed and apparent developmental abnormalities manifested in oocytes and early preimplantation stage human embryos may be iatrogenic rather than caused by pre-existing biological dysfunctions that have specific molecular, biochemical or cellular origins. This notion repeats throughout the course of IVF investigations that seek to identify factors that predict competence, as described below.

Microscopically detectable determinants of competence in the mature human oocyte: imaging spindle microtubule birefringence by polarizing light microscopy

The introduction of polarizing optics and computer-enhanced imaging has enabled non-invasive detection of the meiotic MII spindle in living oocytes such that its relative state of organization and location with respect to the first polar body can be identified prior to fertilization [26–28]. For clinical IVF, one suggested advantage of spindle imaging during ICSI was that it enabled placement of the sperm injection micropipet in order to avoid the potential disruption of the MII spindle during cytoplasmic aspiration and sperm insertion, and thus reduce the possibility of inducing iatrogenic chromosomal defects [29]. Whether this methodology is of benefit in this specific respect is controversial, but its utility has been demonstrated in regard to the following: (1) the MII spindle cannot be assumed to be positioned in the pericortical cytoplasm beneath the first polar body [30]; (2) spindle organization is altered when human MII oocytes are maintained and observed at subnormal temperatures but usually returns to normal when

37 °C is restored [31]; (3) some proportion of oocytes characterized as MII owing to the presence of a first polar body have no detectable spindle when viewed by polarizing light microscopy [32–34]. However, most oocytes have a detectable MII spindle and its apparent "absence" is likely due to the transient loss of birefringence during polar body formation.

To date, the clearest indication of the value of applying polarizing microscopy to competence assessment of human MII oocytes is the reported association between the level of light retardation by birefringent spindles and pronuclear score indicated by the spatial alignment and organization of primitive nuclei termed nuclear precursor bodies (NPBs) [35]. In this multicenter study, quantitative analysis of the relative magnitude of polarized light retardation of MII spindle birefringence, which is a function of the density and higher-order alignment of spindle microtubules, was suggested to indicate the normality of spindle organization. Pronuclear morphology indicated by the number and equatorial alignment of NPBs (see below) was correlated with normal development in vitro and implantation after transfer. High levels of retardance were correlated with higher frequencies of normal development in vitro and implantation after transfer than for oocytes with lower retardance, which showed subsequent pronuclear morphology indicative of poor competence. The reduced levels of spindle birefringence are associated with a lower microtubular density and indicative of an aberrant state of spindle organization that could lead to chromosomal segregation defects, such as those detectable after fertilization and associated with specific pronuclear phenotypes. What is unclear and warrants further investigation is the underlying biology that associates microtubular dynamics, spindle organization, NPBs and pronuclear morphology. In this regard, Shen *et al.* [35] are most likely correct in assuming that molecular and biochemical processes that characterize the preovulatory cytoplasmic maturation of the oocyte are defective in promoting the formation of a normal spindle, i.e., one that exhibits high (light retardation) birefringence when viewed under polarizing light.

While the details of the molecular interaction between cytoplasm and spindle need clarification, additional outcome results from a larger patient population will be required to demonstrate that this non-invasive method is of clear benefit in oocyte selection for ICSI, and that with respect to competence can provide a high level of certainty needed to distinguish between oocytes that appear equivalent by conventional light microscopy.

A potentially important finding to come from polarization imaging of human oocytes has been the detection of differential birefringence in the zona pellucida that in early reports appears to correlate well with the developmental competence of the resulting embryo [36–38]. Embryos derived from MII oocytes with high zona birefringence appear more capable of developing to the blastocyst stage and implanting after uterine transfer than siblings with comparatively lower birefringent values. While the origin of differential birefringence remains to be determined, it seems likely that if the described changes in birefringence are confined to the innermost aspect of the zona, the agent of change may be the oocyte itself. In this regard, imaging with polarized light optics may provide both empirical and quantifiable indicators of the normality of preovulatory cytoplasmic maturation. An understanding of the etiology of differential birefringence with respect to stage of maturation and the biochemistry involved may also provide the biological basis for experimental investigations of whether molecular differences between oocytes can have critical downstream influences on the normality of development during the preimplantation stages. Studies of this type should also indicate the extent to which birefringent characteristics of the meiotic spindle and zona pellucida are related and, when used in combination, are truly predictive of embryo competence [37]. The findings may also indicate whether putative downstream influences of oocyte cytoplasmic maturation indicated by spatial changes in the organization of the zona pellucida extend to the normality of hatching at the late blastocyst stage. If confirmed, such information may be an important aspect of oocyte selection for insemination and the identification of specific embryos that may bene-fit from assisted hatching. Positive correlations with the normality of cytoplasmic maturation, embryo developmental competence, or hatching potential would warrant the added expense to the IVF lab-oratory of microscopic systems that use polariz-ing optics and computer-enhanced imaging [38]. The combination of this biometric with biochemical markers and physiological characteristics of follic-ular development that have been related to oocyte and embryo competence, as discussed below, is a particularly attractive approach to competence assessment because it is non-invasive and based on independent parameters. This approach would be especially applicable where the number of oocytes that can be inseminated and the duration of embryo culture prior to transfer is proscribed by law.

Competence indicators at the one-cell stage

Garello *et al.* [39] described spatial aspects of jux-taposed human pronuclei in which a largely per-pendicular alignment, with respect to the first and second polar bodies, seemed to be highly predica-tive of developmental potential and therefore out-come. This orientation was relatively easy to deter-mine and calibrate up to the stage of pronuclear membrane dissolution (a process that is commonly, and perhaps incorrectly for the human, termed syngamy). The prognostic value of pronuclear ori-entation diminished somewhat for the purposes of competence assessment after time-lapse studies showed that opposed pronuclei that initially devi-ated from the perpendicular could rotate prior to nuclear membrane dissolution and become aligned in a largely perpendicular orientation [40]. How-ever, significant deviations from the perpendicular were reported to diminish competence [39] and, although controversial, this characteristic is still used by some as one of the parameters for com-petence assessment. The importance of pronuclear orientation may be related to how the normally meridional plane of the first cleavage division in the human bisects the cell to produce daughter blas-

tomeres that are mostly equivalent in size. The pos-sibility that abnormal pronuclear orientation could have adverse downstream developmental conse-quences by virtue of putative regulatory molecules or domains inherited from the oocyte and mald-istributed between daughter cells has also been suggested [39].

The notion that developmental determinants pre-exist and are spatially compartmentalized in the oocyte and newly fertilized mammalian egg is con-troversial [39–47]. Recently, much excitement in the field of early mammalian embryology was gen-erated by the report that *Cdx2*, a transcription factor associated with trophectodermal develop-ment [48], had a unique and polarized distribu-tion in the mouse oocyte and after fertilization was unequally distributed between daughter cells [49]. These authors reported that experimental inactiva-tion of *Cdx2* in the mouse with interference RNA (RNAi) resulted in loss of the capacity to generate a normal trophectoderm. This finding led to the pos-sibility that the spontaneous absence or maldistri-bution of *Cdx2* in some blastomeres, perhaps owing to abnormal planes of cleavage, could have adverse consequences for the human with respect to the derivation of one of the two basic cell lineages of the early embryo, the trophectoderm (trophoblast) and the inner cell mass. If anomalies in *Cdx2* distri-bution at the 2-cell stage were associated with the pattern of pronuclear alignment, it could begin to explain the apparent reduction in competence that had been reported for embryos in which pronuclear orientation deviated significantly from the perpen-dicular, as described above.

For clinical IVF, a unique cell lineage deter-minant such as *Cdx2*, if present at the earliest stages of development, has the potential to provide the first definitive molecular marker of competence. For example, analytical studies with discarded embryos could have the potential to correlate *Cdx2* distribution with specific morphological aspects and patterns of embryo performance in vitro currently used for competence assessment (e.g., non-uniform cleavages, fragmentation, numer-ically insufficient or disorganized blastocyst).

Unfortunately, the use of this marker in clinical IVF suffered a significant setback with the disclosure in 2007 that results central to the conclusions and interpretations in the original publication were likely fabricated, and the paper was retracted [50]. However, the search for similar markers of preimplantation human embryogenesis that could provide molecular clues to defects or abnormalities in early development is a continuing process that, if successful, could yield new insights into the heterogeneous patterns of early development common in our species.

Identification and characterization of morphodynamic activities

For clinical relevance, examinations of dynamic activities that use a specific method to predict competence, such as the spatial organization or reorganization of cellular components (e.g., orientation of pronuclei), should incorporate a standard protocol and timing. This would support contentions that the observations are developmentally relevant and comparable between operators and programs. For example, in conventional IVF, but not ICSI, the actual time of sperm penetration and pronuclear evolution can differ between oocytes, and, owing to the relatively narrow temporal windows during which certain morphodynamic activities occur, differences of 2 or 3 hours could lead to different interpretations, especially if only a single time point is used. For example, time-lapse studies of human pronuclear eggs reveal intracytoplasmic motion that often creates a zone of translucency in the pericortical cytoplasm. This dynamic process has been described as a wavelike activity, or "cytoplasmic flare" [51] that progresses around the pericortical cytoplasm during the peri-syngamic stage to form a circumferential "halo". The occurrence of a flare that leads to a halo, which in some fertilized eggs is associated with a pronounced region of cytoplasmic translucency, was proposed to be a normal activity at the 1-cell stage and a visible marker of the developmental activation of the oocyte and competence

for the embryo [39, 51, 52]. Consequently, the inclusion of the cytoplasmic halo and a perpendicular pronuclear alignment, if based on a single observation, could lead to the elimination of an embryo(s) for transfer if, according to a program's standard timing of inspection, these characteristics are absent at the time of inspection. Their occurrence some time later, owing to later penetration or oocyte-specific timing of activation, might go unnoticed and, based on the stringency of selection criteria, an otherwise competent embryo may not be considered appropriate for transfer or cryopreservation. The predictive value of these two morphodynamic features of the 1-cell human embryo requires further validation and in our unreported experience, normal outcomes are common with embryos that at the pronuclear stage showed no cytoplasmic flare or halo. In contrast, a significant deviation from a largely perpendicular pronuclear alignment at "syngamy" has often been followed by an asymmetric first cleavage division that produces blastomeres unequal in size, and the subsequent cell divisions during cleavage have usually resulted in embryos at the 6- to 10-cell stage whose blastomeres are disproportionate with respect to size. With continued culture, these embryos rarely develop to the expanded blastocyst stage. The relative position of the pronuclei during the peri-syngamic stage seems to be a useful first marker of competence and suggests that their position and orientation may be determinants of the plane of the first cell division. The normality with which this plane bisects the 1-cell embryo may be the first critical developmental determinant of competence that is embryo- rather than oocyte-derived.

The number, size and organization of NPBs in the pronuclear stage human embryo is another morphological feature that has been related to competence, and one that is clearly detectable by routine light microscopy. Scott and Smith [52] proposed NPB scoring systems based on the number and spatial distribution of these entities within each pronucleus, and reported outcome results with each pronuclear phenotype. This scoring system was modified by Tesarik and Greco [53], and subsequent outcome reports with both scoring systems demonstrated that certain configurations, such as an equatorial alignment at the region of pronuclear opposition, were associated with high implantation potential and ongoing pregnancy rates [54–57]. The predictive value of an NPB score that is number- and distribution-based has been controversial with respect to embryo selection at the pronuclear stage and equivocal with respect to outcome [58]. However, NPB scoring has largely persisted in evaluation schemes, especially where selection must be made at the 1-cell stage owing to prohibitions on further embryo culture [59]. The utility of competence selection by pronuclear morphology has been supported by cytogenetic findings demonstrating that certain NPB phenotypes are associated with high frequencies of chromosomal defects and disorders after fertilization [60–63]. With respect to competence, an equatorial alignment appears to be the most positive configuration of NPBs and is evident by the accumulation of these structures on either side of the apposed pronuclei. Prior to the introduction of scoring systems, this orientation was reported to be associated with the spatial distribution and alignment of replicating DNA in each pronucleus [64]. These authors reported that replicating and condensing chromatin (i.e., condensing into mitotic chromosomes) was co-localized (spatially polarized) in each pronucleus at the site of their opposition and co-localized with NPBs, especially between the latter stages of pronuclear evolution and pronuclear membrane dissolution (syngamy). It was suggested that an equatorial co-localization facilitated the appropriate attachment of spindle kinetochore microtubules to the nascent mitotic chromosomes, leading to their normal segregation at the first mitotic (cleavage) division. Spatial abnormalities in the distribution of NPBs in either the maternal or the paternal pronucleus, or both, were associated with corresponding spatial abnormalities in chromatin orientation. Although untested, it was suggested that DNA distributions that showed spatially significant deviations from a largely equatorial alignment could increase

the probability of chromosomal malalignment and lead to aneuploidies or chromosomal mosaicism in early blastomeres.

Differences in the number, location and orientation of NPBs at the peri-syngamic stage are readily identifiable, which makes these characteristics attractive for morphology-based competence assessment. As noted above, a normal NPB complement showing an equatorial alignment is generally considered a positive indicator of competence. Complicating the use of this dynamic activity for diagnostic purposes in early embryo selection are time-lapse findings showing NPBs' movements [64], perhaps reflecting the progressive polarization of chromatin and its condensation into chromosomes in proximity to their respective pronuclear membranes. The importance of sequential inspections of dynamic activities, such as those involving NPBs, is that an alignment considered negative for competence at one time may become positive in this regard only a short time later and could go unnoticed if selection was based on a single observation.

Our unpublished experience with NPB activity and location is generally supportive of NPB characterizations when done during the peri-syngamic period, which is usually between 18- and 24-hours post-insemination. In this regard, we have found the following phenotypes are consistently negative factors with respect to outcome: (1) numerous, small NPBs scattered throughout either or both pronuclei, and (2) a single, large, centrally located NPB in one or both pronuclei. Nuclear precursor bodies of an equivalent size and shape that are largely equatorially aligned appear to be a generally favorable indicator of competence likely owing to the corresponding polarized distribution of replicated DNA in both pronuclei. However, while this configuration tends to be a positive indicator, subsequent cleavages can produce embryos that (1) have multinucleated blastomeres, (2) arrest development during cleavage, or (3) show irregular patterns of cell division, but at collective frequency that in our experience is considerably lower ($< 8\%$, $n = 1600$) than observed when one or both pronuclei contain a single, large NPB ($> 60\%$; $n = 450$), or numerous, small structures scattered within the nucleoplasm (~40%, $n = 370$). At present, pronuclear morphology is used in our program as one of several characteristics for selection. However, where embryo culture beyond the 1-cell stage is prohibited, selection based on pronuclear morphology alone can provide a positive bias with respect to competence, especially for the two negative phenotypes described above which are likely to be most robust indicators of the NPB phenotypes reported.

Fragmentation during cleavage

The degree of fragmentation during the early cleavage stages is another example of a morphodynamic metric that is nearly universally used to assess human embryo competence. While a large descriptive literature exists on extents and patterns of fragmentation, a definitive biological basis for this phenomenon and why it affects only some embryos in cohorts remains to be established [65–67]. It is also unclear whether fragmentation in general is related to inherent development defects that are embryo- or blastomere-specific, and, if so, should have an identifiable molecular or cellular origin. In this regard, fragmentation has largely been assumed a consequence of the apoptotic elimination of blastomeres with genetic or molecular defects [67, 68]; however, this notion is controversial [67, 69] and recent evidence does not support apoptosis as a common etiology of spontaneous fragmentation observed during the cleavage stages of in vitro cultured human embryos [70, 71].

It has also been suggested that for some embryos fragmentation is a normal aspect of early development and, therefore, may be unavoidable during culture if the in vitro situation largely reflects in vivo conditions [66]. Unfortunately, information about human preimplantation development in vivo is scarce and insufficient to validate this assumption. Alternatively, the extent and pattern of fragmentation can be viewed in terms of the often-stated developmental heterogeneity of early human embryos that in this instance may reflect

the unique ability of each to adapt to culture. Consequently, the occurrence, pattern and extent of fragmentation may have iatrogenic origins, rather than being the result of naturally occurring physiological differences that influence performance. Evidence in support of this notion comes from reports of reduced rates of fragmentation in different culture media formulations used for clinical IVF [72]. In this respect, our unpublished experience indicates that relatively minor changes in medium composition and culture conditions can virtually eliminate the occurrence of fragmentation in general, and for patients whose embryos showed high frequencies of fragmentation in previous cycles that used different media, in particular. The possibility that common patterns of fragmentation displayed by human embryos in vitro are not unavoidable or natural phenomena will be confirmed if the progressive optimization of culture conditions largely eliminates fragmentation or shows a significant reduction in frequency and severity.

Until such optimized culture conditions exist, fragmentation will remain in competence assessment schemes that derive a score or grade that signifies extent or pattern, or both. While heavily weighted with respect to fragmentation, these schemes also consider other performance variables such as timing and uniformity of cleavages and the presence or absence of blastomere multinucleation. Yet, few scoring systems that include fragmentation evaluations are truly quantitative or employ a common biometric that, if used by others, would reliably come to similar objective conclusions. As a result, most scoring for fragmentation is empirically based and subjective estimates of the degree of cytoplasm that may be lost to affected blastomere(s) are usually presented in terms of a percent [65–67]. Clearly, when the extent of fragmentation is so severe that individual blastomeres can no longer be identified, the loss of competence for the affected embryo is not in question. However, such instances are less common than previously in contemporary IVF, perhaps because of improvements in culture media and conditions, and when detected are largely embryo-specific rather than cohort-wide.

It is the competence of embryos in which intact blastomeres are decorated by a small number of fragments that vary in size and density that can be the most difficult to assess with respect to developmental viability for the embryo. However, based on outcomes, these common patterns are mostly developmentally benign [65–67, 71]. Indeed, time-lapse analysis of affected embryos demonstrates that such "fragments" often arise rapidly and subsequently disappear by resorption into the underlying blastomere some hours later [67, 73]. This raises the question of whether light microscopy affords the level of resolution necessary to distinguish between "apparent fragments" and true cytoplasts that are detached from the plasma membrane. We have previously shown by confocal fluorescent [74] and transmission electron microscopy [70] that cytoplasmic structures characterized as extracellular by light microscopy can occur in the form of columns of spherical protrusions in which cytoplasmic continuity exists between the apparent fragments and the underlying blastomere. Thus, a cellular basis for resorption exists, and recent experimental findings with early cleavage stage human embryos indicate that true cytoplasts (fragments) elaborated from one blastomere can be resorbed by a different cell within the same embryo [73]. These findings may explain why early human embryos can undergo a change in "grade" during culture, from a classification of "developmentally questionable" to "high-grade", especially when the grading system is heavily biased to deselection with respect to the presence of clusters of fragments, despite stage-appropriate cell numbers.

The above findings indicate some of the limitations of morphology-based competence assessment and support the necessity for sequential and timed observations of embryos when morphodynamic activities are involved. These limitations are also evident when normal outcomes occur with embryos judged low grade and likely incompetent at the 2-, 4- or 8-cell stage. Figure 2.1 shows examples from our own experience where normal births occurred from known embryos that, based on morphological characteristics and performance during early

cleavage, were judged highly unlikely to progress or implant in vivo. The importance of determining the extent to which fragmentation in general, or specific patterns of fragmentation in particular, are naturally occurring physiological processes such as apoptosis, or are iatrogenic in origin, cannot be overstated because much of the decision-making in embryo selection is based on this performance characteristic.

Prolongation of development to the blastocyst stage

Extending human embryo culture to days 5 or 6, at which time normally progressing embryos should be at the expanded blastocyst stage, has generally been thought to be a strong indicator of competence because it is based on the assumption that extended culture will largely self-select embryos on their ability to develop to the peri-implantation stage. The culture medium composition and requirements needed by the human embryo to progress to the expanded blastocyst stage are similar to those developed for other mammals [72], and the availability of commercial media stated to be optimized for the human has facilitated this method of culture in many IVF programs [75]. Although several morphologically based scoring systems are used to evaluate the developmental potential of the human blastocyst, they all share common characteristics such as apparent cell numbers in the trophectoderm and the presence, size and organization of the inner cell mass [76]. Current grading systems are largely derived from early studies of human blastocyst development in vitro, which demonstrated the occurrence of embryos with an absent or disorganized inner cell mass, and for the trophectoderm, cell numbers that were significantly below normal for day 5 or 6 [77–79]. For programs that must limit the number of replaced embryos to one or two, prolongation of culture to the blastocyst stage has become the procedure of choice and improved viability after cryopreservation has also contributed to the acceptance of prolonged culture.

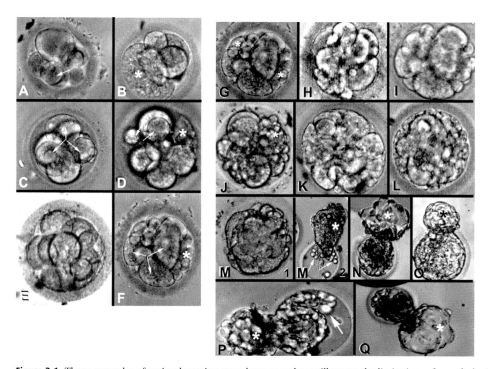

Figure 2.1 These examples of preimplantation stage human embryos illustrate the limitations of morphological assessments of competence and, with noted exceptions shown here, each has resulted in the birth of a normal child conceived after conventional IVF or ICSI. Morphological criteria of competence typically include stage-appropriate cell numbers, uniformity of cell divisions, mononucleation and the absence of cytoplasmic fragments or their occurrence at low density. However, while these characteristics are widely accepted as optimal in the selection of embryos for transfer (e.g., Figure E), and represent reasonably good indicators of embryo performance that can be readily assessed during the cleavage stages, their predictive power with respect to embryo implantation potential and ability to develop progressively through gestation to birth is limited. This limitation is demonstrated by the transfer of morphologically equivalent, stage-appropriate embryos that can be classified as 'high grade' but, after the replacement of multiple embryos, only one implants or progresses to birth. Irregular cleavage divisions resulting in blastomeres of very different diameters (Figure A), or where a blastomere fails to divide or spontaneously degenerates (asterisk, Figure B) are features usually associated with developmental incompetence. In the same respect, the presence of fragment clusters at the free margins of blastomeres is generally considered to be indicative of compromised developmental potential and, depending upon extent, largely signifies a poor post-transfer prognosis. The cleavage stage embryos shown in Figures F–L displayed varying degrees of fragmentation at the time of transfer on day 3, yet each developed normally to term. In these instances, transfers involved one to three morphologically similar embryos. The presence of an irregular blastomere (arrows, Figures C, D) does not necessarily compromise developmental competence if the size differential is relatively small and the affected cells continue to divide. Embryos with fragments and blastomeres of different sizes could seem to have two major competence-related characteristics that would suggest a very low probability of producing normal outcomes after transfer. Yet, the embryos shown in Figures G–L produced normal outcomes after single embryo transfer on day 3.

Progression from the morula to hatched blastocyst stage is generally assumed to be an important and positive indicator of competence. Here too, morphological characteristics of embryo performance in vitro, when used for selection, can be misleading. Figures M1 and M2 show an embryo that developed slowly to the morula stage, while its sibling was in the process of hatching on day 6. Yet, the transfer of both resulted in a normal twin pregnancy. Figures N–Q are examples of blastocysts that showed an apparent arrest in hatching for approximately 16 to 18 hours after it was initiated on day 6, and where complete emergence from the zona pellucida would have normally been expected. In each instance, normal outcomes after transfer indicate that a delay or putative arrest of hatching in vitro may not be synonymous with or predictive of developmental incompetence at the last stage of preimplantation embryogenesis.

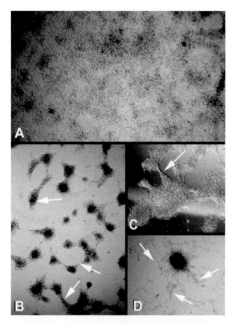

Figure 2.2 Approximately 16 to 24 hours after conventional IVF, distinct oocyte-specific phenotypes of cumulus oophorus cell outgrowths are evident. Figures A–C show three common phenotypes observed in the same culture dish. A rapid and highly proliferative pattern of outgrowth and cell division, as shown in Figure A, results in the rapid formation of a relatively dense cellular monolayer. This pattern has been suggested to be a positive and independent indicator of developmental competence for the corresponding oocyte and embryo. Figure B is a second distinct phenotype in which small clusters of cells are well spaced and inter connected by cellular bridges (arrows). After two days of culture, continued cell division is associated with the merging of clusters, although the cellular bridges are still evident (arrow, Figure C). For a third common phenotype, the cumulus oophorus remains largely unattached or only scattered clusters of cells attach and divide. As shown in Figure C, linear cellular extensions develop from the periphery of these scant and isolated cellular clusters in a manner similar to interconnected bridges shown in Figures B and C. As discussed in the text, each phenotype has been suggested to be related to the developmental competence of the corresponding oocyte and, as such, may provide a criterion for selection that is independent of embryo performance during the cleavage stages.

However, whether development to the blastocyst universally improves outcome when compared to transfers of cleavage stage embryos selected after multiple inspections with strict morphological- and performance-based guidelines remains controversial [80, 81]. Similar to their cleavage stage counterparts, the occurrence of a normal appearing and stage-appropriate blastocyst is not synonymous with normal ploidy [82–84].

Whether certain embryos that failed to progress to the blastocyst or are characterized as stage-inappropriate on days 5 or 6 would have implanted and developed to term had they been transferred on day 3 is also a topic of continuing controversy. While it might seem intuitive that prolongation of culture provides a direct benefit for embryo self-selection, at present, clinical IVF programs that have achieved similar outcomes with the same number of transferred cleavage- or blastocyst-stage embryos form opposite poles of an ongoing debate that centers on the use of morphology for selection, and whether prolongation of culture affords a significant benefit with respect to competence assessment.

The prevailing notion that development to the blastocyst is the most visible evidence of competence was succinctly summed up in a single statement by Behr [85], who concluded that "no blastocyst development in vitro is equivalent to a negative pregnancy test several days early," i.e., had the same embryos been replaced during the cleavage stages. This is an important concept that still forms the basis for the prolongation of culture to the blastocyst. In this context, it can be difficult to understand the rationale behind reported protocols for embryo culture that require a threshold number of stage-appropriate embryos on day 3 (e.g., > 6 or ≥ 8, 8-cell, embryos) as the sole determining factor in whether culture should be continued for an additional 2 or 3 days [80]. Why should thresholds be employed if, by virtue of developmental self-selection, the blastocyst stage provides a demonstrable level of competence? If the confidence level for a positive outcome is significantly increased by the prolongation of embryo culture, then shouldn't the same paradigm be applied regardless of the number of stage-appropriate embryos that exist on day 3, even if it's only one? In reality, after the considerable expense, effort and anguish by the patients undergoing IVF, few clinical IVF programs want to face the situation of not having any embryos to replace because of failure to develop to the blastocyst, or of having a single blastocyst that is morphologically inappropriate with respect to the organization of the trophectoderm or inner cell mass. In this instance, whether inherent physiological differences between embryos manifest in culture with respect to a differential ability to adapt to in vitro conditions and progress to the blastocyst cannot be determined. Therefore, whether stage-appropriate embryos that failed to develop to the blastocyst would have been competent if transferred on day 2 or 3 is unknown when extended culture to day 5 is used [86]. While one interpretation of numerical thresholds as a determinant of the culture protocol would imply a level of uncertainty in the actual predictive value of culture to the blastocyst, embryos that progress normally to this stage clearly demonstrate an inherent competence that is often not shared by their siblings that appeared normal on day 2 or 3 [86], but developed abnormally or arrested cell division thereafter. Thus, blastocyst culture is an appropriate protocol for selection, especially when only single embryos are transferred, but it does not necessarily prove that embryos that failed to progress in vitro beyond day 3 or 4 of culture would have a similar fate in vivo had the transfer been performed earlier. It seems likely that the developmental heterogeneity expressed by human embryos in vitro reflects two important issues: (1) inherent molecular, cellular or genetic differences between embryos may be non-permissive for development beyond cleavage and would have occurred in vivo, and (2) an embryo-specific ability to maintain competence over prolonged culture periods. Gene expression and proteomic analyses may be the most effective approach to distinguish between these possibilities if unique and subtle differences between embryos can be detected and associated with embryo performance and competence. In this respect, it may be that no single culture system in

current use will be able to address inherent differences related to adaptability.

The inherent failings of embryo morphology as applied to the prediction of human embryo viability have led to the investigation of other potential developmental markers that can be assessed in conjunction with performance. In this respect, non-invasive assessments of competence have taken two directions: (1) the evaluation of growth factors and intrafollicular conditions to which the preovulatory oocyte is exposed during the follicular and early luteal phases and (2) biochemical, metabolic and gene expression patterns in oocytes and early embryos that could provide a profile of bioactivities that are consistent with competence. Although these evaluative directions are not mutually exclusive, each is based on different assumptions concerning influences on competence.

The intrafollicular milieu and perifollicular blood flow as determinants of developmental competence

The search for markers of embryo competence directed to molecular and physiological aspects of follicular biology is based on two underlying assumptions: (1) that the developmental competence of the early embryo can be influenced by stage-specific molecular, cellular and nuclear (i.e., chromosomal) processes that occur in the fully grown oocyte during follicular growth and preovulatory maturation and (2) that the normality of these stage-specific activities can be influenced by intrafollicular conditions. From the earliest days of clinical IVF, quantitative measurements of follicle-specific levels of steroid hormones, such as estrogen and progesterone, and gonadotropins (follicle-stimulating hormone [FSH], luteinizing hormone [LH]) have used follicular aspirates obtained during ovum retrieval. However, despite the existence of a sizeable literature in this regard, evidence that relates specific levels to outcome for the corresponding oocyte has not been sufficiently compelling to warrant their analysis on a follicle-specific basis for gamete or embryo selection. With respect to steroid biology, a strong association seems to exist between follicular cortisol:cortisone ratios and oocyte competence, as indicated by outcome after IVF [87, 88]. Because quantitation of these molecules requires both technical expertise and analytical equipment that may not be routinely available in most clinical IVF laboratories, measurements of follicle-specific cortisol and cortisone levels have been not been adopted. However, with increasing awareness of the biochemical complexity of the follicular milieu to which the oocyte is exposed, the notion that markers of competence may exist has gained currency and intrafollicular levels of growth factors such as leptin, vascular endothelial growth factor (VEGF) and inhibin A and B have been suggested to correlate with outcome [89–91]. However, a clear correspondence between level and outcome has yet to be established to the point that follicle-specific measurements for these factors are warranted for the purpose of oocyte and early embryo selection.

One protein growth factor that currently does show promise in this regard is Müllerian inhibiting hormone (homologous to its male counterpart, anti-Müllerian hormone, or AMH), a dimeric glycoprotein member of the tumor growth factor-β (TGF-β) superfamily. As a granulosa cell product, levels of AMH measured in serum during follicular stimulation are predictive of the number of preovulatory follicles that should be responsive to ovulation induction [92, 93], or when measured the day of ovulation induction, seem to correlate well with normal, stage-appropriate embryo development in vitro [94]. At aspiration, AMH levels in follicular fluid also seem to be highly predictive of competence for the corresponding oocyte and resulting embryo [95]. These results have led some to conclude that of all the bioactive molecules identified in follicular fluid and suggested to date to be markers of competence, AMH may be the only one with sufficient reliability to actually serve as a predictor of outcome [96]. The utility of AMH as a competence marker based on follicle-specific levels requires quantitative assays to be available in routine clinical IVF laboratories. For selective purposes, levels for each follicular aspirate would have to be obtained within the relatively narrow time frame between ovum retrieval and insemination (typically, 1 to 4 hours) by conventional IVF or ICSI. In addition, follicles would have to be individually aspirated with rinses between follicular punctures, which would add additional time to the ovum retrieval procedure. These conditions could be problematic for IVF programs, but not insurmountable if follicular fluid-specific levels are confirmed to be competence-associated at high certainty.

Measurements of perifollicular blood flow velocity by two-dimensional and three-dimensional color pulsed Doppler ultrasonography, and determinations of the degree of expansion of the perifollicular microvasculature during stimulation by digital power angiography, have received a recent resurgence of interest as a non-invasive method of assessing oocyte competence. The introduction of new digital platforms for high-resolution ultrasonographic analysis and display has been especially important in this regard, as it has enabled patterns and velocities of blood flow around the circumference of the follicular wall to be examined at a level of detail significantly finer than afforded by previous generations of Doppler ultrasound instruments. Present versions permit real-time analysis with background subtraction such that the dynamic characteristics of individual follicles can be studied in isolation. Current interest in whether perifollicular blood flow characteristics reflect the normality of the intrafollicular milieu that can be related to the competence of the corresponding oocyte are largely based on earlier Doppler studies of human follicles that suggested such a relationship [89, 97, 98, for reviews]. A significant correspondence between oocyte and embryo competence and high blood flow velocities was reported to be associated with reduced frequencies of aneuploidy [99] and higher rates of implantation and term development with oocytes that originated from follicles with high blood flow velocities [100, 101]. Van Blerkom *et al.* [99] reported that differences in perifollicular blood flow rates also correlated with the degree of oxygenation of the follicular fluid measured at aspiration. These authors proposed that follicle-specific differences in oxygen perfusion from the perifollicular capillary bed could directly influence the biosynthetic activity of the mural and cumulus granulosa cells and, indirectly, an intrafollicular biochemistry consistent with oocyte competence [97].

Follicle-specific differences in perifollicular blood flow rates have been suggested to result from the relatively rapid expansion of the perifollicular capillary bed during the follicular phase of stimulation, or from an increased patency of the existing vasculature, or both. The level of expansion may be related to the ability of FSH-sensitized granulosa cells to respond to hypoxia by upregulating hypoxia-induced transcription factor (HIF) pathway [89, for review] that in turn upregulates the expression of several potent angiogenesis-promoting factors, such as VEGF [102]. The presence of elements of the HIF pathway within human follicular granulosa cells has been demonstrated at the mRNA [97] and protein levels [89], and differences in expression levels have been detected between follicles characterized by Doppler ultrasonography as high or low flow [97]. Increased perifollicular flow rates and the number of follicles experiencing this rise during follicular stimulation may be associated with corresponding follicle-specific levels of growth factors such as AMH that, as noted above, have been purported to predict the number of fully grown preovulatory follicles that should be present at ovum retrieval and, possibly, oocyte competence, although the latter notion requires additional validation. Although speculative, it is a testable hypothesis that the stimulation of angiogenesis may facilitate increased oxygen perfusion into the follicle and positively influence the biosynthetic activity of steroid- and protein growth factor-producing granulosa cells. The progressive increase in perifollicular blood flow may be associated with a corresponding increase in the circulating levels of exportable factors produced by granulosa cells and measured in serum. Confirmation of this notion will require studies that determine levels in circulation and correlate

these values with the number of high flow follicles detectable during follicular stimulation. A positive association would provide further support for measurements of perifollicular vascularity and perhaps reduce the need to measure levels of AMH or other competence-associated markers.

At present, it seems that the competent oocytes are more likely to originate from follicles where relatively high rates of perifollicular flow occur around the entire circumference of the follicle rather than in local "hot spots" of apparent elevated velocity [89]. Doppler imaging of ovarian follicles has been suggested to be particularly valuable in poor responder IVF patients where outcomes after embryo transfer have been reported to occur at the same frequency as in the so-called "normal" responder, if one or more follicles show high flow [103]. Indeed, high rates of pre- and postimplantation failure observed in patients with undetectable or "low-grade" flow led these authors to suggest that such cycles should be canceled prior to ovulation induction. Although most studies have largely supported a clinically relevant association between perifollicular blood flow rates, levels of intrafollicular oxygenation and oocyte competence, embryo performance in vitro and outcome after transfer [103–107], it remains unclear what specific biochemical or physiological conditions occur between high and low flow follicles that could influence the subsequent developmental viability of the intact (cumulus-enclosed) oocyte and embryo. The suggestion that persistent intrafollicular hypoxia can reduce oocyte cytoplasmic pH (pHi) during meiotic maturation and adversely affect the organization of spindle microtubules [97], leading to aneuploidy from chromosomal malalignment and segregation, warrants investigation and imaging of spindle birefringence may be especially applicable in this regard, as discussed above. While these are intriguing notions, they will remain speculative until more is known about the molecular biology of the human follicle, how biochemical differences between follicles arise, and whether and how such differences can influence the establishment of developmental competence in the corresponding oocyte.

Metabolic and molecular approaches to assessment

A second direction in the non-invasive assessment of human oocyte and early embryo competence uses molecular markers (proteomic) or metabolic parameters (metabolomic) that are largely independent of morphological considerations. While proteomic technology can display arrays of hundreds of proteins separated by their physical characteristics, such as molecular weight and charge, clinical application requires that the identification and characterization of putative stage-specific markers of competence be limited to secreted polypeptides that can be detected in culture medium at quantifiable levels. This approach would exclude the analysis of cytoplasmic proteins involved in critical cellular activities such as (1) the formation of the meiotic and mitotic spindles, (2) the normality of DNA replication, repair and chromosomal segregation, (3) intracellular signal transduction pathways, (4) the regulation of the cell cycle and cleavage divisions and (5) metabolism. Quantitation of expression levels for both specific mRNAs and proteins is amenable for experimental analysis where the oocyte or early embryo is destroyed in the process, but not for clinical purposes which would require some form of "molecular sampling" of cytoplasmic extracts removed by mechanical means.

The detection of certain bioactive molecules secreted by early embryos at levels that can be measured in culture medium has the potential to add a second and independent dimension to competence assessment schemes that are primarily morphology- and performance-based, if expression levels can be correlated with competence in vitro and outcome in vivo. The search for and analysis of such proteins has been an ongoing process that began in the early days of clinical IVF with levels of platelet-activating factor (PAF) and human chorionic gonadotropin (hCG) suggested to be viability markers [108, 109]. However, the inclusion of quantitative assays to measure levels in culture medium has not been widely used because, as shown in these early reports, their concentration can vary considerably between embryos that appear equivalent in competence. Threshold levels associated with successful outcomes have been difficult to establish, especially for the earliest stages of development, when selection may be necessary. For example, in the case of hCG, the molecule is not secreted at levels that could be meaningful for competence until the peri-implantation period, which is problematic where current restrictions exist on the length of culture [e.g., 110].

More recently, human leukocyte antigen-G (HLA-G) has received considerable attention as a competence marker for the early preimplantation stage human embryo [111]. This is a non-classical major histocompatibility complex (MHC) ligand that is expressed on the surface of the trophoblast shortly after implantation and is thought to act as an immunosuppressive agent that regulates cytokine production by uterine natural killer (uNK) cells, which can participate in the rejection of the embryo [112]. The HLA-G gene is expressed in multiple isoforms because of alternative splicing, and occurs in membrane-bound (HLA-G 1–4) and soluble forms (sHLA-G; HLA-G 5–7) [113]. It is the soluble form(s) that has been quantified in the spent human embryo culture medium and reported to be a potent biomarker of competence and outcome in clinical IVF [111, 114, 115].

While some studies have reported that a developmentally significant correspondence exists between sHLA-G levels and outcome, others have not [116–118] and at present it is unclear whether the failure to detect sHLA-G is indicative of incompetence, regardless of normal morphology and stage-appropriate performance. Further complicating the issue of whether sHLA-G levels are a clear predictor of competence are questions concerning the origin of this molecule and whether levels measured in culture medium are reflective of embryonic translation capacity. For example, Blaschitz et al. [119] reported that the source of sHLA-G in blastocyst culture medium was not from an alternatively spliced mRNA but rather from the cleavage of a membrane-bound HLA-G1 isoform. Yao et al. (113) reported that HLA-G5 mRNA was undetectable in single 2- to 8-cell human embryos and was expressed in only 20% of embryos at the morula and blastocyst stage. In contrast, the sHLA-G protein was detected immunologically in most embryos between the 2- and 8-cell stage and in all blastocysts studied, which led these authors to suggest that the source of the HLA-G protein detected in the absence of corresponding transcripts was from maternal stores that were either produced or incorporated into the oocyte prior to embryonic genomic activation. The validity of sHLA-G levels measured for competence was further questioned by Menezo *et al.* [120], who calculated that virtually all of the translational activity of the early cleavage stage human embryo would have to be devoted to the production of sHLA-G in order to support the concentrations measured in culture medium and associated with developmental competence for the corresponding embryo. Because important molecular, genetic and physiological issues have been raised concerning the use of sHLA-G for diagnostic purposes in clinical IVF, the questions of whether it "really exists" [116] and whether levels measured in culture medium are more than an "interesting artifact" [120] and "worth measuring" [121], need to be resolved with a standardized bioassay that provides sufficient specificity and sensitivity [118] to allow replication between laboratories and threshold levels to be determined. If the presence of sHLA-G in culture medium for the early cleavage stage human embryos is confirmed and threshold levels can be correlated with outcome, its inclusion as a criterion for embryo assessment would become a very powerful tool for selection where development beyond this stage is not permitted. At present, the absence of detectable sHLA-G in spent culture medium in which the corresponding embryo(s) were known to develop normally after uterine transfer calls into question its diagnostic capacity for embryo selection in clinical IVF.

While the utility of sHLA-G for embryo selection in clinical IVF remains to be determined conclusively, another immune protein, the stress-inducible soluble MHC Class I chain-related molecule (sMIC),

has been very recently reported to be a potent biomarker of outcome [122]. Unlike sHLA-G, which for diagnostic purposes requires levels to be measured in spent culture medium, sMIC is measured in serum prior to the initiation of IVF. These authors reported levels consistent with a term pregnancy (< 2.45 ng/ml), or indicative of a significant risk of spontaneous abortion (> 3.0 ng/ml), and proposed that specific threshold levels of sMIC existed, above which term pregnancies never occurred during natural pregnancy or with IVF after controlled ovarian hyperstimulation. The mechanism of sMIC activity in early pregnancy may involve its influence on NK cell function, which is mediated by a cell surface receptor, the G2D receptor (NKG2D); at high level, the production of cytotoxic (embryotoxic) factors by uNK cells is upregulated. However, NKG2D activity is also downregulated by sMIC, which indicates a potential suppressive role for this molecule in contributing to maternal immuno-tolerance and fetal survival during early pregnancy, i.e., it inhibits the production of embryotoxic cytokines and chemokines [123]. The role of uNK cells in pregnancy has emerged as both important and complex in the creation of an "immunologically privileged" environment for embryo implantation, and for the production of a wide variety of growth factors and cytokines, including angiogenic promoters, involved in implantation and normal placentation [124].

While it is not atypical for a ligand to have stimulatory and inhibitory effects, the mechanism by which certain threshold levels of sMIC may be associated with outcome remains to be determined. However, what makes the possibility that sMIC could be highly predictive of outcome in IVF is that critical levels are measured in maternal blood prior to IVF and in this instance outcome is independent of normal ("high-grade") morphological parameters or stage-appropriate in vitro performance during the preimplantation stages. Similar to the suggested use of perifollicular blood flow characteristics (see above) in deciding whether a stimulated cycle should proceed to follicular aspiration and IVF, confirmation that certain sMIC levels are indeed prognostic for women at higher risk of a spontaneous abortion can have important implications in the management of IVF cycles. Rather than stopping a cycle prior to retrieval, oocytes or embryos could be cryopreserved and thawed for fertilization or transfer when levels consistent with term gestation are detected. Indeed, if the predictive power of sMIC levels is validated and assays can be developed that are applicable for use in most clinical IVF laboratories, its combination with routine follicular monitoring by three-dimensional Doppler ultrasonography may provide two embryo-independent measures of competence and the probability of a normal outcome. This level of assessment could become a very significant factor in designing new paradigms to measure the risk of failure in IVF, as well as determining the suitability of a single embryo transfer, or transfer at all, on the fresh cycle.

Proteomic and genomic mining for competence biomarkers

Genomic (mRNA) analyses of complex cellular systems have become relatively adaptable to single oocytes and preimplantation stage embryos primarily because of the availability of commercial systems for sequence amplification and gene detection in microarrays. It remains to be seen whether the application of modern proteomic analysis to spent embryo culture medium in which mass spectroscopy is used for protein identification will have a similar sensitivity for the detection of novel proteins that may be secreted in a stage-specific manner and, if defined, worthy of study with respect to competence. However, some intriguing findings from studies of human cumulus cells suggest that the expression levels of certain genes may be related to the competence of the corresponding oocyte [125, 126]. For example, McKenzie et al. [125] reported that the expression levels of three genes, cyclooxygenase 2 (COX2), hyaluronic acid synthetase (HAS2) and gremlin (GREM1), were associated with the normality of human embryo performance in vitro to day 3, as based on standard morphological parameters such as blastomere number, shape, size, degree of fragmentation and certain cytoplasmic characteristics. The association between upregulated expression levels of GREM1 and HAS2 by cumulus cells and normal, stage-appropriate development in vitro that resulted in a "high-grade" classification on day 3 has also been reported by Cillo et al. [126]. Although outcomes for the corresponding embryos were not reported, these types of studies demonstrate that subtle differences in expression levels within the cumulus oophous that surrounds the oocyte can have a significant downstream influence on the apparent normality of early embryogenesis and, presumably, their competence to develop progressively after transfer.

The specialized instrumentation required for detection by proteomic and genomic analysis is generally unavailable in clinical IVF laboratories [127], and while molecular analyses are attractive in concept, their introduction could add an unnecessary level of complexity, especially if the results are equivocal with respect to outcome. A genomic- or proteomic-based diagnostic test for competence assessment that could be suitable for clinical IVF would be one containing a panel of markers whose developmental functions are understood, clearly relatable to the normality of early development and which occur in individual cumulus masses, or in culture medium containing single embryos, at levels that can be meaningfully quantified. In this regard, while molecular and genetic analyses can be powerful tools for oocyte and embryo selection, it should be considered that "molecular bullets" that can unambiguously predict competence may not exist. This is most obvious in instances of normal implantation potential and developmental competence after transfer of embryos with certain chromosomal abnormalities, whose performance and viability is equal to their euploid counterparts. Genomic and proteomic analysis of expression at the mRNA and protein levels that are focused on the identification of molecules known to be the products of genes located on specific chromosomes would be a boon to embryo selection for ploidy defects, especially if putative marker proteins occur in spent culture medium and at levels that can be determined in a bioassay applicable to clinical IVF laboratories. In the context of embryo selection for transfer, it will also be important to determine whether such markers can be related to specific morphological (e.g., fragmentation, multinucleation) and performance characteristics (e.g., stage-appropriates rates and uniformity of cell division) currently used for selection purposes. The above caveats are formidable barriers to the goal of using protein biomarkers derived from culture medium to assess competence for the corresponding embryo. In the same respect, why normal outcomes occur with embryos whose performance in vitro leads to a "low-grade" morphological classification or a poor prognosis designation with regard to developmental competence needs to be understood in the context of expression levels for proposed marker genes and proteins.

At present, the identification of proteins that may be secreted by the granulosa cells surrounding an oocyte could be a more productive avenue of investigation if outcome results can clearly demonstrate that the presence or levels of specific proteins are associated with competence for the corresponding oocyte. Reason for optimism in this regard comes from the characterization of specific patterns of human cumulus cell attachment, growth and expansion during the first 24 hours of culture. Gregory *et al.* [128] and Van Blerkom [129] described distinct cumulus cell phenotypes that were oocyte-specific and, in these preliminary studies, were suggested to be predictive of the subsequent developmental normality for the corresponding embryo when cultured in their absence (Figure 2.2). If an association between outcome and cumulus cell behavior in vitro can be confirmed, proteins secreted or shed by these cells, under culture conditions standardized for cell density, could provide independent biomarkers of competence based on phenotype (i.e., morphological) and molecular analysis. This approach to selection may be particularly relevant where the preferred or

mandated protocol requires embryo transfer during the early cleavage stages. In this regard, stage-appropriate and morphologically equivalent cleavage stage embryos can occur in instances where their separately cultured cumulus cell component exhibits a phenotype suggested to be a positive or negative indicator of competence [128, 129]. Ideally, the occurrence of marker proteins combined with cumulus cell phenotype may be one basis for selection where embryos have similar morphological characteristics or where morphology is equivocal for this purpose.

The extent to which outcome and cumulus behavior in vitro are related is currently under investigation with respect to the level of certainty this approach can provide. Because the biology of cumulus cells in vivo is associated with the normality of oocyte growth, preovulatory maturation and development after fertilization, as discussed above, follicle-specific differences in cumulus cell bioactivity that could have downstream influences on embryo development [89, 97] may persist in vitro for a time sufficient for unique phenotypes to manifest (∼24 hours). Our preliminary findings in this regard support the notion of phenotype-specific cumulus cell protein profiles, as determined by S^{35}-methionine incorporation into nascent proteins followed by high-resolution two-dimensional polyacrylamide gel electrophoresis and autoradiography. Cumulus masses mechanically divided shortly after aspiration into two fragments, one of which is incubated in the presence of radiolabeled amino acids, including S^{35}-l-methionine, while the other is radiolabeled after phenotype was evident (18–24 hours), indicates that the unique elements of the protein synthetic profile in the intact mass persist in vitro. If current efforts successfully verify the specificity of the phenotype-specific proteins and confirm their occurrence in culture media, their identification from proteomic databases could provide the first step needed for this type of correlative protocol. While potential application in a fresh cycle is apparent, such a protocol could be important in oocyte cryopreservation, where freezing is done before cumulus behavior in vitro is known. Once determined for each oocyte, the findings could be used to prioritize selection for thawing. At present, the extent to which conditions unique to each follicle, such as differential levels of intrafollicular dissolved oxygen, could influence cumulus cell gene expression for molecules that have important downstream developmental effects on oocyte and embryo competence is unclear. Because important changes in follicular physiology, granulosa cell function and activity, and the acquisition of competence for the oocyte are developmentally coordinated and interactive processes [130], it seems reasonable to speculate that studies which examine follicle-specific characteristics (e.g., perifollicular blood flow velocities or AMH levels) may detect corresponding differences in cumulus cell gene expression that are associated with competence. For clinical purposes, the value of such studies may lie in the detection of marker proteins and the identification of their function or activities, that can provide a biological understanding of the developmental origins of competence and which would increase the level of confidence in non-invasive methods of selection.

Genomic analysis using commercially available microarrays allows thousands of genes to be detected simultaneously and, as with somatic cell research, is becoming a powerful tool to study the "topology" of gene expression during oogenesis and early embryogenesis that may provide competence markers [131]. This approach allows families of genes (e.g., regulatory, signaling, cell cycle, metabolic, enzymatic, structural, biosynthetic) to be examined in terms of expression levels and in the context of developmental stage, duration of expression and relation to abnormal development in vitro. Differences in the topology of gene expression (duration and levels) between oocytes grown in vivo and in vitro may provide clinically relevant insights that could aid in the optimization of culture systems designed to produce competent oocytes after growth in vitro from early stages. Differences in gene expression between embryos fertilized in vivo and in vitro [132] and the responses of early embryos to different culture conditions or medium formulations [133] can also be monitored

at this level. However, the comparative enormity of the data generated can make it difficult to distinguish between changes that reflect the ability of the embryo to adapt to in vitro conditions [127] from those that may be developmentally significant or have beneficial or adverse downstream consequences. It is also important to consider that small changes in culture conditions (e.g., percent oxygen) could be developmentally benign despite an apparent effect on expression levels (Van Blerkom, unpublished). A similar situation applies to embryos in culture, where differences detected by microarray analysis may reflect normal heterogeneity in molecular expression levels or inherent differences related to how each embryo adapts to in vitro culture, which, as noted above, may or may not be of developmental significance. Human embryos develop successfully in different media formulations and atmospheric conditions, (e.g., room air vs. 5% O_2), yet it is likely that microarray analysis would indicate differences in expression levels [134].

These caveats raise an important issue with respect to the utility of microarray and proteomic analyses for the selection of human oocytes and embryos, especially where specific genes are initially assumed to be competence-related in experimental studies. Findings from the study of single human oocytes and preimplantation stage embryos within the same or different cohorts may be more difficult to interpret owing to inherent heterogeneity that may create "background noise" at the level of gene detection. Indeed, for the purpose of selection based on findings from genomic analyses, it is possible that no clinically *useful* signal or signals will be detected. This is not to say that such signals don't exist, only that their detection by non-invasive means may not be realistic or practical for most clinical IVF programs. On the other hand, the combination of proteomic and genomic analyses offers the very real potential to investigate causes of developmental incompetence and differential performance of human oocytes and embryos that are manifested in vitro. This may be especially evident with respect to the following common problems in early development: (1) premature meiotic arrest, (2) fertilization failure (e.g., inability to evolve pronuclei), (3) arrest at the pronuclear and cleavage stages, (4) aberrant performance (toxic levels of fragmentation, blastomere multinucleation, asymmetric divisions), (5) abnormalities in cell allocation between the inner cell mass and trophectoderm during blastocyst formation and (6) failure of apparently normal-appearing expanded blastocysts to emerge from the confines of the zona pellucida (i.e., "hatch") or attach to the endometrium after hatching.

The metabolic approach to selection

The notion that the differential developmental competence of human embryos cultured under identical conditions and manifested by morphological and performance heterogeneity has a metabolic basis dates to the earliest days of clinical IVF. Early reports of oxygen consumption by single human oocytes and embryos [135] showed wide differences in uptake levels that may be related to developmental potential. Later studies examined other metabolic parameters, such as substrate utilization and metabolite and amino acid turnover (depletion from or secretion into culture medium) [136–139], and came to similar conclusions, namely, (1) that bioenergetic status was largely oocyte- and embryo-specific and (2) as energy availability is a primary engine of stage-specific developmental and morphogenetic change during the preimplantation stages, it was likely to be a critical determinant of competence.

Analysis of metabolic parameters suggested to be competence-related has yet to be widely used for oocyte or embryo selection because the quantitative methodology requires analytical instrumentation and expertise not usually available in clinical IVF programs, especially those not affiliated with major research institutions. This may change with the development of instrumentation capable of measuring oxygen levels and uptake rates in microliter volumes, and designed for clinical IVF laboratories where oocytes or embryos can be cultured

individually [140]. The ability to monitor and record coincident morphological and performance characteristics is an especially important feature in this regard, as it enables metabolic and developmental parameters during the preimplantation stages to be assessed simultaneously and later correlated with embryo-specific outcome. However, to achieve a high level of certainty for selection, it will be necessary to understand the cellular basis of the differential bioenergetic state that exists between human oocytes and embryos, particularly those that display similar morphological and performance characteristics during the preimplantation stages. Likewise, threshold levels of oxygen consumption and substrate utilization measured on the single oocyte or embryo level and suggested to be diagnostic of competence will require extensive multicenter validation. The introduction of instrumentation designed to measure metabolic and performance characteristics at the single cell or embryo level is a necessary first step in designing new competence assessment paradigms [140]. In this respect, selection in clinical IVF may transition rapidly from an endeavor that is largely empirical to one that includes developmentally relevant physiological and molecular information for each stage.

Mitochondria and competence

Because mitochondria are the principal source of energy in the preovulatory oocyte and preimplantation stage embryo, by virtue of their ability to generate ATP, the extent to which these elements are proximal determinants of competence has become a recent focus of interest in clinical IVF [141–143]. Earlier studies of the net cytoplasmic ATP content of morphologically normal-appearing MII human and mouse oocytes suggested that energetic capacity for the early embryos is largely established in the mature oocyte, and that certain levels of ATP generation may represent competence thresholds [144]. The notion of bioenergetic thresholds was supported in later work by Van Blerkom et al. [145], who described the phenomenon of (spontaneous) disproportionate mitochondrial segregation during early human cleavage that resulted in mitochondrial underrepresentation (i.e., numerical) in some blastomeres. The affected cells were shown to have significantly reduced ATP contents with different levels having different developmental effects, such as arrested cytokinesis or lysis.

The introduction of methods to quantify the number of mitochondrial DNA (mtDNA) copies in single human oocytes has facilitated investigations of the apparent developmental association between mitochondria and the performance of human embryos in vitro and outcome in vivo. Initial reports of the mtDNA content of oocytes routinely obtained for IVF after ovarian hyperstimulation seemed to show a correspondence between copy number and the normality of meiotic maturation, fertilizability, and the capacity of the embryo to develop progressively and normally in vitro [141, 146, 147]. These findings tend to support the notion that rates or levels of mitochondrial replication during the growth phase of oogenesis may be oocyte-specific and after fertilization could contribute to bioenergetic differences that have developmental consequences. As additional quantitative analyses of human oocytes were undertaken, the reported mtDNA contents of MII oocytes within and between cohorts showed huge variability, ranging from the tens of thousands to well over a million [141, 142, 148]. If, as is generally assumed, each oocyte mitochondrion contains one or two mitochondrial genomes [149], then the size of the actual organelle complement in similarly appearing oocytes at the same stage of meiotic maturation (e.g., MII) would, based on reported mtDNA contents, range from $\leq \sim 20\,000$ to $> 1\,000\,000$, or by nearly two orders of magnitude [148]. Indeed, inherent differences in mitochondrial complement size would support the use of metabolic indicators based on measurements of substrate utilization by individual MII oocytes or early embryos.

The relationship between oocyte-specific variability in mtDNA content, actual organelle numbers and bioenergetic capacity needs to be better understood [149] in the context of differential rates of substrate utilization, oxygen consumption or metabolite/amino acid turnover if they are to provide important diagnostic information that can serve as an independent indicator of competence. This approach would require only that embryos be cultured individually and the analytical means to assess bioenergetic capacity is available and does not add significant complexity to routine IVF protocols. In this regard, new generations of instruments that use microelectrodes capable of detecting small changes in oxygen tension in microliter volumes [140] may provide a means for analyses that can be used in most clinical IVF laboratories. However, the physiological basis of what oocyte- or embryo-specific differences reflect, or whether threshold levels exist that can accurately predict competence, will have to be clearly validated with respect to outcome. It is important to emphasize that relative certainty is the central issue at each level of selection, and is one that repeats in every scheme advanced to date for this purpose. As noted above, subjective morphological criteria can fail in this regard, as often evidenced by normal outcomes with embryos judged "poor quality," "low-grade" or "stage-inappropriate" at transfer, or where "objective" criteria are used. This is also the case with biomarkers such AMH, sMIC and sHLA-G, as normal outcomes have occurred when levels measured in circulation (sMIC, AMH), follicular fluid (AMH), or spent embryo culture medium (sHLA-G) suggested poor competence or developmental potential.

Because of the current emphasis on metabolic parameters as predictors of competence, special attention needs to be paid to what these levels actually reflect in developmental terms, the extent to which, if any, extrinsic and intrinsic factors regulate bioenergetic status, and what metabolic thresholds are permissive or consistent with normal development. The last is presently controversial but is among the most important aspects of early development if this selection approach is to be used in clinical IVF laboratories. Zeng *et al.* [34] examined the extent to which the bioenergetic capacity of human oocytes was related to developmental competence by measuring mtDNA copy numbers and ATP concentrations in human oocytes classified as MII owing to the presence of a first polar body (after maturation in vitro from the germinal vesicle stage). They further subdivided these oocytes into those with or without a meiotic spindle detectable by polarizing light imaging. They compared these values with mtDNA and ATP levels measured in normally fertilized eggs that arrested development in vitro or showed abnormal patterns of cleavage. Fifty percent of MII oocytes had a detectable metaphase spindle and an average mtDNA copy number of $\sim$ 637 K ($+$238 K) and ATP content of $\sim$ 1.97 pmol ($+$0.38 pmol). These values were significantly higher than for sibling oocytes with a first polar body but with no detectable MII spindle, where the average mtDNA copy number was $\sim$ 491 K ($+$153 K) and the net average ATP content was 1.65 pmol ($+$0.32 pmol). They concluded that a low mtDNA copy number was indicative of a reduced organelle complement and the corresponding reduction in cytoplasmic ATP content was related to a subnormal bioenergetic capacity. This notion was suggested further by fertilization results using ICSI with MII oocytes with and without detectable spindles. In the absence of a detectable MII spindle, fertilization rates were lower and the frequency of arrested or abnormal embryonic development during the early preimplantation stages was significantly higher than in sibling MII oocytes with detectable spindles. A similar relationship between mtDNA content and outcome after conventional IVF and ICSI was described by Santos *et al.* [150], who found that the mean mtDNA copy number in fertilized human oocytes was $\sim$ 250K, while for unfertilized oocytes, the mean number was $\sim$ 164K. These two studies indicate one of the current problems in assessing competence by relating developmental performance in vitro with biological indicators (mtDNA copy numbers) and physiological characteristics (ATP content). The mtDNA copy number reported as normal for human MII oocytes by Santos *et al.* is well below the competence threshold described by Zeng *et al.*

Determinations of how levels of oxygen consumption or substrate utilization relate to actual organelle content will be required to validate the efficacy of such measurements for selection. In addition, the potential relevance of developmentally significant phenomena, such as disproportionate mitochondrial segregation during cleavage, which can have demonstrable effects on blastomere-specific ATP contents and fate, needs to be addressed with respect to frequency and impact if the quantitation of metabolic parameters is to have a high level of certainty. In this instance, a normal bioenergetic condition might be expected for embryos experiencing disproportionate mitochondrial segregation because the factors measured in culture medium relate to the entire embryo and not to unique conditions in individual cells. This notion is supported by Shoubridge and Wai [147], who suggested that a numerical mitochondrial deficit in the oocyte might be the most important determinant of embryo competence, not because of adverse effects on oocyte metabolism, but because too few organelles would result in "maldistribution" in the blastomeres of the early embryo. As shown for the human [145] and pig [151, 152], mitochondrial maldistribution between blastomeres during early cleavage can have variable adverse developmental consequences for the affected cells, despite an apparently normal numerical complement of organelles in the embryo.

Non-invasive microscopic methods, such as laser illumination at near infra red wavelengths (1003 nm) that detects mitochondrial autofluorescence [153], if developed for clinical IVF laboratories, could be used to identify and quantitate levels of disproportionate mitochondrial segregation, and to correlate estimates of mitochondrial content with (1) metabolic parameters, (2) embryo performance in vitro, (3) morphology, (4) ploidy determined by preimplantation genetic diagnosis and, most importantly, (5) outcome. However, it is unlikely that any microscopic method could address the question of bioenergetic thresholds, i.e., how much ATP is required to drive early human development. For example, both Van Blerkom *et al.* [144] and Zeng *et al.* [34] suggested that a net cytoplasmic ATP content of around 2 pmol for the MII human oocyte might be an optimal level for competence.

However, the developmental ability of the oocytes or early embryos used in these studies is unknown because the analytical methods required their destruction. Van Blerkom *et al.* [144] reported that mouse oocytes matured to MII from the germinal vesicle stage in vitro at high frequency despite a net cytoplasmic ATP content that had been experimentally reduced by nearly 50%. More recently, Van Blerkom and Davis [154] described similar results for sperm penetration, pronuclear formation and the initial cleavage divisions of mouse embryos, in which the net cytoplasmic ATP contents were experimentally reduced to ~50% to 60% of normal.

Local regulation of mitochondrial activity: mitochondrial microzonation in the oocyte and early embryo

The respiratory role of mitochondria in energy production in oocytes and early embryos tends to be viewed at the level of the entire cytoplasm, which is not surprising since substrate, metabolite and ATP measurements involve whole oocytes or embryos. However, energy levels that drive developmentally significant activities and processes may be under local control and within the cytoplasm spatial differences in ATP generation may be a more critical determinant of competence than net cytoplasmic content. In somatic cells, passive mitochondrial redistribution by intracytoplasmic circulation [155], or active translocation along a microtubular array [156], allows changing energy demands within the cytoplasm to be met by increasing the local concentration of mitochondria. Mitochondrial redistributions that primarily involve a periodic perinuclear accumulation and dispersion during the meiotic maturation of the oocyte, and at the pronuclear and early cleavage stages for the embryo, have been described for several species, including the human [148, for review]. Similar to cytoplasmic remodeling in somatic cells, mitochondria in oocytes and early embryos are translocated to perinuclear regions along microtubular arrays

[148, 157–159]. It is generally thought that transient mitochondrial translocations serve to increase ambient ATP levels to meet focal energy demands that are stage-specific, and abnormalities in this dynamic activity, or its failure to occur, can be correlated with developmental incompetence for both oocyte and embryo [148, for review].

In somatic cells, certain patterns of mitochondrial aggregation have been shown to create microzones of differential cytoplasmic physiology (e.g., ambient levels of free calcium, intracellular pH) (microzonation) that lead to functional compartmentalization of biosynthetic and regulatory activities within the cytoplasm [160]. The normal occurrence of mitochondria in small clusters, as well as their active redistribution in oocytes and preimplantation embryos, may create "microzones" that permit a similar type of functional compartmentalization [148, 154], which may be especially relevant in the oocyte and newly fertilized egg if it permits autonomous regulation of development activities that are spatially distant in the largest cells in the body. Several lines of investigation provide preliminary support for this notion. The polarity ($\Delta\Psi$m) of mitochondria localized in small clusters in the subplasmalemmal cytoplasm is normally higher than that detected in their cytoplasmic counterparts [161]. The level of $\Delta\Psi$m is an important determinant of several important mitochondrial functions, including respiratory activity that generates ATP [141, 148]. Van Blerkom and Davis [154] reported that the presence of a microdomain of high-polarized mitochondria in the subplasmalemmal cytoplasm was associated with sperm penetration and cortical granule exocytosis. While the number of mitochondria in this domain are a very small fraction of the total complement, they are spatially stable and remained so during early cleavage, such that loss by minor fragmentation in early cleavage stage embryos results in arrested cell division for the affected cell(s) [162]. Earlier studies indicated that they may also be involved in the regulation of calcium homeostasis in the pericortical cytoplasm [163] and for thawed MII human oocytes, loss of high $\Delta\Psi$m was a suggested factor in penetration failure after conventional IVF [164]. Van Blerkom [148] proposed that this domain of high-polarized mitochondria may be an example of microzonation and, given the influence of $\Delta\Psi$m in different mitochondrial activities [154], could indicate a level of functional compartmentalization within the cytoplasm of the oocyte and early embryo. For example, focally elevated levels of ATP generation by a microzone of high-polarized mitochondria along the circumference of the oocyte may be required to drive developmental processes such as cortical granule exocytosis that are co-localized in the same region.

A second line of support for local regulation of ATP generation in the oocyte and early embryo comes from the studies of Dumollard *et al.* [165, 166], who reported that small changes in ambient free calcium can regulate levels of mitochondrial ATP production. In particular, calcium released by or sequestered into elements of the endoplasmic reticulum was shown to up- or downregulate levels of mitochondrial ATP production in organelles located in proximity to these elements. They proposed that ionic crosstalk between these organellar systems allows focal energy demands to be met locally rather than requiring a general increase in mitochondrial respiratory activity throughout the cytoplasm. An attractive feature of this interpretation is that ATP is largely used by activities (e.g., protein phosphorylation and enzymatic/biosynthetic processes) that occur in close proximity to the site of its generation. They also suggested that focal regulation of ATP production reduced the potential for generating increased levels of damaging reactive oxygen species (ROS) that could result if the upregulation of mitochondrial ATP generation occurred throughout the cytoplasm. We have proposed that the co-localization of elements of the endoplasmic reticulum and high-polarized mitochondria in the subplasmalemmal cytoplasm of the oocyte and early embryo may involve a similar metabolic regulatory mechanism that is confined to a spatially distinct microzone [148, 154, 163]. The finding that certain early events in fertilization, such as sperm

penetration, cortical granule exocytosis and pronuclear formation, can occur at subnormal ATP levels [154] supports the possibility that focal bioenergetic differences may be of greater developmental significance than average values measured for a whole oocyte or embryo. The value of metabolic assessments for selection that are based on measurements of metabolic and bioenergetic characteristics of whole oocytes or embryos (e.g., oxygen and substrate uptake and utilization) could be complicated if a spatial aspect for differential ATP generation and use is confirmed and shown to be developmentally relevant.

Is there an optimal scheme for selection?

The search for validated biomarkers of competence that provide an acceptable level of certainty is a necessary endeavor if single embryo transfers are to become the standard of practice. While the use of morphological criteria is often criticized because it is empirical and often provides information that is equivocal for selection, it should be noted that other means of assessment, such as perifollicular blood flow rates, levels of certain molecules in serum or culture medium, or metabolic and performance parameters (e.g., blastocyst development), each has a failure rate indicated by normal pregnancies with values or characteristics suggested to be indicative of low competence or subsequent failure after transfer. If confidence in a biomarker is to be achieved, it is important to understand why normal outcomes occur in these instances.

For assessment and selection purposes, it may be too much to expect that any of the markers or protocols described above has sufficient "stand alone" diagnostic power to serve as a sole predictor of competence. A more practical and effective approach may be one based on a series of markers that reflect different maternal and embryological aspects associated with success and which are based on known biological functions. While more labor intensive, the use of screening methods during ovarian stimulation may bias the order of aspiration to first retrieve oocytes from follicles with perifollicular blood flow characteristics indicative of competence for the corresponding oocyte. If oocytes are first segregated after retrieval according to the characteristics of the follicles of origin, specific morphological cues presently considered consistent with competence may be applied with greater effect. However, Doppler ultrasonographic imaging of individual follicles is problematic when stimulation produces large numbers of fully grown antral follicles that (1) can change grade designation during stimulation or after ovulation induction, and (2) make it difficult to identify selected follicles from one day to another. An assessment protocol that surveys each ovary for the presence of high-grade follicles could provide information related to how many to expect and where they are likely to be located at ovum retrieval. At retrieval, the brief application of Doppler ultrasonography could be used to identify high-grade follicles, as they would be the first set aspirated. Follicles classified as low or moderate flow, or which are ambiguous in this regard, would be aspirated next.

Levels of other markers such as serum sMIC and AMH may become standard determinants used to decide whether a cycle should begin. Because Doppler imaging can distinguish between follicles based on their unique physiological properties, and current evidence suggests these differences are relevant with respect to the competence of the corresponding oocyte, its application can have the dual use of (1) determining whether a cycle with appropriate sMIC and AMH levels should proceed to ovulation induction and aspiration and (2) providing a positive bias in the choice of oocytes for insemination, as noted above. This "holistic" approach to outcome assessment with independent determinants of whether to stop or proceed with treatment could be particularly important where restrictions or prohibitions exist on the number of oocytes that can be inseminated, the duration of embryo culture, the number of embryos that can be transferred and whether cryopreservation or preimplantation genetic diagnosis is permitted.

Can morphology retain a role in selection?

Morphological assessments for competence are often considered more "art" than science by those whose emphasis is on molecular or biochemical signals. For clinical embryologists responsible for the generation of embryos, the ability to use morphology for selection is largely a function of their individual experience based on direct observations of oocyte and embryo performance combined with knowledge of outcome after transfer. The experiential component should not be casually dismissed simply because of its descriptive foundation. In this regard, Arce *et al.* [167] reported a remarkable consensus of opinion between experienced embryologists who used morphologically based competence grading to independently evaluate over 4000 cleavage stage human embryos provided as digital images for this study. As the use of molecular and metabolic biomarkers enter the clinical IVF laboratory, it can be anticipated that their relative weight in the decision-making process will increase. However, morphology and performance are always evident in IVF, and, regardless of stage, difficult not to take into consideration for selection. The potential for conflict between direct observation and indirect biochemical or molecular indicators will become especially evident (and important) when they differ with respect to competence decisions. If the detection of subtle differences between oocytes and embryos that may provide a positive or negative bias for selection is too dependent upon the experience of the observer, knowledge about the underlying biological causes of different oocyte and embryo phenotypes and how they relate to competence will become essential. For example, do they reflect significant differences in critical developmental pathways and processes, or are they simply manifestations of the differential ability of embryos to adapt to in vitro conditions. The latter notion is currently supported by differential rates and extents of fragmentation reported for different culture environments and media, suggesting that fragmentation may not be an inherent and unavoidable aspect of development, as noted above.

The future of competence selection and single embryo transfers

The present course of research related to the origins of heterogeneity at the earliest stages of human development will undoubtedly benefit from the type of information that metabolic, genomic and proteomic investigations can provide. The extent to which this information can readily translate to the clinical IVF laboratory for purposes of selection remains to be seen. However, because it is ever-present, increased confidence in morphological assessments can come by making them less subjective and operator dependent. Objective evaluations that are biometric-based could incorporate existing image recognition and analysis algorithms in which stage-specific characteristics (e.g., NPB number and distribution, pronuclear orientation, blastomere geometry and volume) and aspects of performance (e.g., amount of cytoplasm lost to fragments, uniformity of cell divisions) are correlated with outcome, and the findings periodically contributed by IVF programs to a common database that is universally accessible. The inclusion of cumulus complex-specific phenotype manifest during the first 24 hours of culture may also be considered if a relationship to competence for the corresponding oocyte is confirmed. Early steps in this direction were taken by Hnida and Ziebe [168] who, for the early cleavage stage embryo, used computerized image analysis to relate certain biometric parameters of individual blastomeres with subsequent performance in vitro and outcome. The capacity to perform simultaneous (non-invasive) assessments of mitochondrial density and distribution at the pronuclear stage and between blastomeres during early cleavage would add an important dimension to objective competence determinations of this type.

It can be anticipated that sufficient outcome results will accumulate to correlate objective determinations of embryo morphology and performance with metabolic values related to bioenergetic capacity, and possibly, biochemical and molecular indicators of competence. Investigations of this type will test the merits of each and their diagnostic power in combination. The fundamental importance for human IVF that would derive from demonstrating the occurrence of specific genetic or chromosomal defects by virtue of an association with morphological characteristics or levels of molecular or metabolic biomarkers is self-evident albeit hypothetical at present. Thus, it is not difficult to envisage that the selection of specific oocytes for insemination, single embryos for transfer, or competent oocytes and embryos for cryopreservation, will involve a series of characteristics and biomarkers whose relative importance is likely to be determined in an operator-independent manner and evaluated by a standard algorithm. The predictive power of competence assessments at the follicular level, whether based on physiology (e.g., perifollicular blood flow velocity) or biochemistry (e.g., AMH levels) needs further validation with respect to embryo performance and outcome. Indeed, this may become the most effective means for selection where the number of oocytes that can be inseminated is proscribed by law or culture beyond the 1-cell stage is prohibited. Where such restrictions do not exist or are more relaxed and related to patient circumstances, its combination with biometric, metabolic and molecular evaluations of embryos should afford the high level of certainty required for single embryo transfers to become the accepted standard in clinical IVF.

REFERENCES

1. P. Steptoe and R. Edwards, Birth after the reimplantation of a human embryo. *Lancet*, **2** (1978), 366.
2. H. Foulot, C. Ranoux, J. Dubuisson *et al.*, In vitro fertilization without ovarian stimulation: a simplified protocol applied in 80 cycles. *Fertil. Steril.*, **52** (1989), 617–621.
3. M. Pelinek, A. Hoek, A. Simmons and M. Heineman, Efficacy of natural cycle IVF: a review of the literature. *Hum. Reprod. Update*, **8** (2002), 129–139.
4. J. Gerris, Reducing the number of embryos to transfer after IVF/ICSI. In J. Van Blerkom and L. Gregory, eds.,

Essential IVF, Basic Research and Clinical Applications (Boston: Kluwer Academic Publishers, 2004), pp. 505–554.

5. R. Edwards, Causes of early embryonic loss in human pregnancy. *Hum. Reprod.*, **1** (1986), 185–198.

6. J. Van Blerkom (ed.), *The Biological Basis of Early Human Reproductive Failure: Applications to Medically-Assisted Conception.* (New York: Oxford University Press, 1994)

7. J. Boue, A. Boue and P. Lazar, Retrospective and prospective epidemiological studies of 1500 karyotyped spontaneous human abortions. *Teratology*, **12** (1975), 11–26.

8. P. Burgoyne, K. Holland and R. Stephens, Incidence of numerical chromosome abnormalities in human pregnancy: estimation from induced and spontaneous abortion data. *Hum. Reprod.*, **6** (1991), 555–564.

9. H. Wramsby, K. Fredga and P. Leidholm, Chromosomal analysis of human oocytes recovered from preovulatory follicles in stimulated cycles. *N. Engl. J. Med.*, **316** (1987), 121–124.

10. R. Angell, W. Ledger, E. Yong, L. Harkness and D. Baird, Cytogenetic analysis of unfertilized human oocytes. *Hum. Reprod.*, **6** (1991), 568–573.

11. J. Van Blerkom, Developmental failure in human reproduction associated with chromosomal abnormalities and cytoplasmic pathologies in meiotically mature oocytes. In J. Van Blerkom, ed., *The Biological Basis of Early Human Reproductive Failure: Applications to Medically-Assisted Conception* (New York: Oxford University Press, 1994), pp. 283–326.

12. J. Van Blerkom and G. Henry, Cytogenetic analysis of living human oocytes: cellular basis and developmental consequences of perturbations in chromosomal organization and complement. *Hum. Reprod.*, **3** (1988), 777–790.

13. A. Viega, G. Calderon, J. Santalo, P. Barri and J. Egozcue, Chromosome studies in oocytes and zygotes from an IVF programme. *Hum. Reprod.*, **2** (1987), 425–430.

14. L. Veeck, *An Atlas of Human Gametes and Conceptuses: An Illustrated Reference for Assisted Reproductive Technology* (New York: Parthenon Publishing Group, 1998).

15. J. Van Blerkom, Occurrence and developmental consequences of aberrant cellular organization in meiotically mature human oocytes after exogenous ovarian hyperstimulation. *J. Electron Microsc. Tech.*, **16** (1990), 324–346.

16. J. Van Blerkom and G. Henry, Oocyte dysmorphism and aneuploidy in meiotically mature human oocytes after ovarian stimulation. *Hum. Reprod.*, **7** (1992), 379–390.

17. J. Otsuki, K. Okada, Y. Morimoto *et al.*, The relationship between pregnancy outcome and smooth endoplasmic reticulum clusters in MII human oocytes. *Hum. Reprod.*, **19** (2004), 2334–2339.

18. J. Meriano, J. Alexis, S. Visram-Zaver *et al.*, Tracking of oocyte dysmorphisms for ICSI patients may prove relevant to outcome in subsequent patient cycles. *Hum. Reprod.*, **16** (2001), 2118–2123.

19. A. Mikkelsen and S. Lindenberg, Morphology of invitro matured oocytes: impact on fertility potential and embryo quality. *Hum. Reprod.*, **16** (2001), 1714–1718.

20. P. De Sutter, D. Dozortsev, C. Qian *et al.*, Oocyte morphology does not correlate with fertilization rate and embryo quality after intracytoplasmic sperm injection. *Hum. Reprod.*, **11** (1996), 595–597.

21. B. Balaban, B. Urman, A. Sertac *et al.*, Oocyte morphology does not affect fertilization rate, embryo quality and implantation rate after intracytoplasmic sperm injection. *Hum. Reprod.*, **13** (1998), 3431–3433.

22. M. Alikani, G. Palermo, A. Adler *et al.*, Intracytoplasmic sperm injection in dysmorphic human oocytes. *Zygote*, **3** (1995), 283–288.

23. J. Van Blerkom, G. Henry and R. Porreco, Preimplantation human embryonic development from polypronuclear eggs after in vitro fertilization. *Fertil. Steril.*, **41** (1984), 686–696.

24. J. Osborn and R. Moor, An assessment of the factors causing embryonic loss after fertilization in vitro. *J. Reprod. Fertil.*, **36**: Suppl. (1988), 59–72.

25. J. Van Blerkom and G. Henry, Dispermic fertilization of human oocytes. *J. Electron Microsc. Tech.*, **17** (1991), 437–449.

26. L. Liu, R. Oldenbourg, J. Trimarchi *et al.*, A reliable, noninvasive technique for spindle imaging and enucleation of mammalian oocytes. *Nat. Biotechnol.*, **18** (2000), 223–225.

27. L. Liu, J. Trimarchi, R. Oldenberg *et al.*, Increased birefringence in the meiotic spindle provides a new marker for the onset of activation in living oocytes. *Biol Reprod.*, **63** (2000), 251–258.

28. D. Keefe, W. Liu, W. Wang *et al.*, Imaging meiotic spindles by polarizing light microscopy, principles and applications to IVF. *Reprod. Biomed. Online*, **7** (2003), 24–29.

29. U. Eichenlaub-Ritter, Y. Shen and H. Tinneberg, Manipulation of the oocyte, possible damage to the spindle apparatus. *Reprod. Biomed. Online*, **5** (2002), 117–124.

30. L. Rienzi, F. Ubaldi, F. Martinez *et al.*, Relationship between meiotic spindle location with regard to polar body position and oocyte developmental potential after ICSI. *Hum. Reprod.*, **18** (2003), 1289–1293.

31. W. Wang, L. Meng and R. Hackett, Limited recovery of meiotic spindles in living human oocytes after cooling-rewarming observed using polarized light microscopy. *Hum. Reprod.*, **16** (2001), 2374–2378.

32. W. Wang, L. Meng, R. Hackett *et al.*, Developmental ability of human oocytes with or without birefringent spindles imaged by PolScope before insemination. *Hum. Reprod.*, **16** (2001), 1464–1468.

33. L. Rienzi, F. Ubaldi, M. Iacobelli *et al.*, Meiotic spindle visualization in living human oocytes. *Reprod. Biomed. Online*, **10** (2005), 192–198.

34. H. Zeng, Z. Ren, S. William *et al.*, Low mitochondrial DNA and ATP contents contribute to the absence of birefringent spindle imaged with PolScope in in vitro matured human oocytes *Hum. Reprod.*, **22** (2007), 1681–1686.

35. Y. Shen, T. Stalf, C. Mehnert *et al.*, Light retardance by human oocyte spindle is positively related to pronuclear score after ICSI. *Reprod. Biomed. Online*, **12** (2006), 737–751.

36. Y. Shen, T. Stalf, C. Mehnert *et al.*, High magnitude of light retardation by the zona pellucida is associated with conception cycles. *Hum. Reprod.*, **20** (2005), 1596–1606.

37. G. Rama Raju, G. Prakash, K. Krishna and K. Madan, Meiotic spindle and zona pellucida characteristics as predictors of embryonic development: a preliminary study using PolScope imaging. *Reprod. Biomed. Online*, **14** (2007), 166–174.

38. M. Montag, T. Schimming, M. Koster *et al.*, Oocyte zona birefringence is associated with implantation potential in ICSI cycles. *Reprod. Biomed. Online*, **16**, 239–244.

39. C. Garello, H. Baker, J. Rai *et al.*, Pronuclear orientation, polar body placement, and embryo quality after intracytoplasmic sperm injection and in-vitro fertilization: further evidence for polarity by single human preimplantation embryos. *Hum. Reprod.*, **14** (1999), 2588–2595.

40. J. Van Blerkom, Clinical applications of symmetry, asymmetry and polarity in early human development. In A. Trounson and R. Gosden, eds., *Biology and Pathology of the Oocyte: Role in Fertility and Reproductive Medicine* (Cambridge: Cambridge University Press, 2003), pp. 163–181.

41. R. Edwards and H. Beard, Oocyte polarity and cell determinaiton in early mammalian embryos. *Mol. Hum. Reprod.*, **3** (1997), 863–905.

42. M. Antczak and J. Van Blerkom, Oocyte influences on early development: the regulatory proteins leptin and STAT3 are polarized in mouse and human oocytes and differentially distributed within the cells of the preimplantation stage embryo. *Mol. Hum. Reprod.*, **3** (1997), 1067–1086.

43. R. Edwards and H. Beard, Hypothesis: sex determination and germline formation are committed at the pronuclear stage in mammalian embryos. *Mol. Hum. Reprod.*, **5** (1999), 595–606.

44. T. Hiiragi and D. Solter, First cleavage plane of the mouse egg is not predetermined but defined by the topology of the two apposing pronuclei. *Nature*, **430** (2004), 360–364.

45. J. Rossant and P. Tam, Emerging asymmetry and embryonic patterning in early mouse development. *Dev. Cell*, **7** (2004), 155–164.

46. R. Gardner, Specification of embryonic axes begins before cleavage in normal mouse development. *Development*, **128** (2001), 839–847.

47. K. Piotrowska-Nitshe, A. Perea-Gomez, S. Haraguchi and M. Zernicke-Goetz, Four-cell stage mouse blastomeres have differential developmental properties. *Development*, **132** (2005), 479–490.

48. D. Strumpf, C. A. Mao, Y. Yamanaka, *et al.*, Cdx2 is required for corrrect cell fate specification and differentiation of trophectoderm in the mouse blastocysts. *Development*, **132** (2005), 2093–2102.

49. K. Deb, M. Sivaguru, H. Yong and R. Roberts, Cdx2 gene expression and trophectoderm lineage specification in mouse embryos. *Science*, **311** (2006), 992–996.

50. R. Roberts, M. Sivaguru and H. Yong, Retraction of Cdx2 gene expression and trophectoderm lineage specification in mouse embryos. *Science*, **317** (2007), 450.

51. D. Payne, S. Flaherty, M. Barry and C. Mathews, Preliminary observations on polar body extrusion and pronuclear formation in human oocytes using time-lapse video cinematography. *Hum. Reprod.*, **12** (1997), 532–541.

52. L. Scott and S. Smith, The successful use of pronuclear embryo transfer the day following oocyte retrieval. *Hum. Reprod.*, **13** (1998), 1003–1013.

53. J. Tesarik and E. Greco, The probability of abnormal preimplantation development can be predicted by a single static observation on pronuclear stage morphology. *Hum. Reprod.*, **14** (1999), 1318–1325.

54. L. Scott, R. Alvero, M. Leondires and B. Miller, The morphology of human pronuclear embryos is positively related to blastocyst development and implantation. *Hum. Reprod.*, **15** (2000), 2394–2403.

55. L. Scott, Pronuclear scoring as a predictor of embryo development. *Reprod. Biomed. Online*, **6** (2003), 201–204.

56. L. Scott, The biological basis of oocyte and embryo competence: morphodynamic criteria for embryo selection in in vitro fertilization. In J. Van Blerkom and L. Gregory, eds., *Essential IVF: Basic Research and Clinical Applications* (Boston: Kluwer Academic Publishers, 2004), pp. 333–376.

57. J. Tesarik, A. Junca, A. Hazou *et al.*, Embryos with high implantation potential after intracytoplasmic sperm injection can be recognized by a single, non-invasive examination of pronuclear morphology. *Hum. Reprod.*, **15** (2000), 1396–1399.

58. M. Lundqvist, U. Johansson, Q. Lundqvist *et al.*, Does pronuclear morphology and/or early cleavage rate predict embryo implantation potential? *Reprod. Biomed. Online*, **2** (2001), 12–16.

59. U. Zollner, K. Zollner, G. Hartl *et al.*, The use of a detailed zygote score after IVF/ICSI to obtain good quality blastocysts, the German experience. *Hum. Reprod.*, **17** (2002), 1327–1333.

60. S. Kahraman, Y. Kumtepe, S. Sertyel *et al.*, Pronuclear morphology scoring and chromosomal status of embryos in severe male factor infertility. *Hum. Reprod.*, **17** (2002), 3193–3200.

61. C. Chen, G. Shen, S. Horng *et al.*, The relationship of pronuclear stage morphology and chromosome status at cleavage stage. *J. Assist. Reprod. Genet.*, **20** (2003), 413–420.

62. L. Gianaroli, M. Magli, A. Ferraretti *et al.*, Pronuclear morphology and chromosomal abnormalities as scoring criteria for embryo selection. *Fertil. Steril.*, **80** (2003), 343–349.

63. W. Edirisinghe, R. Jemmott, C. Smith *et al.*, Association of pronuclear Z score with rates of aneuploidy in in-vitro fertilised embryos. *Reprod. Fertil. Dev.*, **17** (2005), 529–534.

64. J. Van Blerkom, P. Davis, J. Merriam and J. Sinclair, Nuclear and cytoplasmic dynamics of sperm penetration, pronuclear formation, and microtubule organization during fertilization and early preimplantation development in the human. *Hum. Reprod. Update*, **1** (1995), 429–461.

65. M. Alikani, J. Cohen, G. Tomkin *et al.*, Human embryo fragmentation in vitro and its implications for pregnancy and implantation. *Fertil. Steril.*, **71** (1999), 836–842.

66. M. Alikani, The origins and consequences of fragmentation in mammalian eggs and embryos. In K. Elder and J. Cohen, eds., *Human Preimplantation Embryo Selection* (London: Informa Press, 2007), pp. 51–77.

67. J. Van Blerkom, The enigma of fragmentaton in early human embryos: possible causes and clinical relevance. In J. Van Blerkom and L. Gregory, eds., *Essential IVF: Basic Research and Clinical Applications* (Boston: Kluwer Academic Publishers, 2004), pp. 377–421.

68. K. Hardy, Apotosis in the human embryo. *Rev. Reprod.*, **4** (1999), 125–134.

69. A. Juriscova, S. Varmuza and R. Casper, Programmed cell death and human embryo fragmentation. *Mol. Hum. Reprod.*, **2** (1996), 93–98.

70. J. Van Blerkom, P. Davis and S. Alexander, Human embryo fragmentation: A multifaceted microscopic, biochemical and experimental study of fragmentation in early human preimplantation stage embryos *Hum. Reprod.*, **16** (2001), 719–729.

71. A. Jurisicova and B. Acton, Deadly decisions: the role of genes regulating programmed cell death in human preimplantation embryo development. *Reproduction*, **128** (2004), 281–291.

72. J. Biggers, Fundamentals of the design of culture media that support human preimplantation development. In J. Van Blerkom and L. Gregory, eds., *Essential IVF: Basic Research and Clinical Applications* (Boston: Kluwer Academic Publishers, 2004), pp. 291–332.

73. J. Van Blerkom, Spontaneous and experimental translocation of the subplasmalemmal cytoplasm within and between blastomeres in early human embryos: possible effects on the redistribution and inheritance of regulatory domains. *Reprod. Biomed. Online*, **14** (2007), 191–200.

74. M. Antczak and J. Van Blerkom, Temporal and spatial aspects of fragmentation in early human embryos: possible effects on developmental competence and association with the differential elimination of

regulatory proteins from polarized domains. *Hum. Reprod.*, **14** (1999), 429–447.

75. D. Gardner and M. Lane, Towards a single embryo transfer. *Reprod. Biomed. Online*, **6** (2003), 470–481.

76. L.Veeck and N. Zaninovic, *An Atlas of Human Blastocysts*. (Boca Raton: Parthenon Publishing Group, 2003).

77. K. Hardy, A. Handyside and R. Winston. The human blastocyst: cell number and allocation during late pre-implantation development in vitro. *Development*, **107** (1989), 597–604.

78. N. Winston, P. Braude, S. Pickering *et al.*, The incidence of abnormal morphology and nucleo-cytoplasmic ratio in 2, 3- and 5-day human pre-embryos. *Hum. Reprod.*, **6** (1991), 17–24.

79. J. Van Blerkom, Development of human embryos to the hatched blastocyst stage in the presence and absence of a monolayer of VERO cells. *Hum. Reprod.*, **8** (1993), 1525–1539.

80. C. Racowsky, K. Jackson, N. Cekleniak *et al.*, The number of eight-cell embryos is a key determinant for selecting day 3 or day 5 transfer. *Fertil. Steril.*, **73** (2000), 558–564.

81. J. Gerris, D. De Neubourg, K. Mangelschots *et al.*, Elective single day 3 embryo transfer halves the twinning rate without decrease in the ongoing pregnancy rate of an IVF/ICSI programme. *Hum. Reprod.*, **16** (2002), 626–631.

82. M. Sandalinas, S. Sadowy, M. Alikani *et al.*, Developmental ability of chromosomally abnormal human embryos to develop to the blastocyst stage. *Hum. Reprod.*, **16** (2001), 1954–1958.

83. J. Derhaag, E. Coonen, M. Bras *et al.*, Chromosomally abnormal cells are not selected for extra-embryonic compartment of the human preimplantation embryo at the blastocyst stage. *Hum. Reprod.*, **18** (2003), 2565–2574.

84. S. Evsikov and Y. Verlinsky, Mosaicism in the inner cell mass of human blastocysts. *Hum. Reprod.*, **13** (1998), 3151–3155.

85. B. Behr, Blastocyst culture and transfer. *Hum. Reprod.*, **14** (1999), 5–6.

86. R. Edwards and H. Beard, Is the success of human IVF more a matter of genetics and evolution than growing blastocyst? *Hum. Reprod.*, **14** (1999), 1–4.

87. S. Keay, C. Harlow, P. Wood *et al.*, Higher cortisol:cortisone ratios in the preovulatory follicle of unstimulated IVF cycles indicates oocytes with increased pregnancy potential. *Hum. Reprod.*, **17** (2002), 2003–2008.

88. A. Michael, Do biochemical predictors of IVF outcome exist? In J. Van Blerkom and L. Gregory, eds., *Essential IVF: Basic Research and Clinical Applications* (Boston: Kluwer Academic Publishers, 2004), pp. 81–109.

89. J. Van Blerkom and S. Trout, Oocyte selection in contemporary clinical IVF: do follicular markers of oocyte competence exist? In K. Elder and J. Cohen, eds., *Human Preimplantation Embryo Selection* (London: Informa Press, 2007), pp. 301–323.

90. M. Antczak, The synthetic and secretory behaviors (nonsteroidal) of ovarian follicular granulosa cells: parallels to cells of the endothelial cell lineage. In J. Van Blerkom and L. Gregory, eds., *Essential IVF: Basic Research and Clinical Applications* (Boston: Kluwer Academic Publishers, 2004).

91. A. Malamitsi-Puchner, Novel follicular fluid factors influencing oocyte developmental potential in IVF: a review. *Reprod. Biomed. Online*, **12** (2006), 500–506.

92. S. Hirobe, W. He, M. Gustafson *et al.*, Mullerian inhibiting substance gene expression in the cycling rat ovary correlates with recruited or Graafian follicle selection. *Biol. Reprod.*, **50** (1994), 1238–1243.

93. I. van Rooij, F. Broekmans, E. te Velde *et al.*, Serum anti-Mullerian hormone levels: a novel measure of ovarian reserve. *Hum. Reprod.*, **17** (2002), 3065–3071.

94. T. Silberstein, D. MacLaughlin, I. Shai *et al.*, Mullerian inhibiting substance levels at the time of HCG administration in IVF cycles predicts both ovarian reserve and embryo morphology. *Hum. Reprod.*, **21** (2006), 159–163.

95. M. Falla, Y. Siow, M. Marra *et al.*, Mullerian-inhibiting substance in follicular fluid and serum: a comparison of patients with tubal factor infertility, polycystic ovary syndrome, and endometriosis. *Fertil. Steril.*, **67** (1997), 962–965.

96. A. Hazout, P. Bouchard, D. Seifer *et al.* Serum anti-mullerian hormone/mullerian-inhibiting substance appears to be a more discriminatory marker of assisted reproductive technology outcome than follicle-stimulating hormone, inhibin B, or estradiol. *Fertil. Steril.*, **82** (2004), 1323–29.

97. J. Van Blerkom, Follicular influences on oocyte and embryo competence. In C. De Jonnge and C. Barrat, eds., *Assisted Reproductive Technology: Accomplishments and New Horizons* (Cambridge: Cambridge University Press, 2002), pp. 81–105.

98. L. Gregory, Peri-follicular vascularity: a marker of follicular heterogeneity and oocyte competence and a predictor of implantation in assisted conception cycles. In J. Van Blerkom and L. Gregory, eds., *Essential IVF: Basic Research and Clinical Applications* (Boston: Kluwer Academic Publishers, 2004), pp. 59–79.

99. J. Van Blerkom, M. Antczak and R. Schrader, The developmental potential of the human oocyte is related to the dissolved oxygen content of follicular fluid: association with vascular endothelial growth factor levels and perifollicular blood flow characteristics. *Hum. Reprod.*, **12** (1997), 1947–1955.

100. P. Bahl, N. Pugh, D. Chui *et al.*, The use of transvaginal power Doppler ultrasonography to evaluate the relationship between perifollicular vascularity and outcome in in-vitro fertilization treatment cycles. *Hum. Reprod.*, **14** (1999), 939–945.

101. C. Coulam, C. Goodman and J. Rinehart, Color Doppler indices of follicular blood flow as predictors of pregnancy after in-vitro fertilization and embryo transfer. *Hum. Reprod.*, **14** (1999), 1979–1982.

102. G. Semenza, Regulation of mammalian O2 homeostasis by hypoxia-inducible factor 1. *Annu. Rev. Cell Dev. Biol.*, **15** (1999), 551–578.

103. H.-A. Pan, M.-H. Wu, Y.-C. Cheng, L. H. Wu and F. M. Chang, Quantification of ovarian stromal Doppler signals in poor responders undergoing in vitro fertilization with three-dimensional power Doppler ultrasonography. *Am. J. Obstet. Gynecol.*, **190** (2004), 338–344.

104. S. Palomba, T. Russo, A. Falbo *et al.*, Clinical use of the perifollicular vascularity assessment in IVF cycles: a pilot study. *Hum. Reprod.*, **21** (2006), 1055–1061.

105. S. Shrestha, M. Costello, P. Sjoblom *et al.*, Power Doppler ultrasound assessment of follicular vascularity in the early follicular phase and its relationship with outcome in in vitro fertilization. *J. Assist. Reprod. Genet.*, **23** (2006), 161–169.

106. K. Kim, D. Oh, J. Jeong *et al.*, Follicular blood flow is a better predictor of the outcome of in vitro fertilization-embryo transfer than follicular fluid vascular endothelial growth factor and nitric oxide concentrations. *Fertil. Steril.*, **82** (2004), 586–592.

107. L. Merce, S. Bau, M. Barco *et al.*, Assessment of the ovarian volume, number and volume of follicles and ovarian vascularity by three-dimensional ultrasonography and power Doppler angiography on the HCG

day to predict outcome in IVF/ICSI cycles. *Hum. Reprod.*, **21** (2006), 1218–1226.

108. M. Collier, C. O'Neil, A. Ammit and D. Saunders, Measurements of human embryo-derived platelet-activating factor (PAF) using a quantitative bioassay of platelet aggregation. *Hum. Reprod.*, **5** (1990), 323–328.

109. A. Lopata and K. Oliva, Chorionic gonadotrophin secretion by human blastocysts. *Hum. Reprod.*, **8** (1993), 932–938.

110. G. Benagiano and L. Gianaroli. The new Italian IVF legislation. *Reprod. Biomed. Online*, **9** (2004), 117–125.

111. G. Sher, L. Keskintepe, M. Nouriani *et al.*, Expression of sHLA-G in supernatants of individually cultured 46-h embryos: a potentially valuable indicator of 'embryo competency' and IVF outcome. *Reprod. Biomed. Online*, **9** (2004), 74–78.

112. T. Hviid, HLA-G in human reproduction: aspects of genetics, function and pregnancy complications. *Hum. Reprod. Update*, **12** (2004), 209–232.

113. Y. Yao, D. Barlow and I. Sargent, Differential expression of alternatively spliced transcripts of HLA-G in human preimplantation embryos and inner cell masses. *J. Immunol.*, **175** (2005), 8379–8385.

114. I. Noci, B. Fuzzi, R. Rizzo *et al.*, Embryonic soluble HLA-G as a marker of developmental potential in embryos. *Hum. Reprod.*, **20** (2005), 138–146.

115. S. Yie, H. Balakier, G. Motamedi and C. Librach, Secretion of human leukocyte antigen G by human embryos is associated with a higher in vitro fertilization pregnancy rate. *Fertil. Steril.*, **83** (2005), 30–36.

116. L. Sargent, Does 'soluble' HLA-G really exist? Another twist to the tale. *Mol. Hum. Reprod.*, **11** (2005), 695–698.

117. M. van Lieropl, Y. Ijnands, P. Loke *et al.*, Detection of HLA-G by a specific sandwich ELISA using monoclonal antibodies G233 and 56B. *Mol. Hum. Reprod.*, **8** (2002), 776–784.

118. C. Warner, M. Comiskey, P. Clisham and C. Brenner, Soluble HLA-G (sHLA-G) a predictor of IVF outcome? *J. Assist. Reprod. Genet.*, **21** (2004), 315–316.

119. A. Blaschitz, H. Juch, A. Volz *et al.*, The soluble pool of HLA-G produced by human trophoblast does not include detectable levels of the intron 4-containing HLA-G5 and HLA-G6 isoforms. *Mol. Hum. Reprod.*, **11** (2005), 699–710.

120. Y. Menezo, K. Elder and S. Viville, Soluble HLA-G release by the human embryo: an interesting artefact? *Reprod. Biomed. Online*, **13** (2006), 763–764.

121. G. Sher, L. Keskintepe and M. Ginsburg, sHLA-G expression, is it really worth measuring? *Reprod. Biomed. Online*, **14** (2007), 9–10.

122. G. Porcu-Buisson, M. Lambert, L. Lyonnet *et al.*, Soluble MHC class I chain-related molecule serum levels are predictive markers of implantation failure and successful term pregnancies following IVF. *Hum. Reprod.*, **22** (2007), 2261–2266.

123. L. Mincheva-Nilsson, O. Nagaeva, T. Chen *et al.*, Placenta-derived soluble MHC class I chain-related molecules down-regulate NKG2D receptor on peripheral blood mononuclear cells during human pregnancy: a possible novel immune escape mechanism for fetal survival. *J. Immunol.*, **176** (2006), 3585–3592.

124. J. Hanna, D. Goldman-Wohl, Y. Hamani *et al.*, Decidual NK cells regulate key developmental processes at the human fetal-maternal interface. *Nat. Med.*, **12** (2006), 1065–1074.

125. L. McKenzie, S. Pangas, A. Carson *et al.*, Human cumulus granulosa cell gene expression: a predictor of fertilization and embryo selection in women undergoing IVF. *Hum. Reprod.*, **19** (2004), 2869–2874.

126. F. Cillo, A. Tiziana, L. Brevini *et al.*, Association between human oocyte developmental competence and expression levels of some cumulus genes. *Reproduction*, **134** (2007), 645–650.

127. Y. Menezo and P. Guerin. Preimplantation embryo metabolism and embryo interaction with the in vitro environment. In K. Elder and J. Cohen, eds., *Human Preimplantation Embryo Selection* (London: Informa Press, 2007), pp. 191–200.

128. L. Gregory, A. Booth, C. Wells and S. Walker, A study of the cumulus-corona cell complex in in-vitro fertilization and embryo transfer: a prognostic indicator of the failure of implantation. *Hum. Reprod.*, **9** (1994), 1308–1317.

129. J. Van Blerkom, Epigenetic influences on oocyte developmental competence. Follicular oxygenation and perifollicular vascularity. *J. Assist. Reprod. Genet.*, **15** (1998), 226–234.

130. F. Diaz, K. Wigglesworth and J. Eppig, Oocytes determine cumulus cell lineage in mouse ovarian follicles. *J. Cell Sci.*, **120** (2007), 1330–1340.

131. S. Gasca, F. Pellestor, S. Assou *et al.*, Identifying new human oocyte marker genes: a microarray approach. *Reprod. Biomed. Online*, **14** (2007), 175–183.

132. G. Giritharan, S. Talbi, A. Donjacour *et al.*, Effect of in vitro fertilization on gene expression and development of mouse preimplantation embryos. *Reproduction*, **134** (2007), 63–72.

133. P. Lonergan, T. Fair, D. Corcoran and A. Evans, Effect of culture environment on gene expression and developmental characteristics of IVF-derived embryos. *Theriogenology*, **65** (2006), 137–152.

134. A. Harvey, K. Kind, M. Pantaleon *et al.*, Oxygen-regulated gene expression in bovine blastocysts. *Biol. Reprod.*, **71** (2004), 1108–1119.

135. C. Magnusson, T. Hillensjo, L. Hamberger and L. Nilsson, Oxygen consumption by human oocytes and blastocysts grown in vitro. *Hum. Reprod.*, **1** (1986), 183–184.

136. D. Gardner, T. Pool and M. Lane, Embryo nutrition and energy metabolism and its relationship to embryo growth, differentiation, and viability. *Semin. Reprod. Med.*, **18** (2000), 205–218.

137. H, Leese, What does an embryo need? *Hum. Fertil.*, **6** (2003), 180–185.

138. F. Houghton, J. Hawkhead, P. Humpherson *et al.*, Non-invasive amino acid turnover predicts human embryo developmental capacity. *Hum. Reprod.*, **17** (2002), 999–1005.

139. D. Brison, F. Houghton, D. Falconer *et al.*, Identification of viable embryos in IVF by non-invasive measurement of amino acid turnover. *Hum. Reprod.*, **19** (2004), 2319–2324.

140. A. Lopes, L. Larsen, N. Ramsing *et al.*, Respiration rates of individual bovine in vitro-produced embryos measured with a novel, non-invasive and highly sensitive microsensor system. *Reproduction*, **130** (2005), 669–679.

141. J. Van Blerkom, The role of mitochondria in human oogenesis and preimplantation embryogenesis: engines of metabolism, ionic regulation and developmental competence. *Reproduction*, **128** (2004), 269–280.

142. C. Brenner, What is the role of mitochondria in embryo competence? In J. Van Blerkom and L. Gregory, eds., *Essential IVF: Basic Research and Clinical Applications* (Boston: Kluwer Academic Publishers, 2004), pp. 273–290.

143. P. May-Panloup, M. Chretien, Y. Malthiery and P. Reynier, Mitochondrial DNA in the oocyte and the developing embryo. *Curr. Top. Dev. Biol.*, **77** (2007), 51–83.

144. J. Van Blerkom, P. Davis and J. Lee, ATP content of human oocytes and developmental potential and outcome after in-vitro fertilization and embryo transfer. *Hum. Reprod.*, **10** (1995), 415–424.

145. J. Van Blerkom, P. Davis and S. Alexander, Differential mitochondrial distribution in human pronuclear embryos leads to disproportionate inheritance between blastomeres: relationship to microtubular organization. ATP content and competence. *Hum. Reprod.*, **15** (2000), 2621–2633.

146. P. Reynier, P. May-Panloup, M. Chretien *et al.*, Mitochondrial DNA content effects the fertilizability of human oocytes. *Mol. Hum. Reprod.*, **7** (2001), 425–429.

147. E. Shoubridge and T. Wai, Mitochondrial DNA and the mammalian oocyte. *Curr. Top. Dev. Biol.*, **77** (2007), 87–111.

148. J. Van Blerkom, Mitochondria as regulatory forces in oocytes, preimplantation embryos and stem cells. *Reprod. Biomed. Online*, **16** (2008), 553–569.

149. R. Jansen, Germline passage of mitochondria: quantitative considerations and possible embryological sequelae. *Hum. Reprod.*, **15** (Suppl 2) (2000), 112–128.

150. T. Santos, S. El Shourbagy and J. St John, Mitochondrial content reflects oocyte variability and fertilization outcome. *Fertil. Steril.*, **85** (2006), 584–591.

151. M. Katayama, Z. Zhong, L. Lai *et al.*, Mitochondrial distribution and microtubule organization in fertilized and cloned porcine embryos: implications for developmental potential. *Developmental Biology*, **299** (2006), 206–220.

152. S. H. El Shourbagy, E. C. Spikings, M. Freitas and J. C. St. John, Mitochondria directly influence fertilisation outcome in the pig. *Reproduction*, **131** (2006), 233–245.

153. J. Squirrell, R. Schramm, A. Paprocki, D. L. Wokosin and B. D. Bavister, Imaging mitochondrial organization in living primate oocytes and embryos using multiphoton microscopy. *Microsc. Microanal.*, **9** (2003), 190–201.

154. J. Van Blerkom and P. Davis, Mitochondrial signaling and fertilization. *Mol. Hum. Reprod.*, **13** (2007), 759–777.

155. P. Hockachka, The metabolic implications of intracellular circulation. *Proc. Natl. Acad. Sci. USA*, **96** (1999), 12233–12239.

156. T. Misgeld, M. Kerschensteiner, F. Mareyre *et al.*, Imaging axonal transport of mitochondria in vivo. *Nat. Methods*, **4** (2007), 559–561.

157. J. Van Blerkom, Microtubule mediation of cytoplasmic and nuclear maturation during the early stages of resumed meiosis in cultured mouse oocytes. *Proc. Natl. Acad. Sci. USA*, **88** (1991), 5031–5035.

158. D. Barnett, J. Kimua and B. Bavister, Translocation of active mitochondria during hamster preimplantation embryo development studied by confocal laser scanning microscopy. *Dev. Dyn.*, **205** (1996), 64–72.

159. M. Katayama, Z. Zhong, L. Lai *et al.*, Mitochondrial distribution and microtubule organization in fertilized and cloned porcine embryos: implications for developmental potential. *Dev. Biol.*, **299** (2006), 206–220.

160. T.-Y. Aw, Intracellular compartmentalization of organelles and gradients of low molecular weight species. *Int. Rev. Cytol.*, **192** (2000), 223–253.

161. J. Van Blerkom, P. Davis, V. Mathwig and S. Alexander, Domains of high-polarized and low-polarized mitochondria may occur in mouse and human oocytes and early embryos. *Hum. Reprod.*, **17** (2000), 393–406.

162. J. Van Blerkom and P. Davis, High-polarized ($\Delta\Psi m_{HIGH}$) mitochondria are spatially polarized in human oocytes and early embryos in stable subplasmalemmal domains: developmental significance and the concept of vanguard mitochondria. *Reprod. Biomed. Online*, **13** (2006), 246–254.

163. J. Van Blerkom, P. Davis and S. Alexander, Inner mitochondrial membrane potential ($\Delta\Psi m$), cytoplasmic ATP content and free Ca^{2+} levels in metaphase II mouse oocytes. *Hum. Reprod.*, **18** (2003), 2429–2440.

164. A. Jones, J. Van Blerkom, P. Davis and A. Toledo, Cryopreservation of metaphase II human oocytes effects mitochondrial membrane potential: implications for developmental competence. *Hum. Reprod.*, **19** (2004), 1861–1866.

165. R. Dumollard, K. Hammar, M. Porterfield *et al.*, Mitochondrial respiration and Ca^{2+} waves are linked during fertilisation and meiosis completion. *Development*, **130** (2003), 683–692.

166. R. Dumollard, M. Duchen and J. Carroll, The role of mitochondrial function in the oocyte and embryo. *Curr. Top. Dev. Biol.*, **77** (2007), 21–49.

167. J. Arce, S. Ziebe, K. Lundin *et al.*, Interobserver agreement and intraobserver reproducibility of embryo quality assessments. *Hum. Reprod.*, **21** (2006), 2141–2148.

168. C. Hnida and S. Ziebe, Morphometric analysis of human embryos. In K. Elder and J. Cohen, eds., *Human Preimplantation Embryo Selection* (London: Informa Press, 2007), pp. 89–99.

SECTION 2

Clinical aspects

3

Single embryo transfer: concepts and definitions

Jan Gerris and Petra De Sutter

Introduction: to define is to limit

The transfer of one embryo, single embryo transfer (SET), refers to the simple idea of replacing just one embryo into the uterus during an in vitro fertilization/intracytoplasmic sperm injection (IVF/ICSI) cycle. In bovine reproductive medicine, where high quality offspring is created for consumption reasons, it is the standard. The main reason for this is that bovine twins are often freemartins. Bovine blastocysts obtained through uterine lavage from superovulated donor cows inseminated with top bulls implant in almost 100% of transfers. Economics dictates everything. Human reproductive medicine tries to remediate involuntary childlessness. At first sight, all that counts is to create the highest chance to obtain a pregnancy. Transfers are crowned with success in between 10% and 60% of transfers only, and are highly dependent on female age, which is the main determinant of embryo implanting capacity.

A workable, uniform and strict definition of SET, and especially of *elective* SET (eSET), is not as easy as it seems. Embryos are usually transferred at the cleavage stage (both day 2 and day 3) or at the blastocyst stage (day 5 and day 6). Occasionally they have been transferred at the two pronuclei stage or at the day 4 or morula stage. A wide variation in methods of embryo selection has resulted in a wide variation in the results after SET [1]. One SET does not equal another. It is therefore very difficult to compare results from one center to another and even more so from one country to another. Results from particular centers in a particular country may be excellent, whereas overall national data will not reveal this because other centers perform poorly. There is also a lag time between the introduction of SET and its impact on national, regional or global data. This is clearly visible in the progressive, but slow, shift towards more SET as witnessed in Europe [2].

Throughout the literature, the abbreviations of SET and eSET are often used confusedly. The main reason for this is that eSET *implies* a (validated) form of embryo selection, which is not always fully appreciated or implemented. Embryo selection criteria based on cleavage speed and morphological characteristics cannot simply be extrapolated from one center to another, because of differences in the many variables that determine the mean embryo implantation potential of a center, such as the culture media that are used, the frequency and assiduity with which embryos are checked (e.g., for multinucleation) and differences in sheer expertise. Ideally, each center would have to substantiate its own particular validation. Moreover, the correlation between morphology and implantation potential *is* intrinsically a poor one, which further contributes to differences in opinion regarding SET.

Single Embryo Transfer, ed. J. Gerris, G. D. Adamson, P. De Sutter and C. Racowsky. Published by Cambridge University Press.
© Cambridge University Press 2009.

All of this explains the wide differences in the perception of SET and the enthusiasm with which it is met by different practitioners worldwide.

The target: the twin-prone patient

One way to define SET is by describing it as a way to serve its target population: in this view, SET is the appropriate approach in women who either do not *want* more than one embryo replaced or in women where most clinicians would agree that the chance for a (multiple) pregnancy is very high indeed or perhaps even low but medically undesirable. There are many retrospective analyses that have identified the robot photo of the twin-prone patient. In this definition, it is the definition of the target group that determines whether SET is appropriate or not.

The first group (women who do not *want* more than one embryo to be replaced) is small but not all that small as may be supposed and its size is very variable between different parts of the world. Much depends on the counseling patients receive regarding the risks of multiple pregnancy, which is time-consuming. Most of the European randomized trials comparing SET with double embryo transfer (DET) had difficulties, near the end of the trial, to recruit patients agreeing to expose themselves to the risk of twin pregnancy by being randomized into the DET arm of the study. Moreover, women coming back for a second IVF/ICSI pregnancy, especially if pregnant in a first or second trial and even more so if pregnant after SET, will request a single (frozen-thawed or fresh) embryo when they recommence treatment to obtain a second child. So do patients who already have twins and come back for a third baby! This group of patients is growing. The reputation of a center also comes into play. Patients talk to other patients and this provides a fertile ground for new approaches in assisted reproductive technology (ART).

By defining SET through the group it is intended to serve, one acknowledges the fact that SET is not a must for all patients. Patients who are clearly at the other end of the spectrum, with a "never-pregnant-prone" profile, are not served by SET.

Of course, the challenge to define what a "twin-prone patient" is remains. Efforts have been made to define that patient [3] and it seems accepted now that they are young women (≤ 36 years of age according to Belgian law; < 35 years of age according to American Society for Reproductive Medicine [ASRM] recommendations) [4, 5] in their first or second IVF/ICSI trial, who have at least some good quality embryos to choose from (alternatively, who have embryos to freeze) and who have preferably another cause of infertility than tubal disease. Although some degree of individual prognosis overlap remains, this profile differs widely from that of the 41-year-old woman in her fifth treatment cycle who despairs – with good reason. It also differs from the young, first-cycle testicular sperm extraction (TESE) + ICSI patient with restricted financial means, in whose husband a mere 11 sperm cells are detected but who happens to end up at transfer with two nice embryos. It is likely that this woman should receive both embryos. Other examples can be given to show that defining SET as a solution for particular groups of patients is a sound way to define its possibilities and limits. In all cases, the application of SET must be *judicious* and that will at the same time define and limit its applicability.

SET (single embryo transfer)

As mentioned before, SET simply means the transfer of one embryo but that does not *signify* very much. For SET to be judiciously applied, it has to be linked to embryo selection, to the possibility of identifying the embryo with the highest projected implantation capacity from the available cohort. Even such a vague and deliberately wide definition does not prevent all apprehension. In Germany, the term "selection" is neutral neither in political circles nor in the population at large. In Italy, there is no question of considering the total cohort, since only three oocytes can be (and, if available, must be) fertilized. In Belgium, in women ≤ 36 years of age, no more than one embryo can be transferred, irrespective of morphological characteristics. This does not mean that selection does not take place, but even if no good qualities embryos are available SET is legally mandatory.

Hence, the term SET does not convey anything else than the intention to (= intended SET) or the fact of having transferred (= factual SET) one single embryo.

A comparison between two cases will serve as an example to illustrate the kind of differences that should be considered. In the first, a woman of 28 years in a first ICSI cycle has obtained 18 metaphase II-oocytes out of a total of 21 oocytes punctured, 17 of which are normally fertilized, 16 have cleaved and 5 of which have followed the ideal cleavage pattern (4 cells on day 2; 8 cells on day 3) with < 10% fragments and no multinucleation. In the second, a 29-year-old polycystic ovary syndrome (PCOS) patient had a first IVF cycle with 10 metaphase II-oocytes from a grand total of 26 oocytes, just one of which has reached the ideal non-fragmented, 8-cell stage on day 3, all other embryos being either retarded to a maximum of 6 cells or fragmented up to 70%. In the first patient, SET will become eSET, whereas in the second it really is compulsory SET (cSET). This may result in a lower chance for a pregnancy in the second patient, even though they both receive a high implantation potential embryo. Describing both transfer situations as SET is correct but does not convey the huge difference between both clinical situations. In reality, there probably is no system of abbreviations or acronyms which is subtle enough to convey such differences. It remains imperative for a physician to "know" his or her patient and be able to take an individualized approach towards each couple.

eSET (elective single embryo transfer)

Any *judicious* implementation of SET, apart from looking at the twin-proneness and the specific clinical details of a particular patient, should ideally be linked to some form of quantification of the projected implantation potential of each available embryo. One of the important things to realize is that, at present, there is no single simple method that can be applied with similar efficacy in all

centers to perform this quality choice of *the* best embryo. Many different approaches have been suggested and evaluated, ranging from zygote stage morphology to day 1, day 2, day 3–4 (early cleavage embryo) and day 5–6 (blastocyst) morphology. Genetic assessment and measurement of metabolic activity have been considered as well. Therefore, centers will have to make a choice for themselves regarding the criteria they will use for embryo selection. This holds true for non-SET as well, since many centers consider it a great leap already to decrease the number of embryos to transfer to a default number of two. In that case the problem of selection is perhaps somewhat less sharp but nevertheless it exists.

By definition, eSET implies *choice*. The Latin verb eligere means to choose and is encountered in the noun "election." To be able to choose, there must be at least two to choose from. In many cases, the choice goes between many more embryos, especially in good prognosis patients.

Published results of SET/eSET must always be interpreted against the background of to what length a particular group went in applying a strictly defined selection system based on cleavage kinetics, morphological characteristics and the development stage considered optimal for transfer.

Table 3.1 shows both randomized studies and cohort studies comparing SET with DET. Comparisons between eSET (one top embryo) and eDET (two top embryos) in randomized trials indicate, as expected, better results for eDET [6–9]. In the real-life situation where eSET (one top embryo, if available) is compared to DET (two embryos, no further specification) similar results are obtained [10–15]. This is due to the fact that the DET group consists of a small number of transfers of two high quality embryos, a major number of mixed transfers of one high quality and one moderate embryo and a subgroup of DETs of two moderate or poor embryos. In some more recent publications, where very good prognosis patients were included and use was made of blastocyst culture, results were even more impressive [16–19].

In this definition, *elective* SET irrespective of the availability of good quality embryos [20], is a

Table 3.1 Randomized studies and cohort studies comparing SET with DET

Author	N cycles	PR SET (%)	Twins (%)	PR DET (%)	Twins + HOMPs[a] (%)
Randomized trials					
Gerris *et al.*, 1999 [6]	53	10/26 (38.5)	1/10	20/27 (74)	6/20 (30.0)
Martikainen *et al.*, 2001 [7]	144	24/74 (32.4)	1/24	33/70 (47.1)	6/33 (18.2)
Gardner *et al.*, 2004 [8]	48	14/23 (60.9)	0/14	19/25 (76)	9/19 (47.4)
Thurin *et al.*, 2004 [9]	661+ cryo	91/330 (27.6) 131/330 (39.7)	1/91 1/131	144/331 (43.5)	52/144 (36.1)
Total	906	139/453 (30.7)	3/139 (2.16)	216/453 (47.6)	73/216 (33.8)
Cohort studies					
Gerris *et al.*, 2002 [10]	1152	105/299 (35.1)	1/124	309/853 (36.2)	105 + 5/309 (35.6)
De Sutter *et al.*, 2003 [11]	2898	163/579 (28.2)	1/163	734/2319 (31.7)	219 + 4/734 (30.4)
Tiitinen *et al.*, 2003 [12]	1494	162/470 (34.5)	2/162	376/1024 (36.7)	113/376 (30.1)
Catt *et al.*, 2003 [13]	385	49/111 (44.1)	1/49	161/274 (58.8)	71/161 (44.1)
Gerris *et al.*, 2004 [14]	367	83/206 (40.3)	0	65/161 (40.4)	20/65 (30.8)
Martikainen *et al.*, 2001 [7]	1111	107/308 (34.7) 187/308 (60.7)	1/107	255/803 (31.8)	NA
Total	7407	669/1973 (33.9)	6/591 (1.0)	1900/5434 (35.0)	537/1645 (32.6)

PR, pregnancy rate; HOMPs, higher-order multiple pregnancies, NA, not applicable.

[a] Twins only for randomized trials and Twins + HOMPs for cohort studies.

Data for the Martikainen *et al.*, 2001 study [7] and the Thurin *et al.*, 2004 study [9] show both the fresh and the cryoaugmented pregnancy rates.

contradiction in terminis although it is clear that these authors mean well that, even in the absence of a truly high implantation potential embryo (as strictly defined), one should do his/her best at selecting the "least bad" embryo. This paper actually perfectly shows that the Belgian model (see below) is not evidence-based as far as the transfer policy of first cycles are concerned.

Finally, the abbreviation eSFET (elective single frozen embryo transfer) has been used to denote the transfer of one single frozen-thawed embryo in an embryo donation attempt. Embryo donation will be discussed in Chapter 10B.

cSET (compulsory SET)

Compulsory SET is a term reserved for the situation where only one embryo is available for transfer. A number of very different situations may fall under this definition, e.g. the young woman with many mature eggs whose husband has only a couple of sperm from a testicular biopsy; the typical PCOS woman who has many eggs, fertilized with good sperm but ends up with one good embryo only; poor responders; patients with unexpected poor fertilization, etc. This is to say that cSET is again a purely descriptive term, a wide umbrella covering many different situations. Sometimes, cSET may be at the same time as the transfer of a top quality embryo, although it is not clear whether in those circumstances the chance for a pregnancy is similar as it would be in the case of eSET.

The analysis of a large group of cSETs [10–12, 21, 22] (Table 3.2) remains interesting because it made the point that, even in this overall poor prognosis group, there are wide differences in embryo implantation potential which correlate with traditional morphological criteria. This paper cannot be used as an argument against SET *in se*, as has

Table 3.2 Published results of compulsory single embryo transfers

Author, year	*N* of compulsory SETs	*N* of implantations	IR (%)	*N* of live births	LBR (%)
Giorgetti *et al.*, 1995 [21]	858	88	10.3	62	7.2
Vilska *et al.*, 1999 [22]	94	19	20.2	15	16.0
Gerris *et al.*, 2002 [10]	86	26	30.2	19	22.1
Tiitinen *et al.*, 2003 [12]	205	39	19.0	31	15.1
De Sutter *et al.*, 2003 [11]	211	21	10.0	19	9.0
Total	1454	193	13.3	146	10.1

IR, implantation rate; LBR, live birth rate.

been done many times, since precisely no form of embryo selection was possible in these cycles. With hindsight, it confirms rather than refutes the concept of eSET.

mSET (medical SET)

Strictly speaking, *all* eSET is done for medical reasons, since the prevention of the complications of multiple pregnancies also is prevention of an increased incidence of *medical* complications in mother and child(ren). The term mSET, which is not yet frequently used, could be reserved for clinical situations where a multiple gestation is absolutely or relatively contraindicated for pre-existing maternal reasons known to interfere with a good obstetrical outcome rather than for fetal reasons (although healthy women are also at an increased maternal risk in a multiple pregnancy). We exclude here the patient who does not *want* the natural risk for a monozygotic (~1/250 spontaneous births) or a dizygotic (~1/90 spontaneous births) pregnancy to be increased.

Absolute contraindications

• Insulin-dependent diabetes mellitus
• Congenital anomalies of the uterus
• Isthmic insufficiency
• Severe general (cardiac, renal, hepatic, gastrointestinal) diseases
• Severe psychiatric disease
• Previous early loss of a multiple pregnancy

Relative contraindications

• Single mothers
• Older women
• Moderate or mild systemic diseases
• Paraplegic women
• Moderate and mild psychiatric disease
• Thrombo-embolic disorders
• Previous prematurity

Although it may be difficult to predict the risk for early pregnancy loss, in all of these cases a long and serious pretreatment counseling is mandatory. The possibility to reduce a (higher-order or even twin) pregnancy, once it is established, may offer a way out, but the wider application of a preventive attitude using eSET is recommended. Typical results to be expected in the case of mSET are those published by Vilska *et al.*: a pregnancy rate of 29.7% was obtained in the case where there was a possibility to elect the best embryo versus 20.2% if there was only one embryo available [22].

lSET (legally enforced SET)

In Belgium, a law has been implemented since July 2003 which regulates the number of embryos that can legally be transferred as a function of the age of the woman at the time of transfer and of the rank of the attempt. Funding of each cycle is guaranteed if the requirements for the number of embryos to transfer are met. But the law speaks for all patients treated on Belgian soil, even if they pay from their

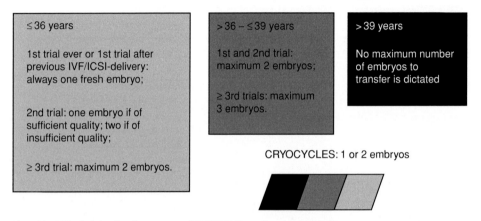

BELGIAN FUNDING REGULATION

• Six IVF/ICSI cycles (= oocyte harvests) funded in a life time
• 1187€ per cycle for laboratory costs (gamete procurement and handling)
• Including cryocycles
• Up to the age of 43 years

Linked to a rational transfer strategy

≤ 36 years	> 36 – ≤ 39 years	> 39 years
1st trial ever or 1st trial after previous IVF/ICSI-delivery: always one fresh embryo;	1st and 2nd trial: maximum 2 embryos;	No maximum number of embryos to transfer is dictated
2nd trial: one embryo if of sufficient quality; two if of insufficient quality;	≥ 3rd trials: maximum 3 embryos.	
≥ 3rd trial: maximum 2 embryos.		

CRYOCYCLES: 1 or 2 embryos

Figure 3.1 The Belgian funding system of IVF/ICSI. See color plate section.

own pockets, e.g. if the six funded cycles in a lifetime have been used up, or if they are foreigners. Since all women ≤ 36 years of age can only receive one embryo in the first two cycles, irrespective of any of the embryo selection possibilities, we must speak of lSET or legally enforced SET.

The Belgian model

It was projected that in Belgium, the savings obtained from halving the number of IVF twin pregnancies and a concomitant near-elimination of triplets would suffice to cover the laboratory cost of the total number of IVF/ICSI cycles in patients who fall under the Belgian reimbursement system. The crux is that a link was made between funding and the number of embryos to be transferred. A total of six cycles can be funded in a lifetime. The number of embryos to be transferred is determined for each of these cycles (Figure 3.1). The law stipulates that in women ≤ 36 years of age, in first IVF/ICSI cycles, only one embryo can be transferred. In second cycles, again only one embryo

should be replaced, unless of insufficient quality (not further specified); from third cycles onwards, a maximum of two embryos can be replaced. In women between 36 and 39 years of age, the law stipulates that from the first cycle onwards a maximum of two embryos can (not: must) be replaced. In women > 39 years of age and up to the age of 43 years, no limitation with respect to the number of embryos is formulated. In women > 43 years of age, there is no funding. In women > 45 years of age, *any* treatment for infertility has become illegal since July 2007. The sole exception is the replacement of thawed embryos created before their 45th birthday, which can be done up to 47 years of age. For each funded cycle, to be carried out in an accredited Centre for Reproductive Medicine, the hospital in which the (laboratory phase) IVF/ICSI treatment takes place receives 1187€. This sum covers all the laboratory costs linked to one oocyte harvest, i.e. the identification and the preparation of the cumulus-oocyte-complexes, insemination or injection of the oocytes and embryo culture, as well as the laboratory phase needed to find sperm after microscopic epididymal sperm aspiration (MESA) and/or TESE and preparing the spermatozoa; freezing supernumerary embryos, thawing them as well as the complete logistics related to all of these (i.e., registration and reporting). The patient is under no circumstances to be charged. This sum is paid directly by the Ministry of Social Affairs to the hospital, where it is booked to the credit of the gynecological department in which the center is embedded. Note therefore that the Belgian system is not a system of reimbursement, because the patient does not pay, hence does not have to be reimbursed. It is a system of state funding of recognized centers. The total amount due is paid following a difficult system of 6-monthly prepayments followed by *post-hoc* adjustments calling for senior accountant expertise. The whole system is completely independent from the payments of the *medical* acts or performances, e.g. consultations, sonographies, oocyte pick-ups and embryo transfers, which fall under the direct application of insurance (called: "mutualities") – mediated reimbursement.

Commentaries to the model

On the upside is the fact that the system exists. It has created access to (repeated) treatments for many couples who previously could not afford it. This is a small measure to cope with the negative demographic evolution in many western European countries. The existence of some link between funding and a limitation of the number of embryos to be transferred guarantees that there will be a decrease in the incidence of multiple pregnancies, improving quality and giving an optimal start in life to IVF children. Twins have dropped dramatically and triplets have almost completely disappeared allowing for persisting underreporting of triplet reductions. Remaining triplets are often dizygotic. Data from the Belgian Registry of Artificial Procreation for the year 2004 illustrate the impact of SET on national results (Figures 3.2 and 3.3). During the first full year of implementation (July 1, 2003 to June 30, 2004), the incidence of twins dropped from a pre-funding 24% to 9.7%. As a consequence of increased access to treatment, the total number of

cycles unexpectedly rose from 11 245 in 2002 to 14 795 during the first full year after the funding law. This effect seems to be levelling off. Interestingly, in women ≤ 36 years of age, second cycles had DET in an unexpected high 60% of cycles.

Funding has been successfully used as a lever to ease psychologically the acceptance of SET in patients who are supposed to otherwise demand more embryos to be replaced.

On the downside are some concerns that perhaps need to be addressed in the future.

The first and foremost is that the law is not taking into account what is known on the (weak but existing) correlation between morphological embryo characteristics and their ongoing implantation potential. In fact *elective* SET only "works" (i.e., leads to a constant ongoing pregnancy rate while approximately halving the twinning rate in the whole program) in the case of transfer of a *top quality embryo* (somehow strictly defined) [23–28]. This fundamental prerequisite for judicious eSET has been "sacrificed" in the political arena because it was feared that a number of centers would try to avoid having to replace only one embryo in a number of cycles by stating they did not have a top quality embryo in those (first) cycles. This is probably what happens for second cycles, in which up to 60% do supposedly not yield one top quality embryo … It illustrates how the notions of SET and eSET are easily mixed up when it comes to hard currency politics. In general, lack of agreement between biologists to come to a strict and reproducible way to select an embryo with a putative high implantation potential has further weakened the applicability of SET. Ironically, in second cycles, the regulation stipulates that two embryos can be replaced if the quality of "the" embryo is considered "insufficient." Therefore, a "shift" of twins from first to second and certainly third attempts is to be expected.

Second, independent of the result of an IVF/ICSI cycle, the number of embryos to be transferred is determined solely by its rank. If a woman of ≤ 36 years got pregnant with a first IVF baby in her fourth cycle, and starts again for a second baby, this "first" cycle will be considered as a fifth cycle and legally speaking two embryos are allowed although

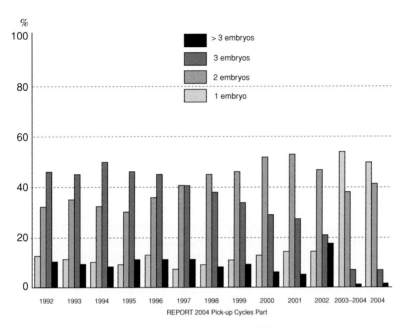

Figure 3.2 Evolution in the number of embryos transferred in Belgium.

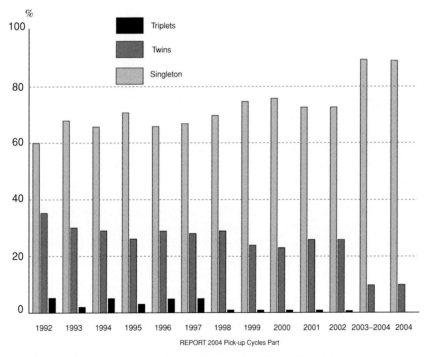

Figure 3.3 Evolution of single and multiple deliveries after IVF/ICSI in Belgium.

eSET is what the spirit of the law intended. When a child was born after a previous attempt the counter is set on zero again. In practice, this is not always easy. A woman who miscarries in a first cycle and who is, in fact, an excellent candidate to become pregnant again [29] is entitled to two embryos in her second attempt. From a biomedical perspective, this is suboptimal, and she should receive SET or at least eSET.

The fact that the whole funding regulation has been given the form of a law rather than an exhortation may be questioned. After all, the "solution" of eSET has come out from the reproductive specialists themselves, who have applied it at a time when no funding existed, out of a genuine sense of medical responsibility. Moreover, no sanction exists to curb those centers who will fail under the new regulation to avoid twins in first cycles. It was Montesquieu who said that useless laws weaken necessary ones.

Exceptions to the model

As suggested earlier, each law creates its own transgressions because the less the law is really needed, the more the risk the law violates common sense and other more fundamental rights than those it tries to protect.

Some examples of clinical situations where eSET can be questioned is the "single attempt" IVF/ICSI. Because of financial constraints and the lack of a funding or reimbursement system, in many countries patients undergo just one single trial of IVF/ICSI. This of course is not favorable to promote SET.

When IVF is performed with almost out-of-stock sperm or if oocyte donation has to be performed in a country where donors are expected to participate without any remuneration and eggs are scarce, the pressure to transfer more than one embryo may be very great.

SBT and eSBT

Single blastocyst transfer (SBT) (purely descriptive of the transfer of one blastocyst, full stop) and elec-tive single blastocyst transfer (eSBT), which is the pendant of eSET at the cleavage stage (day 2 or day 3), have received separate acronyms. This is probably necessary in order to inform the patient or the reader of a paper of the context in which SET (neutral) is performed. Although meta-analysis seems to indicate that eSBT has better results than cleavage stage eSET [19], SBT and eSBT often refer to subpopulations of patients that differ from the subpopulations in whom cleavage stage SET or eSET are performed. In most cases a minimum number of good quality day 3 embryos must be available to perform SBT. Moreover, *all* children that are born pass through the day 2–3 stage, so the real trick is not to perform prolonged blastocyst culture but to recognize the high implantation embryo at an earlier stage. This may be more difficult and require more logistic energy and laboratory expertise than is usually admitted, putting blastocyst culture at an advantage which is the greater as the selection performance at day 2–3 used to be more suboptimal. Single blastocyst transfer and eSBT may also serve as a method to convince patients for SET in countries without funding, just as funding is a lever to convince (by law or otherwise) patients for SET in countries with funding [30]. Both can help but are not the only tool to enhance judiciously applied SET.

DET and eDET (elective double or dual embryo transfer)

Along the same lines of thought as is the case for eSET, double embryo transfer or DET (a purely descriptive term) can be the first step towards a reduction of (mainly high-order) multiples. The same logic applies here: DET should be accompanied by some form of a validated method of choice from among several good quality embryos, in order to become eDET. It has been shown, however, that eDET will reduce the incidence of triplets but not of twins [31, 32], which is logical, since the best two embryos are being replaced and in most cases where there is choice, the implantation potentials of the better embryos in the cohort lie close to each other [25].

TET (triple embryo transfer)

Triple embryo transfer (TET) is a rarely used abbreviation, describing the transfer of three embryos. It is often represented as ≥3ET meaning the transfer of any number of three or more embryos. It is customary and recommendable to indicate multiple embryo transfers by declaring the number of embryos transferred, e.g. 3ET, 4ET, 5ET and so on.

SMET (selective multiple embryo transfer)

Single embryo transfer is rightly becoming the standard of care for those patients whom it was intended for, i.e. the twin-prone patient. This strategy has proven to lower the incidence of multiple pregnancies and improve the outcome of IVF in a specific group of patients. The patients in this group are the relatively young women (< 36 years) in their first or second attempt at IVF, with a good cohort of embryos to choose from and preferably with other causes of infertility than tuboperitoneal problems, the so-called "twin-prone group." However, after the implementation of SET, patients at the other side of the clinical spectrum, i.e. the "never-pregnant-prone" women, tend to receive the same cautious approach as the former group of patients. Typically, these women tend to be older (e.g., > 40 years of age), have poor ovarian response and have already undergone multiple attempts of IVF or ICSI treatment without success. Once these women do get pregnant the abortion rate is high and multiple pregnancies are relatively rare.

Hence, allowing for considerable overlap characteristics in clinical reality, two distinct subgroups should be considered given their different biomedical background and prognosis. In the "never-pregnant-prone" group, adhering too strictly to a low number of embryos to transfer may actually result in a suboptimal treatment of those patients.

The higher aneuploidy rate in women of advanced reproductive age has been used to detect and eliminate from transfer those embryos that are genetically abnormal [33, 34]. However, a randomized controlled trial showed that there is no advantage of aneuploidy screening over no screening [35]. In the screened group both the pregnancy rate and the miscarriage rate were similar as in the non-screened group. Aneuploidy screening only improves the pregnancy per transfer ratio because a number of transfers are "prevented." The value of aneuploidy screening in women with repeated failure of implantation and with recurrent miscarriage still remains to be elucidated.

Furthermore, genetics is important but it is not all that counts. Mitochondrial numbers in oocytes dwindle with age and so does the competence of this unique cell to provide the energy needed for its incredible functions [36]: creating an aster figure from the centriole, splitting the DNA chains, pulling them over the aster figure and arranging for recombination between chromatin pairs. No wonder this process fails in cells that cannot provide the DNA trains with sufficient energy to move this long caravan of nucleotides along the cell's rail system.

For all these reasons, the transfer of a high number or even a maximum number (= all available) embryos in a fresh cycle regains status as the only rational way to increase the chance of pregnancy in this group. The idea is that a larger group of embryos has a higher chance to contain at least one genetically normal embryo than a small group. Heavy load transfer (HLT) trusts the principle of letting nature take care of itself by not allowing abnormal embryos to implant, at least if at present no useful technique exists to do something about it. Clinical research has to find out whether the chance of pregnancy is indeed increased by transferring many embryos over just two or three and whether the effect is at the price of an increased multiple pregnancy rate.

To define extremes is relatively easy, but the majority of patients are somewhere in the middle of the prognostic spectrum and that is what makes the implementation of (e)SET so difficult. When societal factors are added to that, applying (e)SET becomes a really difficult exercise. Both resistance to it or too much enthusiasm ensue. Single embryo transfer is not a dogmatic ideology. Selective multiple embryo transfer, sometimes labelled "heavy load transfer" is not an anathema. Professional judiciousness is the guide. Factors that create professionalism may vary from place to place and from time to time.

The relevance of an agreed set of definitions

The importance of a workable set of definitions regarding the number of embryos to transfer is not purely academic. Several very practical reasons call for a precise terminology.

The first and most important reason is to be able to compare results in a standardized fashion. Results of SET and eSET should not be compared at face value.

When results of eSET *between* centers are compared, not only must the target group of patients be defined, but also and foremost the embryo characteristics on which embryo selection took place, both if transfer is performed at the cleavage stage [24, 27, 28] or at the blastocyst stage [37]. Not all day 2 embryos are similar (especially mononucleation is an overlooked criterion) and not all blastocysts are similar.

When results between eSET and DET *within* a center are compared, it is again important to state very clearly when (in which patient, which embryo) eSET was performed. Never should there be any doubt that the transfer of a single embryo, with say 35% chance of implantation (eSET), results in a lower pregnancy rate than the transfer of two embryos with 35% implantation rate (eDET). From a patient-oriented, evidence-based and quality-concerned point of view, eSET can never be more than an approach to be considered under well-*defined* circumstances. These can be defined very broadly (e.g., real life) or very strictly (e.g., a randomized trial), but should never be absolute. Comparisons must always take into account how strict or how lenient inclusion criteria for SET are. The trade-off where we ourselves put this balance from the beginning was that the *overall* pregnancy rate of

the program should not decline as a consequence of using SET [10]. But it is absolutely clear that the increased effort at optimal embryo selection that has resulted from the concept of SET could also be used to *increase* the pregnancy rate of a program, but it will be at the price of maintaining a (very) high twinning and higher-order multiple rate. Conversely, SET may be used in all cycles, thus avoiding all twins but this will be at the cost of halving the overall pregnancy rate [38]. This is a fascinating dilemma where clinical science fades into ethics and philosophy.

What do we know?
Elective SET is not the same as SET; it means a rational choice of one embryo from among a cohort of a minimum of two embryos with validated morphological (or other) criteria.

What do we need to know?
Which embryo criteria are best to choose *the* highest implantation potential embryo and how can we make embryologists agree on this point?

What should we do?
Enhance the applicability of SET by optimally identifying the ideal patient and the ideal embryo to perform judicious eSET.

REFERENCES

1. J. Gerris, Single embryo transfer and IVF/ICSI outcome: a balanced appraisal. *Hum. Reprod. Update*, **11** (2005), 105–121.
2. European IVF-monitoring programme (EIM) for the European Society of Hum. Reprod. and Embryology (ESHRE). Assisted reproductive technology in Europe, 2002. Results generated from European registers by ESHRE. *Hum. Reprod.*, **21** (2006), 1680–1697.
3. A. Strandell, C. Bergh and K. Lundin, Selection of patients suitable for one-embryo transfer may reduce the rate of multiple births by half without impairment of overall birth rates. *Hum. Reprod.*, **15** (2000), 2520–2525.
4. BELRAP, Report of the College of Physicians for Artificial Reproductive Therapy. *Annual Report 2004* (2007) www.belrap.be.

5. ASRM Practice Committee, Guidelines on the number of embryos transferred. *Fertil. Steril.*, **82** (suppl) (2004), S1–S2.

6. J. Gerris, D. De Neubourg, K. Mangelschots *et al.*, Prevention of twin pregnancy after in-vitro fertilization or intracytoplasmic sperm injection based on strict embryo criteria: a prospective randomized clinical trial. *Hum. Reprod.*, **14** (1999), 2581–2587.

7. H. Martikainen, A. Tiitinen, C. Tomás *et al.*, One versus two embryo transfers after IVF and ICSI: randomized study. *Hum. Reprod.*, **16** (2001), 1900–1903.

8. D. K. Gardner, E. Surrey, D. Minjarez *et al.*, Single blastocyst transfer: a prospective randomized trial. *Fertil. Steril.*, **81** (2004), 551–555.

9. A. Thurin, J. Hausken, T. Hillensjo *et al.*, Elective single-embryo transfer versus double-embryo transfer in in vitro fertilization. *N. Engl. J. Med.*, **351** (2004), 2392–2402

10. J. Gerris, D. De Neubourg, K. Mangelschots *et al.*, Elective single day 3 embryo transfer halves the twinning rate without decrease in the ongoing pregnancy rate of an IVF/ICSI programme. *Hum. Reprod.*, **17** (2002), 2621–2626.

11. P. De Sutter, J. Van der Elst, T. Coetsier and M. Dhont, Single embryo transfer and multiple pregnancy rate reduction after IVF/ICSI: a 5-year appraisal. *Reprod. Biomed. Online*, **6** (2003), 464–469.

12. A. Tiitinen, L. Unkila-Kallio, M. Halttunen and C. Hydén-Granskog, Impact of elective single embryo transfer on the twin pregnancy rate. *Hum. Reprod.*, **18** (2003), 1449–1453.

13. J. Catt, T. Wood, M. Henman and R. Jansen, Single embryo transfer in IVF to prevent multiple pregnancies. *Twin Res.*, **6** (2003), 536–539.

14. J. Gerris, P. De Sutter, D. De Neubourg *et al.*, A real-life prospective health economic study of elective single embryo transfer versus two-embryo transfer in first IVF/ICSI cycles. *Hum. Reprod.*, **19** (2004), 917–923.

15. H. Martikainen, M. Orava, J. Lakkakorpi and L. Tuomivaara, Day 2 elective single embryo transfer in clinical practice: better outcome in ICSI cycles. *Hum. Reprod.*, **19** (2004), 1364–1366.

16. A. Criniti, A. Thyer, G. Chow, N. Klein and M. Soules, Elective blastocyst transfer reduces twin rates without compromising pregnancy rates. *Fertil. Steril.*, **84** (2005), 1613–1619.

17. M. Henman, J. W. Catt, T. Wood *et al.*, Elective transfer of single blastocysts and later transfer of cryo-stored blastocysts reduces the twin pregnancy rate and can improve the in vitro fertilization live birth rate in younger women. *Fertil. Steril.*, **84** (2005), 1620–1627.

18. E. G. Papanikolaou, E. D'haeseleer, G. Verheyen *et al.*, Live birth rate is significantly higher after blastocyst transfer than after cleavage-stage embryo transfer when at least four embryos are available on day 3 of embryo culture. A randomized prospective study. *Hum. Reprod.*, **20** (2005), 3198–3203.

19. E. G. Papanikolaou, E. Kolibianakis, B. Tournaye *et al.*, Live birth rates after transfer of an equal number of blastocysts or cleavage-stage embryos in IVF. A systematic review and meta-analysis. *Hum. Reprod.*, **23** (2008), 91–99.

20. A. P. van Montfoort, A. A. Fiddelers, J. A. Land *et al.*, eSET irrespective of the availability of a good-quality embryo in the first cycle only is not effective in reducing overall twin pregnancy rates. *Hum. Reprod.*, **22** (2007), 1669–1674.

21. C. Giorgetti, P. Terriou, P. Auquier *et al.*, Embryo score to predict implantation after in-vitro fertilization: based on 957 single embryo transfers. *Hum. Reprod.*, **10** (1995), 2427–2431.

22. S. Vilska, A. Tiitinen, C. Hydén-Granskog and O. Hovatta, Elective transfer of one embryo results in an acceptable pregnancy rate and eliminates the risk of multiple birth. *Hum. Reprod.*, **14** (1999), 2392–2395.

23. L. A. Scott and S. Smith, The successful use of pronuclear embryo transfers the day following oocyte retrieval. *Hum. Reprod.*, **13** (1998), 1003–1013.

24. E. Van Royen, K. Mangelschots, D. De Neubourg *et al.*, Characterization of a top quality embryo, a step towards single-embryo transfer. *Hum. Reprod.*, **14** (1999), 2345–2349.

25. E. Van Royen, K. Mangelschots, D. De Neubourg *et al.*, Calculating the implantation potential of day 3 embryos in women younger than 38 years of age: a new model. *Hum. Reprod.*, **16** (2001), 326–332.

26. J. Tesarik, A. M. Junca, A. Hazout *et al.*, Embryos with high implantation potential after intracytoplasmic sperm injection can be recognized by a simple, non-invasive examination of pronuclear morphology. *Hum. Reprod.*, **15** (2000), 1396–1399.

27. K. Lundin, C. Bergh and T. Hardarson, Early embryo cleavage is a strong indicator of embryo quality in human IVF. *Hum. Reprod.*, **16** (2001), 2652–2657.

28. J. Holte, L. Berglund, K. Milton *et al.*, Construction of an evidence-based integrated morphology cleavage score for implantation potential of embryos scored and transferred on day 2 after oocyte retrieval. *Hum. Reprod.*, **22** (2007), 548–557.

29. C. A. Croucher, A. Lass, R. Margara and R. M. Winston, Predictive value of the results of a first in-vitro fertilization cycle on the outcome of subsequent cycles. *Hum. Reprod.*, **13** (1998), 403–408.

30. P. Saldeen and P. Sundström, Would legislation imposing single embryo transfer be a feasible way to reduce the rate of multiple pregnancies after IVF treatment? *Hum. Reprod.*, **20** (2005) 4–8.

31. C. Staessen, C. Janssenswillen, E. Van Den Abbeel, P. Devroey and A. Van Steirteghem, Avoidance of triplet pregnancies by elective transfer of two good quality embryos. *Hum. Reprod.*, **8** (1993), 1650–1653.

32. A. Templeton and J. K. Morris, Reducing the risk of multiple birth by transfer of two embryos after *in vitro* fertilization. *N. Engl. J. Med.*, **339** (1998), 573–577.

33. S. Munné, J. Cohen and D. Sable, Preimplantation genetic diagnosis for advanced maternal age and other indications. *Fertil. Steril.*, **78** (2002), 234–236.

34. Y. Verlinsky, J. Cohen, S. Munné *et al.*, Over a decade of experience with preimplantation diagnosis: a multicenter report. *Fertil. Steril.*, **82** (2004), 292–294.

35. C. Staessen, P. Platteau, E. Van Assche, *et al.*, Comparison of blastocyst transfer with or without preimplantation genetic diagnosis for aneuploidy screening in couples with advanced maternal age: a prospective randomized controlled trial. *Hum. Reprod.*, **19** (2004), 2849–2858.

36. J. Van Blerkom, P. Davis and S. Alexander, Differential mitochondrial distribution in human pronuclear embryos leads to disproportionate inheritance between blastomeres: relationship to microtubular organization, ATP content and competence. *Hum. Reprod.*, **15** (2000), 2621–2633.

37. M. Meintjes, D. M. Bookout, S. J. Chantilis *et al.*, Towards single blastocyst transfers – preliminary experience. *Fertil. Steril.*, **82**: (Suppl.) (2007), S35.

38. A. P. van Montfoort, A. A. Fiddelers, J. M. Janssen *et al.*, In unselected patients, elective single embryo transfer prevents all multiples, but results in significantly lower pregnancy rates compared with double embryo transfer: a randomized controlled trial. *Hum. Reprod.*, **21** (2006), 338–343.

4

Patient selection for single embryo transfer

Ofer Fainaru and Mark D. Hornstein

Introduction

Multiple pregnancies are the most important complication of assisted reproduction technologies due to their impact on obstetrical outcomes and on the associated neonatal complications [1]. In the early days of in vitro fertilization (IVF), multiple pregnancies were thought to be an acceptable cost in order to achieve, by contemporary methods, an acceptable pregnancy rate. With improvements in the IVF laboratory, success rates have increased; however, so has the incidence of multiple gestations [2]. The most important factor influencing the rate of multiple births is the number of embryos transferred [3]. Efforts to reduce high-multiple pregnancies by transferring two instead of three embryos were successful in reducing triplet pregnancies; however, the twinning rate remained fairly unchanged at ∼25% per delivery [2]. It is obvious that transferring only one embryo would result in mainly singletons, but this strategy might also result in a significant decline in the rates of pregnancy and live birth. Already many IVF centers that attain excellent pregnancy rates have incorporated single embryo transfer (SET) into their practice.

While SET has become standard practice in many IVF programs, a key question that remains is which patients would most benefit from this strategy. The aim of this chapter is to briefly review the current literature identifying patients at risk for multiple pregnancies and who thus might benefit from SET, and then review the current data from randomized clinical trials and from observational studies to improve guidelines for patient selection for SET.

Gleicher and Barad [4] described a patient population of potential candidates for SET. Some patients are obvious candidates, as they oppose the risk of twinning for *social* or *economic* reasons. Other patients have a *medical* history that contraindicates multiple pregnancies. These include patients with a previously ruptured uterus or uterine surgery, those with a history of premature labor, or patients with a known Müllerian uterine anomaly. Such patients are more likely to be willing to accept the reduced pregnancy chances that come with SET in exchange for the reduced obstetrical risks of a singleton gestation. However, this describes only a small proportion of the patients in an IVF practice, and better guidelines are needed for administration of SET to a more general patient population to effectively reduce multiple pregnancy rates. These candidates for SET are more controversial of course, as most will decrease their pregnancy chances by switching from double embryo transfer (DET) to SET. In most circumstances, the ideal candidate for SET is therefore the patient who is at high risk for multiple gestations.

Staessen *et al.* [5] defined the IVF population at risk for multiple pregnancies as women younger than 37 years who had at least six good quality

Single Embryo Transfer, ed. J. Gerris, G. D. Adamson, P. De Sutter and C. Racowsky. Published by Cambridge University Press.
© Cambridge University Press 2009.

embryos in the first three IVF cycles. Good quality embryos were in turn defined as those in which the 4-cell stage was reached at 44–48 hours after insemination with less than 20% fragmentation. Coetsier and Dhont [6] considered patients at risk as women younger than 36 years, in their first three IVF cycles, having at least three embryos with a good score. Young age, a higher number of transferred embryos and good transferred embryo quality were also found in other studies to be the best predictors of multiple pregnancies [7, 8]. Interestingly, De Neubourg and Gerris [2] found that 80% of twin pregnancies occur in the first or second IVF/ICSI cycles. The overall implantation rate of all transferred embryos decreased steeply from a stable 23–25% under the age of 38 to 11% above this age. Thus in this study [2], patients older than 38 years are probably not a target group for SET.

Randomized clinical trials

There are data from six randomized clinical trials (RCTs) comparing the results of SET and DET (Table 4.1) in good prognosis patients, utilizing the above selection criteria, namely relatively young age, availability of top quality embryos and first or second IVF cycle. Gerris et al. [9] randomized 53 patients younger than 34 years of age, in their first IVF/ICSI cycle, having at least two excellent quality embryos, to either SET or DET. A significantly higher ongoing pregnancy rate was achieved in the DET group (74.0%) than in the elective SET (eSET) group (38.5%) ($p = 0.013$, relative risk [RR] = 1.9, 95% CI 1.13–3.23). Six twin pregnancies led to a multiple pregnancy rate of 30% in the DET group versus 10% in the SET group. Although the high ongoing pregnancy rates with DET could be attributed to the excellent prognosis predicted for both groups, this RCT showed for the first time that SET could lead to an acceptable conception and ongoing pregnancy rate.

In a Finnish study [10] the patient selection criteria for SET were: age < 36 years, first or second IVF cycle, and at least four good quality embryos.

The ongoing pregnancy rate was 32.4% in the SET group versus 47.1% in the DET group; however, this difference did not reach statistical significance ($p = 0.09$).

Whereas the previous two trials analyzed day 2 or day 3 embryo transfers, Gardner et al. [11] compared single blastocyst transfers with double blastocyst transfers. Patient selection criteria were day 3 FSH < 10 mIU/mL, E2 < 80 pg/mL, hysteroscopically normal endometrial cavity and at least ten follicles >12 mm in diameter on day of human chorionic gonadotropin (hCG) administration. Of the single blastocyst group, 60.9% achieved an ongoing pregnancy versus 76% in the double blastocyst group (difference not significant; 95% CI 0.11–0.41).

The largest multicenter trial from Scandinavia [12] compared two embryo transfer strategies: (1) transferring one single embryo, and if no pregnancy was achieved, a consecutive transfer of one frozen-thawed SET; versus (2) one fresh DET. In this study 661 women were randomized to eSET or DET. Included were women younger than 36 years of age who had at least two good quality embryos undergoing their first or second IVF cycle. The study showed that the live birth rate in the SET group was not substantially lower than the DET group (38.8% vs. 42.9%). However, the live birth rate after only fresh SET was 50% lower in the SET group (27.6% vs. 42.9%, $p < 0.001$) if the frozen-thawed embryos were not taken into account. Predictably, the multiple birth rate was significantly decreased in the SET group. Interestingly, SET was found suitable for many patients, as 37.1% of the IVF cycles at the participating IVF clinics met the inclusion criteria. The authors suggest that this may be a representative estimate for many IVF clinics. This is in contrast to the calculations of Gleicher and Barad [4] that only 10% of their center's patient population was suitable for SET. However, his population in New York was older than that in the Scandinavian study. The results of this trial further emphasize the importance of an established freezing program when considering offering SET to appropriately selected patients.

Table 4.1 Data adapted from randomized and observational trials comparing SET with DET

Patient selection criteria	N SET	DET	Pregnancy rate[a] n (%) SET	DET	Twin pregnancy rate[b] n (%) SET	DET	Delivery rate n (%) SET	DET
Randomized clinical trials								
age < 34 yrs 1st IVF/ICSI cycle ≥ 2 excellent quality embryos (Gerris *et al.*, 1999) [9]	26	27	10(38.5)	20(74.0)	1(10.0)	6(30.0)	NA	NA
age < 36 years 1st/2nd IVF/ICSI cycles ≥ 4 good quality embryos (Martikainen *et al.*, 2001) [10]	74	70	24(32.4)	33(47.1)	1(4.2)	11(39.3)	22(29.7)	28(40.0)
day 3 FSH < 10 mIU/mL E2 < 80 pg/mL 10 follicles > 12 mm[c] (Gardner *et al.*, 2004) [11]	23	25	14(60.9)	19(76.0)	0(0.0)	9(47.4)	NA	NA
age < 36 years 1st/2nd IVF/ICSI cycles ≥ 2 good quality embryos (Thurin *et al.*, 2004) [12]	330	331	94(28.5)	146(44.1)	1(1.1)	47(33.1)	91(27.6)	142(42.9)
age < 35 years basal FSH < 10 IU/L 1st IVF/ICSI cycle/after a successful treatment ≥ 2 embryos, 1 good/excellent quality (Lukassen *et al.*, 2005)[13][d]	54	53	20(37.0)	25(47.0)	0(0.0)	7(37.0)	14(26.0)	19(36.0)
unselected population 1st IVF cycle (van Montfoort *et al.*, 2006) [14]	154	154	33(21.4)	62(40.3)	0(0.0)	13(21.0)	NA	NA
Observational studies								
subject's wish, risk of OHSS, medical reasons (see text) indication for prenatal diagnosis, ≥ 2 good quality embryos (Vilska *et al.*, 1999) [16]	74	742	22(29.7)	218(29.4)	0(0.0)	52(23.9)	18(24.3)	NA
3 groups of patients: 1. age < 34 years, first IVF/ICSI cycle, ≥ 2 top quality embryos 2. age < 38 years, 1st/2nd IVF/ICSI cycles 3. subject's wish (Gerris *et al.*, 2002) [18]	299	853	105(35.1)	309(36.2)	1(1.1)	109(35.3)	NA	NA

(*cont.*)

Table 4.1 (*cont.*)

Patient selection criteria	N		Pregnancy rate[a] n (%)		Twin pregnancy rate[b] n (%)		Delivery rate n (%)	
	SET	DET	SET	DET	SET	DET	SET	DET
risk of severe OHSS, medical reasons, indication for prenatal diagnosis, previous IVF delivery, selection in a randomized study, subject's wish, ≥ 2 good quality embryos (Tiitinen *et al.*, 2003) [17]	470	1024	162(34.4)	376(36.7)	2(1.6)	76(27.6)	128(27.2)	275(26.9)
< 37 years 1st/2nd IVF cycles, ≥ 2 excellent quality embryos (De Sutter *et al.*, 2003) [20]	579	2319	163(28.2)	734(31.7)	1(0.6)	223(30.4)	NA	NA
< 38 years, 1st IVF or after previous delivery, presence of high-competence embryo, favored SET (Gerris *et al.*, 2004) [19]	206	161	83(40.3)	65(40.4)	0(0.0)	20(30.8)	77(37.4)	59(36.6)
< 36 years, 1st/2nd IVF cycles, presence of top quality embryo (Martikainen *et al.*, 2004) [21]	308	803	107(34.7)	255(31.8)	1(1.1)	NA	86(27.9)	NA
age 36–39, good response to stimulation, > one top quality embryo and > one embryo of freezable quality, 1st/2nd IVF cycles (Veleva *et al.*, 2006) [22]	335	585	111(33.1)	175(29.9)	0(0.0)	31(17.7)	87(26.0)	128(21.9)

[a] Clinical pregnancy per transfer (fetal sacs with cardiac activity).

[b] Number of twins per delivery (if available), otherwise twins per ongoing pregnancy.

[c] Criteria of the Colorado Center for Reproductive Medicine for blastocyst stage embryo transfer [23].

[d] Cumulative results after two SET cycles are presented in the text.

NA, not applicable.

ICSI, intracytoplasmic sperm injection; FSH, follicle-stimulating hormone; E2, estradiol; OHSS, ovarian hyperstimulation syndrome.

Lukassen *et al.* [13] conducted a RCT in which they compared two consecutive SET cycles with one DET cycle. They included patients younger than 35 years of age with basal FSH < 10 IU/L; undergoing their first IVF/ICSI cycle ever, or the first cycle after a successful treatment; with at least two available embryos, at least one of which is of excellent or good quality. The cumulative live birth rate in the SET group (22/54; 41%, 95% CI 27–54%) was similar to the live birth rate in the DET group (19/53; 36%, 95% CI 23–49%). After one treatment cycle, however, the live birth rate in the SET group (14/54; 26%, 95% CI 14–38%) approached the rate in the DET group.

Van Montfoort *et al.* [14] performed a randomized clinical trial addressing the applicability of SET in an unselected patient population (i.e., irrespective of the woman's age or embryo quality). The study showed that applying SET in the first cycle of an unselected group of patients led to a twin pregnancy rate of 0%. However, the price to be paid was a reduction of the ongoing pregnancy rate to approximately half of that obtained after DET (21.4% vs. 40.3% respectively), further emphasizing the need for careful patient selection when applying the SET strategy.

Recently, Papanikolaou *et al.* [15] reported the results of a RCT comparing the outcome of the transfer of a single embryo cultured for 3 days (cleavage state) with the transfer of a blastocyst cultured for 5 days. The authors reported significantly higher rates of live delivery in the blastocyst stage group than in the cleavage state group (32.0% vs. 21.6%; RR, 1.48; 95% CI 1.04–2.11). The study again selected for good prognosis patients, i.e., women under 36 years of age with low basal FSH levels and who were undergoing their first or second IVF or ICSI cycle.

The results from the RCTs show that in a carefully selected patient population, i.e., under age 34–36 years, in their first/second IVF/ICSI cycle, having at least two available top quality embryos for transfer, satisfactory pregnancy and delivery rates can be achieved with SET. The lower delivery rate in the SET group might be restored with the addition of either frozen-thawed or a repeated fresh embryo transfer [3, 12]. Single embryo transfer in this selected group of patients results in a significant decrease in the rate of multiple pregnancies.

Observational studies

Though the observational studies comparing SET and DET show promising results in carefully selected patients, they should be interpreted with caution. Methodologically, these studies suffer a selection bias, with good prognosis patients receiving SET and poor prognosis patients receiving DET. Data from observational studies are also summarized in Table 4.1. Vilska *et al.* [16] analyzed all the fresh embryo cycles during 1997 in two clinics in Helsinki and found similar pregnancy rates after SET and DET. The three main indications for eSET were: subject's preference, risk of ovarian hyperstimulation syndrome (OHSS) and various other medical reasons (diabetes mellitus, uterine malformation, history of cervical incompetence or hysterotomy and indication for prenatal diagnosis). The mean age of the women was 35 years (range 24–42 years) in the SET group and 34 years (range 23–42 years) in the DET group. The pregnancy rate after SET when at least two good embryos were available for transfer was 29.7%, similar to that after DET (29.4%). However, when only one embryo was available for transfer, the pregnancy rate for SET was only 20.2%. This study highlights the importance of the availability of at least two good quality embryos as a patient selection criterion.

Tiitinen *et al.* [17] completed a retrospective analysis comparing the results of SET and DET over 4 years (1997–2001). At the beginning of this period, the main indication for SET was a medical reason to avoid a multiple gestation, such as diabetes or other chronic disease, previous hysterotomy, uterine malformation, risk of severe ovarian hyperstimulation or indication for prenatal diagnosis. Later, the number of indications was increased to include previous IVF delivery, selection in a randomized study and the couple's wish to avoid twins. This study again showed good results with similar pregnancy and delivery rates in both SET and DET.

Gerris *et al.* [18] also described their retrospective analysis over a 4-year period (1998–2001). In this study three groups of patients were included. The first group consisted of women under 34 years of age in their first IVF/ICSI cycle who agreed to randomization between the transfer of one top quality embryo versus two top quality embryos. The second group included women under 38 years of age in their first IVF/ICSI cycle ever or after a previous successful IVF/ICSI pregnancy, who could choose between one or two embryos. The third group were women who did not meet the inclusion criteria of either of the two previous studies but nevertheless wanted only one embryo, some of them over 38 years of age. All these patients were considered retrospectively together on the basis of what they actually received at the time of transfer. In this study the authors concluded that when applying SET to approximately one third of all patients, it would be possible to decrease the multiple birth rate by 50% without decreasing ongoing pregnancy rates.

In a later study Gerris *et al.* [19] analyzed data on patients fulfilling the following inclusion criteria: younger than 38 years of age, first IVF/ICSI treatment ever or after a previous delivery, irrespective of whether or not that pregnancy was the result of infertility treatment. The choice between SET or DET was mainly based on embryo morphology. If a high-competence embryo was present, patients generally received SET, otherwise DET was performed. The live birth rate was similar (37.4% for SET and 36.6% for DET). This study further emphasized the importance of the availability of good quality embryos as a major patient selection criterion.

De Sutter *et al.* [20] summarized the largest number of cycles reported (2898) from a Belgian unit over a 5-year period (1997–2002). Elective SET was proposed to patients younger than 37 years old, in their first or second treatment cycle, and who had at least two excellent or good quality embryos. In this study, utilizing these selection criteria, similar pregnancy rates were achieved in the SET and the DET groups (28.2% vs. 31.7%, respectively).

Martikainen *et al.* [21] reported the experience of their unit during the period 2000–2, when SET was routinely carried out among women under the age of 36 in the first or second treatment cycle when a top quality embryo was available. Pregnancy rates were similar between SET and DET (34.7% vs. 31.8%, respectively). Interestingly, in the SET ICSI cycles, the clinical pregnancy rate was significantly higher than in the corresponding IVF cycles (50.6% vs. 28.5%, $p < 0.001$). The authors also found that embryo quality was a more important determinant of outcome than the age of the woman.

Veleva *et al.* [22] addressed the applicability of SET in women older than 35 years (36–39). Interestingly, in this age group the pregnancy rate (33.1% vs. 29.9%, $p = 0.3$) and the live birth rate (26.0% vs. 21.9%, $p = 0.2$) were similar in the SET and DET groups respectively.

The results from the observational studies show that similar pregnancy and delivery rates are achieved with SET and DET in a selected patient population: younger than 39 years; in their first/second IVF/ICSI cycle; with a history of good response to stimulation; having at least two good quality embryos available for transfer; and some at risk for severe OHSS or suffering from various medical conditions. The reason for these good results is most probably the fact that the two groups are not strictly comparable [3], with good prognosis women receiving SET and poor prognosis women receiving DET.

Conclusions

Taken together, the results of both the RCTs and the observational studies point to several groups of patients suitable for SET. Clearly one group would be patients who wish to avoid multiple pregnancies for social or economic reasons or patients with a medical contraindication for multiple gestations. Other appropriate candidates would be young women, in most studies under 36 years. This limitation most probably reflects the difference in applicability of SET between centers with an older [4] and relatively younger population [12], of whom up to 37% of the patients meet the inclusion criteria for SET. Another important selection parameter for SET should be the availability of at least two top quality embryos. Aside from being a good prognostic factor, this will allow the transfer of one fresh embryo and in the absence of a pregnancy the possibility of transfer of a frozen-thawed embryo, a strategy proven to achieve results as good as DET. Finally, data regarding the frequency of multiple pregnancies in the first IVF cycles and the bad prognosis associated with repeated failures point to patients undergoing their first or second IVF cycle as better candidates for SET.

REFERENCES

1. T. Bergh, A. Ericson, T. Hillensjo, K. G. Nygren and U. B. Wennerholm, Deliveries and children born after in-vitro fertilisation in Sweden 1982–95: a retrospective cohort study. *Lancet*, **354** (1999), 1579–1585.
2. D. De Neubourg and J. Gerris, Single embryo transfer – state of the art. *Reprod. Biomed. Online*, **7** (2003), 615–622.
3. C. Bergh, Single embryo transfer: a mini-review. *Hum. Reprod.*, **20** (2005), 323–327.
4. N. Gleicher and D. Barad, The relative myth of elective single embryo transfer. *Hum. Reprod.*, **21** (2006), 1337–1344.
5. C. Staessen, C. Janssenswillen, E. Van den Abbeel, P. Devroey and A. Van Steirteghem, Avoidance of triplet pregnancies by elective transfer of two good quality embryos. *Hum. Reprod.*, **8** (1993), 1650–1653.
6. T. Coetsier and M. Dhont, Avoiding multiple pregnancies in in-vitro fertilization: who's afraid of single embryo transfer? *Hum. Reprod.*, **13** (1998), 2663–2664.
7. A. Strandell, C. Bergh and K. Lundin, Selection of patients suitable for one-embryo transfer may reduce the rate of multiple births by half without impairment of overall birth rates. *Hum. Reprod.*, **15** (2000), 2520–2525.
8. C. C. Hunault, M. J. Eijkemans, M. H. Pieters *et al.*, A prediction model for selecting patients undergoing in vitro fertilization for elective single embryo transfer. *Fertil. Steril.*, **77** (2002), 725–732.
9. J. Gerris, D. De Neubourg, K. Mangelschots *et al.*, Prevention of twin pregnancy after in-vitro fertilization or intracytoplasmic sperm injection based on strict embryo criteria: a prospective randomized clinical trial. *Hum. Reprod.*, **14** (1999), 2581–2587.
10. H. Martikainen, A. Tiitinen, C. Tomás *et al.* One versus two embryo transfer after IVF and ICSI: a randomized study. *Hum. Reprod.*, **16** (2001), 1900–1903.
11. D. K. Gardner, E. Surrey, D. Minjarez *et al.*, Single blastocyst transfer: a prospective randomized trial. *Fertil. Steril.*, **81** (2004), 551–555.
12. A. Thurin, J. Hausken, T. Hillensjo *et al.*, Elective single-embryo transfer versus double-embryo transfer in in vitro fertilization. *N. Engl. J. Med.*, **351** (2004), 2392–2402.
13. H. G. Lukassen, D. D. Braat, A. M. Wetzels *et al.*, Two cycles with single embryo transfer versus one cycle with double embryo transfer: a randomized controlled trial. *Hum. Reprod.*, **20** (2005), 702–708.
14. A. P. van Montfoort, A. A. Fiddelers, J. M. Janssen *et al.*, In unselected patients, elective single embryo transfer prevents all multiples, but results in significantly lower pregnancy rates compared with double embryo transfer: a randomized controlled trial. *Hum. Reprod.*, **21** (2006), 338–343.
15. E. G. Papanikolaou, M. Camus, E. M. Kolibianakis *et al.*, In vitro fertilization with single blastocyst-stage versus single cleavage-stage embryos. *N. Engl. J. Med.*, **354** (2006) 1139–1146.
16. S. Vilska, A. Tiitinen, C. Hydén-Granskog and O. Hovatta, Elective transfer of one embryo results in an acceptable pregnancy rate and eliminates the risk of multiple birth. *Hum. Reprod.*, **14** (1999), 2392–2395.
17. A. Tiitinen, L. Unkila-Kallio, M. Halttunen and C. Hyden-Granskog, Impact of elective single embryo transfer on the twin pregnancy rate. *Hum. Reprod.*, **18** (2003), 1449–1453.
18. J. Gerris, D. De Neubourg, K. Mangelschots *et al.*, Elective single day 3 embryo transfer halves the twinning rate without decrease in the ongoing pregnancy rate of an IVF/ICSI programme. *Hum. Reprod.*, **17** (2002), 2626–2631.
19. J. Gerris, P. De Sutter, D. De Neubourg *et al.*, A real-life prospective health economic study of elective single embryo transfer versus two-embryo transfer in first IVF/ICSI cycles. *Hum. Reprod.*, **19** (2004), 917–923.

20. P. De Sutter, J. Van der Elst, T. Coetsier and M. Dhont, Single embryo transfer and multiple pregnancy rate reduction in IVF/ICSI: a 5-year appraisal. *Reprod. Biomed. Online*, **6** (2003), 464–469.

21. H. Martikainen, M. Orava, J. Lakkakorpi and L. Tuomivaara, Day 2 elective single embryo transfer in clinical practice: better outcome in ICSI cycles. *Hum. Reprod.*, **19** (2004), 1364–1366.

22. Z. Veleva, S. Vilska, C. Hydén-Granskog *et al.*, Elective single embryo transfer in women aged 36-39 years. *Hum. Reprod.*, **21** (2006), 2098–2102.

23. D. K. Gardner, W. B. Schoolcraft, L. Wagley *et al.*, A prospective randomized trial of blastocyst culture and transfer in in-vitro fertilization. *Hum. Reprod.*, **13** (1998), 3434–3440.

5

Perinatal outcome after single embryo transfer

Petra De Sutter and Jan Gerris

Introduction

In vitro fertilization (IVF) and intracytoplasmic sperm injection (ICSI) are now routine treatment methods for longstanding infertility. Worldwide more than 500 000 cycles are performed each year now, and it is estimated that in Western-European countries 2% of all newborn children are conceived through IVF or ICSI [1]. The major problem brought about by these modern reproductive technologies has been a dramatic rise in the incidence of multiple pregnancies in the last two decades. The only way to solve this multiple pregnancy epidemic is to reduce the number of embryos for transfer.

Since the end of the 1990s single embryo transfer (SET) and its clinical implementation and consequences have been the subject of intensive research by many groups. One of the first papers exploring the idea of SET was a paper by Coetsier and Dhont [2], who showed that a reduction in twinning rates could be anticipated if SET was introduced for selected ("twin-prone") patients, without loss of overall pregnancy rates. This theoretical idea was then put into practice and in several papers many authors have proven that elective SET (eSET) could drastically reduce multiple pregnancy rates after IVF/ICSI, while maintaining a stable and acceptable pregnancy rate [3, 4]. A study by Gerris *et al.* [5] analyzed the results of a randomized clinical trial comparing SET and double embryo transfer (DET) of two top quality embryos in first attempts in women younger than 34 years of age; and two observational studies of our group have further investigated the impact of implementing SET in an overall clinical program [6, 7]. These studies were performed even before the Belgian law (see Chapter 3, the Belgian model) was installed, which now requests clinicians to transfer only one embryo in selected cases [8].

Our group has also demonstrated in real-life circumstances that SET was advantageous from a health-economic point of view, because the high cost of twin pregnancies for society can be largely prevented or decreased [9–11]. The latter studies fueled the discussion which ended in the funding regulations granted for IVF and ICSI in Belgium since July 2003. Since the publication of these papers, other groups have confirmed that the SET strategy was more cost-effective than the DET strategy [12–14]. Some authors have also compared different strategies of a combination of ovarian stimulation and embryo transfer with each other from the point of view of efficaciousness and health-economics [15].

Finally, it was also shown that SET could further increase per-cycle pregnancy rates by considering the cryo-augmentation effect, i.e. the additional pregnancies that ensue as the result of subsequent transfers of frozen-thawed embryos [16–18].

The reduction in multiple and especially twinning rates can already be considered to be a major benefit

Single Embryo Transfer, ed. J. Gerris, G. D. Adamson, P. De Sutter and C. Racowsky. Published by Cambridge University Press.
© Cambridge University Press 2009.

of the SET strategy, because of the reduction in the sheer numbers of pregnancies that are complicated by maternal and/or fetal morbidity and even mortality. In addition, we wanted to study perinatal and obstetrical outcome of SET (singleton) pregnancies, on the hypothesis that perhaps SET would not only bring less (complications of) twins (and higher-order multiples), but that, in addition, the transfer of just one embryo should be followed by an optimal early placentation, resulting in a better perinatal outcome of SET singletons when compared with DET or higher-order embryo transfers. Follow-up of IVF/ICSI pregnancies has been of special interest to our team and already in 1999 Dhont et al. demonstrated that for twin pregnancies the outcome after IVF/ICSI was similar to that after spontaneous conception [19]. Paradoxically, IVF/ICSI singletons seemed to have a worse obstetrical and perinatal outcome than singletons after spontaneous conception [20]. This has been puzzling to most authors and has been attributed to either patient characteristics, or to the assisted reproductive technology in se. This worse outcome of IVF/ICSI singletons has been confirmed in many studies since [21, 22] and recently our own group has confirmed that patient characteristics certainly may play a role, because outcome of IVF/ICSI pregnancies is not different from outcome of a comparable infertile population treated with intrauterine insemination [23].

A parallel observation has been a significantly higher non-ongoing pregnancy rate of IVF/ICSI singletons versus twins (expressed per amniotic sac), both before cardiac activity (21.7% vs.17.1%) and after (12.2% vs. 7.3%) [24]. Here again, twins seem to be at an "advantage" over singletons.

Two lines of thought may help explain these observations. One is the hypothesis of the "vanishing twin," the other has to do with population bias.

The latter means that all (meta-)analyses that have been performed so far relate to a very heterogeneous mix of singleton pregnancies whereas the twins are a much more homogeneous group. A large percentage of twins (not to speak of higher-order multiple gestations) occurs during first and

second attempts in younger women, who respond normally to ovarian stimulation and usually produce a cohort of good quality embryos. They are in fact to a large degree good prognosis patients. In contrast, the singleton group contains widely differing patients. On the one hand, there are also a large group of good prognosis patients in their first and second attempts, who happen to have just one evolving fetus after the transfer of perhaps two or three embryos, but on the other hand there are many patients who were in a high rank attempt and received many embryos in an effort to maximize their chances. The profile of these patients (older women, poor responders, unexplained infertility patients) is probably quite different from the typical young early rank ICSI patient. Moreover, it is not known what the percentage of fetal reduction is in this population.

In order to know the full picture, we must study the outcome of singletons after eSET and compare it to the outcome of singletons after the transfer of two or more embryos. In close connection to this population effect comes the former hypothesis of "vanishing twin" syndrome [25]. Indeed, most if not all follow-up studies of assisted reproductive technology (ART) pregnancies and children have studied singletons occurring after transfer of more than one embryo. It may in theory be possible that an early vanishing twin pregnancy may compromise the evolution of the ongoing singleton and lead to a less beneficial perinatal outcome. An incidence of 12.1% of vanishing twins was recorded in the study of our group mentioned earlier [24], which by itself is just the tip of an iceberg, because the authors could only include echographically visible twins, whereas the incidence of incipient twins must be higher. Perhaps comparative analysis of beta-human chorionic gonadotropin (βhCG) curves comparing what happens after the transfer of one top quality embryo versus two embryos will cast more light on this black box of early pregnancy. For the moment, it can not be excluded that the transfer of more than one embryo results in suboptimal nidation and that this may have an effect that can be measured or at least observed by looking at

Table 5.1 Comparison of number of embryos transferred and pregnancy outcome parameters between women with and without first-trimester bleeding

	First-trimester bleeding	Controls	Odds ratio (95% CI) or p-value
Patients	253	1179	
Number of embryos transferred (%)			
1	26 (12.5)	182 (87.5)	χ^2 (d.f. 3) = 14.74
2	129 (16.2)	666 (83.8)	$p < 0.01$
3	75 (21.6)	272 (78.4)	
> 3	23 (28.0)	59 (72.0)	
Percentage of PPROM	7.6	3.2	2.44 (1.83–4.31)
Percentage of preterm contractions	13.9	6.7	2.27 (1.48–3.47)
Percentage of IUGR	3.2	5.5	0.57 (0.270–1.21)
Percentage of intrauterine death	0.8	1.0	0.78 (0.17–3.48)
Percentage of Cesarean section	19	19.4	0.98 (0.69–1.39)
Duration of pregnancy (days)[a]	272 ± 17	275 ± 14	$p = 0.0092$
Percentage of preterm births	11.6	7.4	1.64 (1.05–2.55)
Percentage of very preterm births	2.4	0.8	3.05 (1.12–8.31)
Birth weight (g)[a]	3157 ± 607	3272 ± 559	$p = 0.0038$
Percentage of low birth weight	8.8	7.2	1.24 (0.76–2.02)
Percentage of very low birth weight	2.4	0.7	3.56 (1.28–9.90)
Percentage of 1-min Apgar score < 7	8.1	8.0	1.02 (0.61–1.71)
Percentage of 5-min Apgar score < 7	2.1	2.6	0.80 (0.32–2.03)
Percentage of NICU admission	17.9	11	1.75 (1.21–.54)
Percentage of perinatal deaths	1.2	1.4	0.87 (0.25–3.02)

[a] Fourteen pregnancies ending in intrauterine death have been excluded.

95% CI, 95% confidence interval; IUGR, intrauterine growth retardation; NICU, neonatal intensive care unit; PPROM, preterm prelabor rupture of membranes.

variables such as incidence of first-trimester blood loss, miscarriage and perinatal outcome data. Preliminary data under scrutiny for publication indicate that serum hCG rises more steeply after the transfer of one good quality embryo than after the transfer of two embryos [26].

First-trimester bleeding

Assisted reproductive technology pregnancies are at risk for a common complication, which is first-trimester bleeding. In spontaneous pregnancies this occurs in about 20% of pregnancies [27], but after ART the incidence is increased to between 29% and 36% [28–31]. First-trimester bleeding is corre-

lated with an increased risk for miscarriage both in spontaneous (50%) [27] and in IVF pregnancies (between 25% and 44%) [28–31]. In ongoing spontaneous pregnancies complicated by first-trimester bleeding, lower birth weights have been found, but a direct relationship could not be demonstrated [32]. We recently published a study in which we investigated whether first-trimester bleeding influences the further course and the outcome of the pregnancy after ART if it does not end in a spontaneous abortion [33]. We found that first-trimester bleeding indeed exerts an unfavorable effect on perinatal outcome, as it also does in spontaneous pregnancies (Table 5.1).

Unexpectedly, however, we also discovered that the incidence of first-trimester bleeding increased

Table 5.2 Outcome parameters of SET and DET singleton pregnancies (gestational age, birth weight, preterm birth and low birth weight)

	SET ($n = 404$)	DET ($n = 431$)	Adjusted p-value	Crude OR (CI)	Adjusted OR (CI)
Gestational age (days)	276.2 (± 10.5)	273.4 (± 15.0)	<0.01		
Birth weight (grams)	3324.6 (± 509.7)	3204.3 (± 617.5)	< 0.01		
Preterm birth (<37 weeks)	6.2%	10.4%	1.77 (1.06–2.94)	1.77 (1.06–2.94)	
Low birth weight (<2500 g)	4.2%	11.6%	2.99 (1.69–5.27)	3.38 (1.86–6.12)	

CI, confidence interval; DET, double embryo transfer; OR, odds ratio; SET, single embryo transfer.

Parameters adjusted for maternal age, parity, cycle rank number, indication for assisted reproduction, assisted reproductive method, time of embryo transfer, embryo quality, compulsion to apply SET/DET and sex of the child.

in parallel in a linear fashion with the number of transferred embryos. If one embryo was transferred and an ongoing singleton pregnancy was achieved 12.5% of patients reported first-trimester bleeding. If two embryos were transferred, first-trimester bleeding took place in 16.2% and if three or more than three embryos were transferred, the incidence of first-trimester bleeding was 21.6% and 28.0% respectively. Since most cases of first-trimester bleeding probably find their cause in the mechanism of implantation or placentation, and because also the incidence of vanishing twins increases with the number of embryos transferred, vanishing twins could thus explain in part why more first-trimester bleeding occurs with more embryos transferred. Given the known association between first-trimester bleeding and subsequent complications of pregnancy (second-trimester bleeding, third-trimester bleeding, very low birth weight, severe prematurity…), singleton pregnancies which are the consequence of the transfer of more than one embryo seem to be at a slight disadvantage over singletons after SET, but this has to be confirmed in more studies.

Birth weight comparison between SET and DET

Because first-trimester bleeding and its effects are parameters which are only indirectly correlated with neonatal outcome and birth weight, the really sensible thing to do is to look at birth weights directly. In an earlier study [7] we already noted on a small series that singletons after SET had a higher birth weight than those after DET. In that series the birth weight of the SET singletons was 3303 ± 481 g and of the DET singletons was 3175 ± 641 g (statistically significant difference of 128 g). De Neubourg et al. compared birth weights of a group of 251 SET singletons with those from a large database of spontaneously conceived singletons and they found no difference in birth weight (SET singletons 3322 ± 538 g vs. population-based spontaneous singletons 3330 ± 531 g) [34]. It is interesting to note that these birth weights are remarkably similar to the SET singleton birth weights we recorded in 2003, on a totally different patient set. To study this on a larger group of patients, we conducted a study on more than 800 SET and DET singletons [35]. Because of minor differences in patient and cycle characteristics, we used multivariate statistics and calculated adjusted odds ratios (Table 5.2). Our data showed that SET singletons weighed on average 120 g more than DET singletons. This difference is similar to the one found in our preliminary series from 2003. Again we confirmed the birth weight found by De Neubourg et al. [34]. The difference we observed between SET and DET singletons is a little bit smaller than the difference found a decade ago when DET singletons were compared to spontaneously conceived singletons. For instance, Koudstaal et al. found that the mean birth weight of IVF singletons was 3112 ± 759 g and of spontaneously conceived singletons was 3326 ± 639 g (difference of 214 g, $p < 0.001$) [36].

A third study that compared obstetrical and perinatal outcome of singletons after SET and DET was published recently by Poikkeus et al. [37]. These authors compared 269 SET singletons with 230 DET singletons (including 10% vanishing twins) and found a mean birth weight of 3364 ± 621 g for the SET singletons compared with 3340 ± 668 g for the DET singletons. This difference was not statistically significant, but both birth weights were lower than population controls (3541 ± 547 g). This third study contradicts the findings of the study by De Neubourg et al. [34] and our own study [35]. It has to be noted that the control birth weight in the Scandinavian study is 215 g higher than in the Belgian study, pointing to differences in study groups.

Other obstetrical and neonatal outcome parameters

Table 5.3 shows data from De Neubourg et al. [34], De Sutter et al. [35] and Poikkeus et al. [37] regarding other outcome measures, such as premature birth rate, low birth weight rate, incidence of hypertensive disorders and gestational diabetes during pregnancy, and NICU admission. It seems difficult to compare these data, because of differences in control populations as well as the studied SET and/or DET patients, or in methodology, definitions, design or statistics. It is hard to explain why in the De Neubourg et al. [34] study the prematurity rate in the SET group is the same as for controls and as the SET singletons in our study [35], but only half that of the Poikkeus et al. [37] series. More studies are needed to compare obstetrical and neonatal outcome of SET and DET singletons and to compare them with population controls. From the Poikkeus et al. [37] data, it is clear that there are other issues at stake than only gestational age and birth weight, since these authors have observed a worse outcome for DET as well as for SET singletons compared to controls for variables such as diabetes, hypertension, NICU admission and others. They have postu-

Table 5.3 Comparison of obstetrical and neonatal outcome between SET and DET singletons in De Neubourg et al. [34], De Sutter et al. [35] and Poikkeus et al. [37]

	De Neubourg et al. (34)	De Sutter et al. (35)	Poikkeus et al. (37)
Number of patients			
SET	251	404	269
DET	0	431	230
controls	59535	0	15037
% premature births (< 37 weeks)			
SET	6.1%	6.2%	12.3%
DET	–	10.4%	11.3%
controls	5.1%	–	4.4%
% low birth weight (< 2500 g)			
SET	10.0%	4.2%	5.9%
DET	–	11.6%	9.6%
controls	6.2%	–	3.2%
% hypertensive disorders			
SET	7.6%	–	5.6%
DET	–	–	5.2%
controls	4.6%	–	2.3%
% NICU admission			
SET	4%	–	3.0%
DET	–	–	3.5%
controls	–	–	1.5%
% gestational diabetes			
SET	1.2%	–	10.4%
DET	–	–	7.4%
controls	1.3%	–	6.1%

lated that this can only be attributed to patient characteristics and therefore the infertility in se, which means that SET will not be able to overcome this. The last word has not been said and more analysis is needed. Perhaps SET will serve not only as a target group to be studied but as a model, since singletons after 1, 2, 3 ... n embryos are hardly comparable a priori.

Conclusions

Although there is still controversy in the literature, two out of three published studies have suggested that eSET leads to higher birth weight and longer pregnancy duration in singleton pregnancies than the transfer of two embryos. Both studies undertaken by our own group are intimately connected to each other and provide evidence that eSET is not only successful in lowering the twinning rates after IVF/ICSI, but also may lead to an improved perinatal outcome in singletons, which is then comparable to spontaneous conception. This would mean that the worse outcome (at least the lower birth weights) described in the literature in the last 10 years must be explained by the fact that more than one embryo is transferred in most clinics, at the time these studies were performed. This sheds new light on the risks and complications of assisted reproductive technology and is even a matter of public health. Indeed, by limiting the number of embryos transferred in IVF/ICSI we are able not only to produce "more" singletons, but maybe also "better" singletons. Further research is needed.

What do we know?

SET seems to lead to a higher birth weight and longer pregnancy duration in singleton pregnancies than the transfer of two embryos.

What do we need to know?

These findings have to be confirmed by other studies and the mechanisms by which SET possibly leads to a better perinatal outcome must be unraveled.

What should we do?

We need to start new observational studies and research directed towards implantation and early pregnancy comparing SET with DET.

REFERENCES

1. International Committee for Monitoring Assisted Reproductive Technology (ICMART), G. D. Adamson, J. de Mouzon, P. Lancaster *et al.*, World collaborative report on in vitro fertilization, 2000. *Fertil. Steril.*, **85** (2006), 1586–1622.

2. T. Coetsier and M. Dhont, Avoiding multiple pregnancies in in-vitro fertilization: who's afraid of single embryo transfer? *Hum. Reprod.*, **13** (1998), 2663–2664.

3. S. Vilska, A. Tiitinen, C. Hydén-Granskog and O. Hovatta, Elective transfer of one embryo results in an acceptable pregnancy rate and eliminates the risk of multiple birth. *Hum. Reprod.*, **14** (1999), 2392–2395.

4. H. Martikainen, A. Tiitinen, C. Tomás *et al.*, One versus two embryo transfers after IVF and ICSI: randomized study. *Hum. Reprod.*, **16** (2001), 1900–1903.

5. J. Gerris, D. De Neubourg, K. Mangelschots *et al.*, Prevention of twin pregnancy after in-vitro fertilization or intracytoplasmic sperm injection based on strict embryo criteria: a prospective randomized clinical trial. *Hum. Reprod.*, **14** (1999), 2581–2587.

6. J. Gerris, D. De Neubourg, K. Mangelschots *et al.*, Elective single day 3 embryo transfer halves the twinning rate without decrease in the ongoing pregnancy rate of an IVF/ICSI program. *Hum. Reprod.*, **17** (2002), 2626–2631.

7. P. De Sutter, J. Van Der Elst, T. Coetsier and M. Dhont, Single embryo transfer and multiple pregnancy rate reduction in IVF/ICSI: a 5-year appraisal. *Reprod. Biomed. Online*, **6** (2003), 464–469.

8. Royal Decree of 4 June 2003. Belgisch staatsblad/ Moniteur Belge 16 June 2003 32127. www.juridat. be/cgi_loi/loi_N.pl?cn=2003060431.

9. P. De Sutter, J. Gerris and M. Dhont, A health-economic decision-analytic model comparing double with single embryo transfer in IVF/ICSI. *Hum. Reprod.*, **17** (2002), 2891–2896.

10. P. De Sutter, J. Gerris and M. Dhont, A health-economic decision-analytic model comparing double with single embryo transfer in IVF/ICSI: a sensitivity analysis. *Hum. Reprod.*, **18** (2003), 1361.

11. J. Gerris, P. De Sutter, D. De Neubourg *et al.*, A real-life prospective health economic study of elective single embryo transfer versus two-embryo transfer in first IVF/ICSI cycles. *Hum. Reprod.*, **19** (2004), 917–923.

12. H. G. Lukassen, D. D. Braat, A. M. Wetzels *et al.*, Two cycles with single embryo transfer versus one cycle with double embryo transfer: a randomized controlled trial. *Hum. Reprod.*, **20** (2005), 702–708.

13. A. T. Kjellberg, P. Carlsson and C. Bergh, Randomized single versus double embryo transfer: obstetric and paediatric outcome and a cost-effectiveness analysis. *Hum. Reprod.*, **21** (2006), 210–216.

14. A. A. Fiddelers, A. P. van Montfoort, C. D. Dirksen *et al.*, Single versus double embryo transfer:

cost-effectiveness analysis alongside a randomized clinical trial. *Hum. Reprod.*, **21** (2006), 2090–2097.

15. M. J. C. Eijkemans, E. M. E. W. Heijnen, C. de Klerk, J. D. F. Habbema and B. C. J. M. Fauser, Comparison of different treatment strategies in IVF with cumulative live birth over a given period of time as the primary end-point: methodological considerations on a randomized controlled non-inferiority trial. *Hum. Reprod.*, **21** (2006), 344–351.

16. A. Tiitinen, M. Halttunen, P. Härkki, P. Vuoristo and C. Hyden-Granskog, Elective embryo transfer: the value of cryopreservation. *Hum. Reprod.*, **16** (2001), 1140–1144.

17. J. Gerris, D. De Neubourg, P. De Sutter *et al.*, Cryopreservation as a tool to reduce multiple birth. *Reprod. Biomed. Online*, **7** (2003), 286–294.

18. K. Lundin and C. Bergh, Cumulative impact of adding frozen-thawed cycles to single versus double fresh embryo transfers. *Reprod. Biomed. Online*, **15** (2007), 76–82.

19. M. Dhont, P. De Sutter, G. Ruyssinck, G. Martens and A. Bekaert, Perinatal outcome of pregnancies after assisted reproduction: a case-control study. *Am. J. Obstet. Gynecol.*, **181** (1999), 688–695.

20. F. M. Helmerhorst, D. A. M. Perquin, D. Donker and M. J. N. C. Keirse, Perinatal outcome of singleton and twins after assisted conception: a systematic review of controlled studies. *BMJ*, **328**:7434 (2004), 261.

21. R. A. Jackson, K. A. Gibson, Y. W. Wu and M. S. Croughan, Perinatal outcomes in singletons following in vitro fertilization: a meta-analysis. *Obstet. Gynecol.*, **103** (2004), 551–563.

22. L. Schieve, S. Rasmussen, G. Buck *et al.*, Are children born after assisted reproductive technology at increased risk for adverse health outcomes? *Obstet. Gynecol.*, **103** (2004), 1154–1163.

23. P. De Sutter, L. Veldeman, P. Kok *et al.*, Comparison of outcome of pregnancy after intra-uterine insemination (IUI) and IVF. *Hum. Reprod.*, **20** (2005), 1642–1646.

24. P. Tummers, P. De Sutter and M. Dhont, Risk of spontaneous abortion in singleton and twin pregnancies after IVF/ICSI. *Hum. Reprod.*, **18** (2003), 1720–1723.

25. A. Pinborg, O. Lidegaard, N. Cour Freiesleben and A. N. Andersen, Consequences of vanishing twins in IVF/ICSI pregnancies. *Hum. Reprod.*, **20** (2005), 2821–2829.

26. L. Delbaere, S. Vansteelandt, J. Gerris *et al.*, Human chorionic gonadotropin levels in early IVF/ICSI pregnancies are higher in singletons after single embryo transfer compared with singletons after double embryo transfer. *Hum. Reprod.*, under revision.

27. C. Everett, Incidence and outcome of bleeding before the 20th week of pregnancy: prospective study from general practice. *BMJ*, **315** (1997), 32–34.

28. J. A. Goldman, J. Ashkenazi, M. Ben-David *et al.*, First trimester bleeding in clinical IVF pregnancies. *Hum. Reprod.*, **3** (1988), 807–809.

29. Z. N. Dantas, A. P. Singh, P. Karachalios *et al.*, Vaginal bleeding and early pregnancy outcome in an infertile population. *J. Assist. Reprod. Genet.*, **13** (1996), 212–215.

30. G. Hofmann, C. Gundrun, L. Drake and A. Bertsche, Frequency and effect of vaginal bleeding on pregnancy outcome during the first 3 weeks after positive B-hCG test results following IVF-ET. *Fertil. Steril.*, **74** (2000), 609–610.

31. K. Pezeshki, J. Feldman, D. E. Stein, S. M. Lobel and R. V. Grazi, Bleeding and spontaneous abortion after therapy for infertility. *Fertil. Steril.*, **74** (2000), 504–508.

32. B. Strobino and J. Pantel-Silverman, Gestational vaginal bleeding and pregnancy outcome. *Am. J. Epidemiol.*, **129** (1989), 806–815.

33. P. De Sutter, J. Bontinck, V. Schutysers *et al.*, First-trimester bleeding and pregnancy outcome in singletons after assisted reproduction. *Hum. Reprod.*, **21** (2006), 1907–1911.

34. D. De Neubourg, J. Gerris, K. Mangelschots *et al.*, The obstetrical and neonatal outcome of babies born after single-embryo transfer in IVF/ICSI compares favourably to spontaneously conceived babies. *Hum. Reprod.*, **21** (2006), 1041–1046.

35. P. De Sutter, I. Delbaere, J. Gerris *et al.*, Birth weight of singletons after assisted reproduction is higher after single- than after double-embryo transfer. *Hum. Reprod.*, **21** (2007), 2633–2637.

36. J. Koudstaal, H. W. Bruinse, F. M. Helmerhorst *et al.*, Obstetric outcome of twin pregnancies after in-vitro fertilization: a matched control study in four Dutch University hospitals. *Hum. Reprod.*, **15** (2000), 935–940.

37. P. Poikkeus, M. Gissler, L. Unkila-Kallio, C. Hyden-Granskog and A. Tiitinen, Obstetric and neonatal outcome after single embryo transfer. *Hum. Reprod.*, **22** (2007), 1073–1079.

6

Single embryo transfer as a model for early conception and implantation

Anja Pinborg and Anne Loft

Introduction

This chapter deals with single embryo transfer (SET) as a model for early conception and implantation. The idea is to shed some light on the "black box of early pregnancy" by focusing on what happens after SET and double embryo transfer (DET).

As early as 1945 the vanishing twin phenomenon was recognized for the first time when it was suggested that twins were more often conceived than born [1]. The vanishing twin was described as the presence of a fetus papyraceus and additionally the author proposed that twin material could be reabsorbed due to early death without leaving any trace. Decades later, ultrasound has confirmed beyond doubt the events described by Stoeckel [1], characterized since as the "vanishing twin" phenomenon, which could also be designated as spontaneous reduction. The routine use of ultrasonography has now proved that spontaneous reduction is a relatively frequent event.

The "incipient twin", is not the same as the vanishing twin, but the very early twin gestation which cannot be diagnosed by disappearance of a twin gestation. One simple way to present a quantitative estimate of the "incipient twin" is to measure the difference between the numbers of embryos transferred and the number of implanted embryos, i.e. gestational sacs. As assisted reproductive technology (ART) has been a worldwide contributor to the general increase in twin birth rates, the ART techniques have also increased the number of singletons born after an incipient or a vanishing twin pregnancy.

This chapter briefly deals with the "incipient twin," as the very early, unrecognized twin conception. As an expression for this phenomenon bleeding in early pregnancy will be discussed. The hypothesis is that the "incipient twin" is correlated with poorer outcome, which may constitute another argument in favor of elective SET (eSET). Data on early human chorionic gonadotropin (hCG) levels and curves together with implantation rates after eSET and DET will be presented. The main part of this chapter will focus on the "vanishing twin" phenomenon including pathological considerations of implantation and the possible mechanisms of vanishing twins. Furthermore an overview of the existing data on short- and long-term consequences after vanishing twins will be presented.

The incipient twin

As mentioned in the introduction the incipient twin is the very early, unrecognized twin gestation. This entity is very difficult to quantify as the early implantation of two embryos can only be verified by the presence of two gestational sacs visualized by

Single Embryo Transfer, ed. J. Gerris, G. D. Adamson, P. De Sutter and C. Racowsky. Published by Cambridge University Press.
© Cambridge University Press 2009.

ultrasound. As the number of implanted embryos is less likely to be reported, some authors have looked at the "vanishing embryo syndrome" as the outcome in pregnancies, where the number of embryos transferred goes beyond the number of children born. A hypothetical and very inaccurate indicator of the incipient twin is first-trimester bleeding.

First-trimester bleeding

First-trimester bleeding is present in one third of all ART pregnancies and is associated with a higher rate of miscarriages [2, 3]. Further, disappearance of a fetus or a gestational sac is reported to be associated with vaginal bleeding or spotting, and the clinical presentation of bleeding seems to coincide with the vanishing process [4]. In spontaneously conceived children it has been shown that first-trimester vaginal bleeding was related to adverse obstetric outcome and in a later population-based study, first-trimester vaginal bleeding was an independent risk factor for adverse obstetric outcome, which was directly proportional to the amount of bleeding [5, 6]. Only one report has looked at whether first-trimester bleeding, if not ending in a miscarriage, negatively influences pregnancy outcome in ART singletons [7]. In 1432 ongoing singleton ART pregnancies significantly more with first-trimester bleeding (17.7%) resulted from a vanishing twin pregnancy (22/253, ∼8.7%) than in controls (47/1179, ∼4.0%). A correlation was found between the incidence of first-trimester bleeding and the number of embryos transferred and first-trimester bleeding was more prevalent in ART than in spontaneous pregnancies, which could point to differences in the implantation process after ART. First-trimester bleeding leads to increased risk of various adverse obstetric outcomes including an odds ratio (OR) 3.0 (95% confidence intervals [CI] 1.1–8.3) of extreme preterm birth. Early vanishing twins including incipient twins following transfer of two or more embryos could be an explanation for the increased incidence of first-trimester bleeding in ART pregnancies. Another indicator of the incipient twin in this study was the linear correlation between the incidence of first-trimester

bleeding and the number of embryos transferred, which is very suggestive of the early "vanishing twin" effect. The authors conclude that significantly more embryos were transferred in the first-trimester bleeding group than in controls, which may point to the fact that in part of the patients, this bleeding is associated with both recognized and unrecognized vanishing twins [7].

hCG levels and curves after eSET and DET

Human chorionic gonadotropin is a glycoprotein, which is produced and secreted by the trophoblast, mainly the syncytiotrophoblast. Beta-hCG levels can be detected in maternal serum from about 8 to 9 days after conception and represent the trophoblastic mass and its function [8, 9]. It has been demonstrated that besides the day of assessment after embryo transfer, hCG levels are dependent on the duration of embryo culture and the assay [10]. The results by Hsu *et al.* [9] suggested that various ART protocols with or without a gonadotropin-releasing hormone (GnRH) agonist have no influence on hCG levels, but recently Orasanu *et al.* [11] showed that the hCG levels differ according to the applied culture media. The mechanism for this is unknown, but possible explanations could be alterations in genetic expression, effects on the kinetics of embryo development or influence on the implantation process itself [11]. However, it has consistently been demonstrated that multiple pregnancies have a higher mean level of hCG than singletons, and pathological pregnancies a lower level, but with overlapping confidence intervals between the groups [12]. The doubling time of hCG in normal pregnancies changes according to hCG concentration and gestational age. However, hCG levels increase exponentially in the first 6 weeks and reach a plateau at about 9 weeks of gestation [9, 13]. In early normal pregnancies as well as in ART pregnancies, serum hCG levels double every 1.5–2 days until serum titer exceeds 10 000 IU/L [14, 15]. An early pregnancy serum hCG titer which diverges from this curve is suspicious of abnormality.

In a personal communication from the University Hospital Gent, preliminary results on early hCG curves after eSET and DET were kindly provided to us [16]. This partial analysis of 833 patients (51% eSET and 49% DET) with one to seven hCG assessments in the first 35 days after ovum pick-up showed a tendency that hCG values were higher in eSET than DET patients. However confidence intervals overlapped, suggesting no significant difference in hCG evolution between the two groups ($p = 0.15$). Data were corrected for time interval of hCG assessment, number of fetal sacs at first ultrasound, type of medication used in the luteal phase, indication for infertility treatment, maternal age, child gender, embryo quality and hypertension in pregnancy. Median hCG values in the eSET cohort increased 4% faster per day (95% CI 1.5%–9.0%) (or 40% faster per week) than in the DET cohort. These results point out that large differences may exist between the eSET and DET cohort, but as a result of extreme variability in hCG measurements, more power is needed to further narrow down the confidence intervals.

Implantation rates after eSET and DET

Only randomized controlled trials (RCTs) with well-defined inclusion criteria and strict embryo selection characteristics can elucidate whether implantation rates (IR) after eSET and DET differs. So far only six randomized studies have been published out of which two papers lack information about IR [17, 18].

The first RCT on eSET, which included 53 women below 34 years who had at least two top quality embryos for transfer at day 3, found comparable IR after eSET and DET (42.3% and 48.1%, respectively) [19]. In 2001 Martikainen *et al.* [20] conducted a randomized study, where 144 women, who had at least four good quality embryos for transfer at day 2, were randomized to eSET or DET (mean age 30.8 years and 30.5 years, respectively). In this study IR after eSET and DET were 33.8% versus 30.7%. The only RCT with blastocyst transfer to a highly selected group of women resulted not surprisingly in higher IR rates compared with day 2–3 embryo transfer studies, but again with no difference in IR

between the two groups (60.9% after eSET and 56% after DET) [21].

In a well-conducted, large Nordic multicenter study, where 661 women below 36 years with at least two good quality embryos were randomized to eSET or DET 2–5 days after oocyte retrieval, IR after eSET and DET was 32.6% and 33.6%, respectively [22]. Even though the literature is limited, the results from these four published RCTs agree that IR after eSET and DET are comparable. However, in these randomized studies miscarriage as well as pregnancy rates were higher after DET than eSET. Vanishing twins in the DET group, continuing as singleton pregnancies can, at least partly, explain the difference in miscarriage rates [18].

The vanishing embryo syndrome

While most studies have looked at the vanishing twin syndrome as disappearing gestational sacs [23] or fetal hearts at early ultrasonography [24], only one recent Danish population-based cohort study including 9444 in vitro fertilization/intracytoplasmic sperm injection (IVF/ICSI) children has shown interesting observations regarding "vanishing co-embryos" reflecting the incipient twin [25]. In a Cox regression analysis with all relevant covariates, the authors found that in pregnancies where the number of children at delivery was less than the number of embryos originally transferred the hazard rate ratio of cerebral palsy was 2.3 (95% CI 0.99–5.32) compared to pregnancies with equal number of embryos transferred and number of children at delivery.

One explanation for poorer pregnancy outcome in singleton births with an incipient twin is first-trimester "crowding" of the developing gestations. In addition lack of appropriate sites for placental implantation may be determining factors in placental expansion and ultimate fetal growth.

The vanishing twin

Pathological considerations

In 1979 it was postulated that a collection of blood seen during pregnancy termination represented an earlier sonographic finding of a second sac that had been adjacent to a 6-week viable gestation, which was pathologically confirmed afterwards [26]. In a review on vanishing twins from 1998, Landy and Keith state that several explanations have been proposed to account for the phenomenon of the "vanishing twin" including publications that have convincingly documented histological findings from the fetal surface of placenta including cysts or sacs, degenerated chorion villi, fibrin deposition or fibrinoid degeneration, placental nodules or plaques, embryo remnants, and macerates or stunted fetuses [4]. Further chromosomal abnormalities in one of the twins including trisomy 9 and 16, triploidy, tetraploidy and sex discrepancies have been explained as the cause of the vanishing twin phenomenon [4]. A study from 1989 postulated that trisomy 16 cells arose from residual villi belonging to a trisomic co-twin that never developed. This was supported by a cytogenic analysis of a placental nodule identified at the time of delivery of a healthy infant [27]. The vanishing twin phenomenon could theoretically be responsible for iso-immunization developing during a pregnancy in which a rhesus-positive fetus disappears and a rhesus-negative twin continues in a previously unsensitized rhesus-negative mother [28]. The process of early pregnancy disappearance appears to involve resorption and/or formation of a blighted ovum, but the precise pathophysiological mechanism is still obscure.

Diagnosis and frequency

The extensive use of transvaginal ultrasonography has provided detailed information regarding early resorption in multiple gestations. However it should be noticed that the diagnosis of a vanishing twin conception is highly dependent on the skills of the sonographer and the quality of the ultrasound equipment. Thus both exaggeration and underestimation of the true incidence of vanishing twins can easily be interpreted, as normal early embryonic structures such as amniotic cavity, chorionic sac, yolk sac, extraembryonic coelom and also subchorionic hemorrhage or hydropic changes in chorion villi can be misclassified as additional gestational sacs [4]. In the review by Landy and Keith, the majority of pertinent studies published since 1990 were scrutinized to determine the frequency of resorption in first trimester in ART versus spontaneous pregnancies after early sonography had demonstrated either two sacs or two fetuses. This review including 317 ART pregnancies with initially *two sacs* and a later impressive prospectively designed study by Dickey including a total of 866 ART pregnancies with *two gestational sacs* at early ultrasound showed almost similar results regarding outcome in second trimester with 9% ending up with a miscarriage, 27% with a singleton delivery and 64% with a twin delivery [4, 23]. Thus 27% had a vanishing twin pregnancy in the second trimester after the diagnosis of *two gestational sacs* in early pregnancy.

The frequencies of second-trimester pregnancy outcome after the diagnosis of *two viable fetuses* in 871 early ART pregnancies are less consistent as the frequencies of miscarriage, singleton and twin pregnancy vary from 5% to 12%, 12% to 38% and 57% to 83%, respectively [4, 29, 30]. Our multicenter study of 2137 ART pregnancies on delivery outcome after the diagnosis of *two viable fetuses* in early pregnancy revealed that 4% had a miscarriage, 9% a singleton delivery and 88% a twin delivery [31]. These heterogeneous findings of delivery outcome after two viable fetuses in the first trimester are first attributable to the difficulties in the diagnosis of spontaneous reduction and second to the inter-study variability in gestational age at early ultrasonography.

As mentioned above, the first study on outcome of vanishing twin ART pregnancies found that 27% of ART pregnancies with *two gestational sacs* at early ultrasound (gestational week 6–7) ended up with only one fetus continuing at 12 weeks [23]. Additional analysis presented in a later debate showed that 15% of singleton births following IVF began as a higher-order gestation [23]. A later study included 1200 singleton and 397 IVF/ICSI twin pregnancies followed by transvaginal ultrasound from before week 7 and every second week throughout the first trimester [29]. Of the pregnancies with two gestational sacs 12.1% ended with a vanishing

Table 6.1 Frequency of preterm birth (< 37 gestational weeks) or very preterm birth (< 32 gestational weeks) in IVF singletons after either one or two gestational sacs/embryos had been present at early sonography

Percentage with delivery		< 37 gestational weeks			< 32 gestational weeks		
N of fetuses/sacs		*Two*	*One*	p-*value*	*Two*	*One*	p-*value*
Fetuses	*N*						
Pinborg *et al.*, 2005 [31]	5 879	13.2%	9.0%	< 0.001	3.8%	1.3%	< 0.001
La Sala *et al.*, 2004 [30]	499	19.3%	16.7%	NS	4.8%	2.7%	NS
Gestational sacs							
Lancaster, 2004 [32]	20 183	18.0%	13.7%	S	6.3%	3.3%	S
Dickey *et al.*, 2002 [23]	4 823	11.4%	8.4%	S	4.5%	1.4%	S

NS Non-significant.
S Statistical significant, no p-*value available.*

twin, 5.1% with a complete miscarriage and 82.8% were ongoing. A Danish multicenter cohort study from 1995 to 2001 on 8542 clinical IVF pregnancies detected by week 7 sonography found that 10.4% of live-born IVF/ICSI singletons originated from a twin gestation in early pregnancy [31]. Similarly, a study from the national register of assisted conception in Australia and New Zealand showed that 6.0% of singleton IVF babies were born after *two gestational sacs* at early pregnancy, but no information of gestational age at early sonography was provided [32].

In summary, after double or multiple embryo transfer 6–15% of ART singletons are conceived as a twin gestation. If we consider SET as a model of early conception and implantation vanishing twins will occur only in monozygotic (MZ) twin pregnancies; as the MZ twin rate is very low in ART pregnancies (1–5%), the rate of vanishing twins in SET pregnancies will be negligible [31]. Thus by introducing SET vanishing twin pregnancies can almost be eliminated.

Short- and long-term outcome after a vanishing twin

Obstetric complications

The first studies indicating an influence of double or multiple embryo transfer on the outcome of IVF sin-

gletons showed that the higher the number of gestational sacs the higher the obstetric risks, irrespective of the final birth number [23, 32, 33]. Data on the relationship between the number of sacs or fetuses in early pregnancy and the frequency of preterm and very preterm birth are presented in Table 6.1. Dickey *et al.* found that after spontaneous reduction with two initial gestational sacs, the average length of gestation for singleton births was shortened by 3 days ($p < 0.05$) [23]. Furthermore, the average birth weight for singletons from a single gestation was 3360 g compared with 3200 g in singletons with loss of one gestational sac ($p = 0.002$). In 2004 a national population-based study on 20 183 singleton pregnancies from Australia and New Zealand showed an association between the number of initial gestational sacs and a higher risk of preterm birth particularly extremely preterm born infants, which indicates a causal relationship between the numbers of implanted embryos and later outcome in ART singletons [32]. They elucidated that birth < 37 gestational weeks occurred in 13.7% and 18.0% with initially one and two gestational sacs respectively and birth < 32 weeks occurred in 3.3% and 6.3% with one and two initial gestational sacs respectively [32] (Table 6.1). In a large population-based cohort study on 18 408 singletons it was demonstrated that with one initial live gestation 12.6% were born with low birth weight (< 2500 g), versus 17.6% if two live fetuses had been present in early pregnancy [24].

In coherence with these reports a study on 499 IVF singletons from 2004 showed that the frequency of preterm and very preterm birth was higher, if initially two fetuses were present compared to pregnancies with only one fetus present in early pregnancy [30] (Table 6.1). In our Danish multicenter cohort study on 642 survivors of a vanished co-twin, these survivors carried a 2.3-fold increased risk of very preterm birth (< 32 weeks) and a 2.1-fold increased risk of very low birth weight (< 1500 g) and a mortality rate that was threefold increased [31]. This was the first study to show an inverse correlation between low birth weight and preterm birth and time of onset of spontaneous reduction: the later the gestational age at spontaneous reduction the poorer the outcome. Gestational age at disappearance of a co-twin was subdivided into early (< 8 weeks), intermediate (8–22 weeks) and late (> 22 weeks) vanish [31]. The early and intermediate survivors also had significantly poorer outcome than primary singletons with an odds ratio of child death of OR = 3.3 (1.6–7.3) and even the early survivor cohort had significantly lower mean birth weight than singletons, indicating that disappearance of a co-twin in the very early pregnancy does have influence on the later outcome [31].

Results from the same Danish cohort showed a significant inverse correlation between the frequency of babies born small for gestational age (SGA) and the gestational age at spontaneous reduction [34]. Furthermore after adjustment for maternal age the only significant predictor of SGA in this IVF singleton cohort was *a vanishing co-twin*.

In summary, IVF singletons born after the initial presence of two gestational sacs or fetuses have poorer obstetric outcome than IVF singletons born after one initial gestational sac or fetus. This is seen even in pregnancies with vanish in very early pregnancy; thus with eSET the negative influence of vanishing twins on IVF outcome could be avoided.

Neurological sequelae

The knowledge on neurological sequelae in singleton survivors of a vanished co-twin is very restricted.

Most literature is limited to spontaneously conceived children and to vanish or death of a co-twin late in pregnancy. In a study on spontaneous conceived twins, born in the 1980s and identified from the Western Australian cerebral palsy register, the prevalence of cerebral palsy was 96.2 per 1000 in twins who survived in utero death of a co-twin, 15 times higher than for twins who were both live born (6.4/1000), and 60 times higher than for live born singletons (1.6/1000) [35]. It has later been confirmed that late intrauterine death of one twin has considerable influence on the risk of cerebral palsy and mortality in the surviving co-twin in spontaneously conceived twin pregnancies [36, 37]. Pharoah and Adi [36] found that the live born co-twin of a fetus that died in utero was at a 20-fold increased risk of cerebral impairment compared with the general twin risk and Scher *et al.* [37] found a 4-fold increased risk of cerebral palsy in twin survivors of a stillborn co-twin. However these data relate to death of a co-twin in the third trimester. Only one population-based study has described the risk of cerebral palsy in twins surviving early disappearance of a co-twin and showed that the overall incidence rate of cerebral palsy was 0.8% (5/611) in singletons with a vanished co-twin and 0.4% (22/5237) in singletons with an initial singleton gestation implying a nearly twofold increased risk of cerebral palsy in singleton survivors of a vanished co-twin (OR 1.9, 95% CI 0.7–5.2) [31]. Additionally the Danish study revealed a significant inverse correlation between gestational age at onset of spontaneous reduction and development of neurological sequelae. As previously mentioned the Danish study comprised more than 8000 clinical pregnancies including 642 singleton survivors of a vanished co-twin. Despite a positive correlation between onset of vanish and neurological sequelae being demonstrated, the number of vanishing twins was too low to make specific estimates for single diseases such as cerebral palsy.

Though perinatal outcome in SET pregnancies is not the scope of this chapter, as it is dealt with in the previous chapter, it should briefly be mentioned that data are accumulating of a more favorable outcome in ART singletons, where only one embryo is transferred [38, 39].

Conclusions

From the latest annual European report on ART pregnancies in 2004, IVF newborns account for 1–4% of the national birth cohorts [40]. During recent years large population-based studies have made it evident that IVF singletons compared to their spontaneously conceived counterparts have slightly poorer obstetric outcome including lower birth weight and gestational age and higher risk of perinatal mortality [24, 41, 42]. Furthermore the risk of malformations is 1.3- to 1.4-fold higher in IVF singletons [43, 44] and population-based register studies have shown a higher rate of cerebral palsy [45, 46].

The reasons for this impaired outcome are currently being discussed and apart from the ART methods themselves two plausible explanations have been proposed; the subfertility per se or the underlying characteristics of the infertile couples and the high number of vanishing twins pregnancies as a consequence of the DET policy. Increasing literature has risen on the influence of subfertility on child outcome including a higher risk of preterm birth and low birth weight [47, 48], malformations [49] and neonatal mortality [50, 51]. However studies presented in this chapter also made it evident that a major contributor to the less favorable outcome in ART singletons is incipient and vanishing twin pregnancies as a consequence of the DET policy.

In 2004 55% of all IVF/ICSI treatments in Europe implemented DET, 25% multiple embryo and only 19% single embryo transfers all together with a twin birth rate of 21.5% [40]. Though the rates of eSET are rising in Europe, particularly in Belgium, Sweden and Finland, there is still some way to go before we reach the goal of a markedly reduced twin birth rate. The findings on poorer outcome of vanishing twins make up a further and strong argument for diminishing the double embryo transfers.

What do we know?
Singleton births after a vanishing twin pregnancy account for 6–15% of all IVF singletons and these pregnancies constitute a major contributor to the adverse short- and long-term outcome in ART singletons.

What do we need to know?
Our knowledge about implantation after eSET and DET is limited and the influence of incipient twins on later outcome in pregnancy highly unexplored. Hence studies of the very early implantation process are still needed.

What do we do now?
We should continue and facilitate the process of implementing eSET worldwide.

REFERENCES

1. W. Stoeckel, *Lehrbuch der Geburtshilfe*, (Jena: Gustav Fischer, 1945) (Quoted in S. Levi, Ultrasonic assessment of the high rate of multiple pregnancy in the first trimester. *J. Clin. Ultrasound* **4** (1976), 3–5.)
2. G. Hofmann, C. Gundrun, L. Drake and A. Bertsche, Frequency and effect of vaginal bleeding on pregnancy outcome during the first 3 weeks after positive B-hCG test results following IVF-ET. *Fertil. Steril.*, **74** (2000), 609–610.
3. K. Pezeshki, J. Feldman, D. E. Stein, S. M. Lobel and R. V. Grazi, Bleeding and spontaneous abortion after therapy for infertility. *Fertil. Steril.*, **74** (2000), 504–508.
4. H. J. Landy and L. G. Keith, The vanishing twin: a review. *Hum. Reprod.*, **4** (1998), 177–183.
5. M. A. Williams, R. Mittendorf, E. Lieberman and R. R. Monson, Adverse infant outcomes associated with first-trimester vaginal bleeding. *Obstet. Gynecol.*, **78** (1991), 14–18.
6. J. L. Weiss, F. D. Malone, J. Vidaver *et al.*, Threatened miscarriage: a risk for poor pregnancy outcome, a population based screening study. *Am. J. Obstet. Gynecol.*, **190** (2004), 745–750.
7. P. De Sutter, J. Bontinck, V. Schutysers *et al.*, First-trimester bleeding and pregnancy outcome in singletons after assisted reproduction. *Hum. Reprod.*, **21** (2006), 1907–1911.

8. G. D. Braunstein, J. L. Rasor, E. Engvall and M. E. Wade, Interrelationships of human chorionic gonadotropin, human placental lactogen, and pregnancy-specific beta 1-glycoprotein throughout normal human gestation. *Am. J. Obstet. Gynecol.*, **138** (1980), 1205–1213.

9. M. I. Hsu, P. Kolm, J. Leete *et al.*, Analysis of implantation in assisted reproduction through the use of serial human chorionic gonadotropin measurements. *J. Assist. Reprod. Genet.*, **15** (1998), 496–503.

10. B. Kumbak, E. Oral, G. Karlikaya, S. Lacin and S. Kahraman, Serum oestradiol and beta-HCG measurements after day 3 or 5 embryo transfers in interpreting pregnancy outcome. *Reprod. Biomed. Online*, **13** (2006), 459–464.

11. B. Orasanu, K. V. Jackson, M. D. Hornstein and C. Racowsky, Effects of culture medium on HCG concentrations and their value in predicting successful IVF outcome. *Reprod. Biomed. Online*, **12** (2006), 590–598.

12. M. Fridström, L. Garoff, P. Sjöblom and T. Hillensjö, Human chorionic gonadotropin patterns in early pregnancy after assisted reproduction. *Acta Obstet Gynecol Scand*, **74** (1995), 534–538.

13. D. E. Pittaway, R. L. Reish and A. C. Wentz, Doubling times of human chorionic gonadotropin increase in early viable intrauterine pregnancies. *Am. J. Obstet. Gynecol.*, **152** (1985), 299–302.

14. N. Kadar, M. Freedman and M. Zacher, Further observations on the doubling time of human chorionic gonadotropin in early asymptomatic pregnancies. *Fertil. Steril.*, **54** (1990), 783–787.

15. C. A. Richard, C. J. Kubik and J. A. DeLoia, Physiological range of human chorionic gonadotropin for support of early human pregnancy. *Fertil. Steril.*, **76** (2001), 988–993.

16. I. Delbaere, P. De Sutter, J. Gerris and M. Temmerman, Comparison of HCG – values in early pregnancy between patients who underwent single embryo transfer and patients with double embryo transfer. (2008), *Hum. Reprod.*, under revision.

17. H. G. Lukassen, D. D. Braat, A. M. Wetzels *et al.*, Two cycles with single embryo transfer versus one cycle with double embryo transfer: a randomized controlled trial. *Hum. Reprod.*, **20** (2005), 702–708.

18. A. P. van Montfoort, A. A. Fiddelers, J. M. Janssen *et al.*, In unselected patients, elective single embryo transfer prevents all multiples, but results in significantly lower pregnancy rates compared with double embryo transfer: a randomized controlled trial. *Hum. Reprod.*, **21** (2006), 338–343.

19. J. Gerris, D. De Neubourg, K. Mangelschots *et al.*, Prevention of twin pregnancy after in-vitro fertilization or intracytoplasmic sperm injection based on strict embryo criteria: a prospective randomized clinical trial. *Hum. Reprod.*, **14** (1999), 2581–2587.

20. H. Martikainen, A. Tiitinen, C. Tomás *et al.*, Finnish ET Study Group. One versus two embryo transfer after IVF and ICSI: a randomized study. *Hum. Reprod.*, **16** (2001), 1900–1903.

21. D. K. Gardner, E. Surrey, D. Minjarez *et al.*, Single blastocyst transfer: a prospective randomized trial. *Fertil. Steril.*, **81** (2004), 551–555.

22. A. Thurin, J. Hausken, T. Hillensjö *et al.*, Elective single-embryo transfer versus double-embryo transfer in in vitro fertilization. *N. Engl. J. Med.*, **351** (2004), 2392–2402.

23. R. P. Dickey, S. N. Taylor, P. Y. Lu *et al.*, Spontaneous reduction of multiple pregnancy: incidence and effect on outcome. *Am. J. Obstet. Gynecol.*, **186** (2002), 77–83.

24. L. A. Schieve, C. Ferre, H. B. Peterson *et al.*, Perinatal outcome among singleton infants conceived through assisted reproductive technology in the United States. *Obstet. Gynecol.*, **103** (2004), 1144–1153.

25. D. Hvidtjorn, J. Grove, D. Schendel *et al.*, "Vanishing embryo syndrome" in IVF/ICSI. *Hum. Reprod.*, **20** (2005), 2550–2551.

26. H. J. Finberg and J. C. Birnholz, Ultrasound observations in multiple gestation with first trimester bleeding: the blighted twin. *Radiology*, **132** (1979), 137–142.

27. A. T. Tharapel, S. Elias, L. P. Shulman *et al.*, Resorbed co-twin as an explanation for discrepant chorionic villus results: non-mosaic 47, XX,+16 in villi (direct and culture) with normal (46, XX) amniotic fluid and neonatal blood. *Prenat. Diagn.*, **9** (1989), 467–472.

28. H. J. Landy, S. Weiner, S. L. Corson *et al.*, The "vanishing twin": ultrasonographic assessment of fetal disappearance in the first trimester. *Am. J. Obstet. Gynecol.*, **155** (1986), 14–19.

29. P. Tummers, P. De Sutter and M. Dhont, Risk of spontaneous abortion in singleton and twin pregnancies after IVF/ICSI. *Hum. Reprod.*, **18** (2003), 1720–1723.

30. G. B. La Sala, G. Nucera, A. Gallinelli *et al.*, Spontaneous embryonic loss following in vitro fertilization: incidence and effect on outcomes. *Am. J. Obstet. Gynecol.*, **191** (2004), 741–746.

31. A. Pinborg, O. Lidegaard, N. la Cour Freiesleben and A. N. Andersen, Consequences of vanishing twins in IVF/ICSI pregnancies. *Hum. Reprod.*, **20** (2005), 2821–2829.

32. P. A. L. Lancaster, Number of gestational sacs and singleton IVF preterm birth. *Hum. Reprod.*, **19** (Suppl.1) (2004), Abstract book: O-245 p. i85.

33. L. A. Schieve, S. F. Meikle, C. Ferre *et al.*, Low and very low birth weight in infants conceived with use of assisted reproductive technology. *N. Engl. J. Med.*, **346** (2002), 731–737.

34. A. Pinborg, O. Lidegaard, N. la Cour Freiesleben and A. N. Andersen, Vanishing twins: a predictor of small-for-gestational age in IVF singletons. *Hum. Reprod.*, **22** (2007), 2707–2714.

35. B. Petterson, K. B. Nelson, L. Watson and F. Stanley, Twins, triplets, and cerebral palsy in births in Western Australia in the1980's. *BMJ*, **307** (1993), 1239–1243.

36. P. O. D. Pharoah and Y. Adi, Consequences of in-utero death in a twin pregnancy. *Lancet*, **355** (2000), 1597–1602.

37. A. I. Scher, B. Petterson, E. Blair *et al.*, The risk of mortality or cerebral palsy in twins: a collaborative population-based study. *Pediatr. Res.*, **52** (2002), 671–681.

38. P. De Sutter, I. Delbaere, J. Gerris *et al.*, Birth weight of singletons after assisted reproduction is higher after single- than after double-embryo transfer. *Hum. Reprod.*, **21** (2006), 2633–2637.

39. D. De Neubourg, J. Gerris, K. Mangelschots *et al.*, The obstetrical and neonatal outcome of babies born after single-embryo transfer in IVF/ICSI compares favourably to spontaneously conceived babies. *Hum. Reprod.*, **21** (2006), 1041–1046.

40. A. N. Andersen, V. Goossens, A. P. Ferraretti *et al.*, Assisted reproductive technology in Europe 2004. Results generated from European registers by ESHRE. *Hum. Reprod.*, **23** (2008), 756–771.

41. F. M. Helmerhorst, D. A. M. Perquin, D. Donker and M. J. N. C. Keirse, Perinatal outcome of singletons and twins after assisted conception: a systematic review of controlled studies. *BMJ*, **328** (2004), 261–265.

42. R. A. Jackson, K. A. Gibson, Y. W. Wu and M. S. Croughan, Perinatal outcomes in singletons following in vitro fertilization: a meta-analysis. *Obstet. Gynecol.*, **103** (2004), 551–563.

43. M. Hansen, C. Bower, E. Milne, N. de Klerk and J. J. Kurinczuk, Assisted reproductive technologies and the risk of birth defects – a systematic review. *Hum. Reprod.*, **20** (2005), 328–338.

44. B. Källén, O. Finnström, K. G. Nygren and P. O. Olausson, In vitro fertilization (IVF) in Sweden: risk for congenital malformations after different IVF methods. *Birth Defects Res.*, **73** (2005), 162–169.

45. B. Strömberg, G. Dahlquist, A. Ericson *et al.*, Neurological sequelae in children born after in-vitro fertilisation: a population based study. *Lancet*, **359** (2002), 461–465.

46. Ø. Lidegaard, A. Pinborg and A. N. Andersen, Imprinting diseases and IVF. Danish National IVF cohort study. *Hum. Reprod.*, **20** (2005), 950–954.

47. Z. Pandian, S. Bhattacharya and A. Templeton, Review of unexplained infertility and obstetric outcome: a 10 year review. *Hum. Reprod.*, **16** (2001), 2593–2597.

48. O. Basso and D.D. Baird, Infertility and preterm delivery, birth weight, and Caesarean section: a study within the Danish National Birth Cohort. *Hum. Reprod.*, **18** (2003), 2478–2484.

49. J. L. Zhu, O. Basso, C. Obel, C. Bille and J. Olsen, Infertility, infertility treatment, and congenital malformations: Danish national birth cohort. *BMJ*, **333** (2006), 679.

50. E. S. Draper, J. J. Kurinczuk, K. R. Abrams and M. Clarke, Assessment of separate contributions to perinatal mortality of infertility history and treatment: a case-control analysis. *Lancet*, **353** (1999), 1746–1749.

51. O. Basso and L. Olsen, Subfecundity and neonatal mortality: longitudinal study within the Danish national birth cohort. *BMJ*, **330** (2005), 393–394.

7

Ovarian stimulation, blastocyst culture and preimplantation genetic screening for elective single embryo transfer

Robert P. S. Jansen and Steven J. McArthur

Introduction

This chapter sets out to examine how intrafollicular oocyte preparation and embryo development in the laboratory contribute to successful elective single embryo transfer (eSET) programs and to better birth outcomes. In coming to at least provisional conclusions, the chapter draws on our published and unpublished experience at Sydney IVF as well as the major conclusions published by others. We focus on these questions:

1. To what extent does the degree of follicular stimulation help or jeopardize the provision of a sufficient number of physiologically competent oocytes to foster eSET?
2. To what extent is it helpful to extend culture to day 5 or 6 and thus to demonstrate blastocyst development before selecting the single embryo to transfer?
3. To what extent does preimplantation genetic screening for chromosome numbers help or jeopardize the results from SET?

During the early 2000s, Sydney IVF moved increasingly to eSET as our laboratory moved comprehensively to blastocyst culture and blastocyst stage transfers and cryostorage, with a corresponding increase in take-home baby rates, substantial reductions in multiple pregnancies and reduced rates of miscarriage [1–6]. The principal Sydney IVF-sourced data that led to these changes (and which

will be explored further here) have been published as follows:

- a particularly detailed analysis of all egg retrievals and fresh day 3 transfers performed in the year 1998 and followed by day 3 cryostored embryo transfers over the following five years, to provide baseline *age-dependent cumulative live birth confinements to be expected from single retrieval procedures employing double embryo transfer (DET) practices still widely prevalent* [1], including previously unpublished data relating to stimulation variables;
- an analysis of elective single blastocyst transfers versus double blastocyst transfers in younger women, again including the effects of additional cryostored embryo transfers over several years from one egg retrieval procedure, to provide *cumulative live birth confinements and multiple pregnancy rates when only blastocyst technology is used*; [4]
- a historical but otherwise directly comparable comparison of embryo biopsies performed at the day 3 cleavage stage and followed by blastocyst transfer on day 5 or 6, with embryo biopsies taken at the blastocyst stage and followed by almost immediate transfer, *to examine the efficacy of blastulation as a sign of good embryo potential* and *to determine the effects of day 3 biopsy versus day 5 or 6 on the embryo, while controlling for the embryo's ability to blastulate*; [2, 5, 6] patients in this trial

Single Embryo Transfer, ed. J. Gerris, G. D. Adamson, P. De Sutter and C. Racowsky. Published by Cambridge University Press.
© Cambridge University Press 2009.

had preimplantation genetic diagnosis (PGD) not for infertility or miscarriages but to prevent further propagation of a serious monogenic family disease; and finally

• an analysis of the possible reasons behind an unexpected outcome to a clinical trial employing *blastocyst biopsy for aneuploidy screening to assist in embryo screening for eSET among women under 36*.

Ovarian stimulation issues relevant to eSET

Other things being equal, it is obvious that the more apparently normal embryos one has available to transfer after fertilization of eggs in vitro the greater the chance that a live birth will follow, and that the infertile couple's reproductive ambitions will be realized. The burden of proof must be strong, therefore, in arguing that intentionally producing *fewer* oocytes or embryos can actually improve the outcomes of the elective transfer of just one embryo at a time. Peripheral arguments in favor of lower egg numbers might relate to a couple's ethical preference or to a legal requirement to not produce more embryos than will be given the chance to implant, and thus intentionally to limit the number of available eggs or embryos, but these are not relevant to the biology of eSET and will not be considered further here.

Financial considerations can be relevant

On the other hand, financial considerations for the infertile couple (i.e., their out-of-pocket costs) will play a comprehensive part in conducting practical eSET policies. It is the couple who make the decision and for whom excessive costs are deal-breakers. The most substantial costs in most in vitro fertilization (IVF) markets are: (1) the costs of gonadotropic drugs; (2) medical fees for monitoring, for egg retrievals and for embryo transfers, which can mount up when required repeatedly; and (3) laboratory costs, which will be higher with moves to blas-

tocyst stage cultures, as embryos in culture in the laboratory at any one time can be expected to double compared with an IVF program that runs on day 3 transfers. In many countries patients are protected against the full cost of multiple pregnancies but not the costs of IVF, sending a message that might be logical to the couple but perverse for the community, whether in the form of government assistance or in the hands of private third-party payers. In clinical circumstances where natural cycle IVF is practical, such as in younger women with high fertilization rates, the cause of what might be described as "semi-elective" SET can be well-served, with significant savings in drugs, laboratory overheads and cryostorage costs, and evidence that, in experienced clinicians' hands and flexible egg retrieval timing, embryo quality might suffer less than possibly is the case with ovarian stimulation in comparison with embryos in normal environments in vivo.

Natural cycle IVF – at least in the 80% or so cycles in which egg retrieval can be properly timed in a well-run program, with or without a trigger injection of human chorionic gonadotropin (hCG) that anticipates the luteinizing hormone (LH) surge [7] – is also the situation in which any truth to a hypothesis that minimal stimulation improves embryo quality in a manner that furthers the cause of SET [8] should find its purest form [9].

The remainder of the chapter assumes a context of financial neutrality and controlled ovarian hyperstimulation, and examines the biological principles and evidence in this context.

Ovarian stimulation benchmarks

Many studies and meta-analyses have established that the benchmark for IVF outcomes comes with a "long downregulation regimen" in which a gonadotropin-releasing hormone (GnRH) agonist is commenced a week or more before starting daily injections of follicle-stimulating hormone (FSH) [10, 11]. The purpose of the early start with GnRH is to dispense with the effects of a "flare" in endogenous gonadotropin release, which (because it consists of both FSH and LH) can unpredictably result in a hormonally active follicular or luteal cyst. Less conspicuously, the flare commonly reactivates an ordinarily exhausted corpus luteum to raise progesterone to abnormal levels into the new follicular phase; up to day 6 this is unlikely to affect the endometrium, but if it extends longer will be detrimental. [12] The purpose of the administered FSH is to remove the competition that normally ensues among follicles from about day 7 as serum FSH levels fall and cause the atresia of all but one follicle, which becomes dominant and ovulates [13]. The basis for the competition between follicles during the follicular phase is not known exactly, but is more one of timing than of intrinsic or absolute oocyte quality among recruited follicles or lack of it. Age has a stronger effect on overall egg quality than does any effect of a few days' variation in follicular phase length, judging by the preservation of the mechanism of successful follicular development, dominance and robust, successful ovulation in women for years after most or all eggs have lost their ability to result in a baby (Figure 7.1b) [14, 15].

It has been argued that excessive estradiol levels at the time of egg retrieval might harm pregnancy rates through an effect on the oocyte [16] or the endometrium [17].

Direct harmful effects of estrogen on ovarian follicles and embryos?

A harmful effect of estradiol on the follicular oocyte is on first principles would appear improbable. The extrafollicular concentration (and even more so the intrafollicular concentrations) of estradiol around an ovulating follicle is at least three or four orders of magnitude higher (i.e., 1000–10 000 ×) than serum levels reach [18]. The same is true of progesterone levels [18]. The natural range of estrogen and progesterone exposure leading up to ovulation is so extreme that it would be remarkable if another few-fold increase in these steroids from diffusion from adjacent follicles, follicles at a broadly similar stage of response to the ovulating dose of hCG,

makes any difference to them or the oocyte they contain.

Our unpublished further analyses on stimulation variables performed on our 1998 egg retrievals [1] lend evidence-based support for dismissing the idea of a deleterious effect of high intrafollicular estradiol levels on embryo quality. The most subtle harmful effects of follicular atresia on oocyte quality manifest as a lack of cryostored embryos from the retrieved egg cohort to implant after thawing, and is a more sensitive, if retrospective, indicator of an embryo's potential than its ability to blastulate, to cleave or to fertilize [14, 19]. The data in Figure 7.2 show that the highest cryostored embryo transfer implantations in our series took place in the most extreme stimulations with the highest extant levels of estradiol in the oocytes' immediate milieu.

Indirect harmful effects of a high follicular estradiol response on ovarian follicles have an iatrogenic basis

In attempts to limit the hazard of ovarian hyperstimulation syndrome (OHSS) in young people or in women with polycystic ovary syndrome (PCOS) (these are the groups at special risk of overresponding), there is in practice a likelihood that stimulated follicular phases are cut too short, or that FSH regimens are stopped for several days of "coasting" until estradiol levels start to fall. These are maneuvers that if stretched too far produce follicular atresia of varying but often significant degree, producing suboptimal oocytes and, if fertilization follows, compromised embryos that can, as a cohort, fail to result in ongoing pregnancies [19, 20]. The key to this conundrum may lie in obviating the risk of OHSS by (1) keeping the ovulating dose of hCG strictly to the minimum needed for securing mature oocytes at the retrieval (2500–3000 U is sufficient for most women [21, 22] although for women with body mass indexes over 30 [23] slightly higher doses might be needed); and thus letting the hCG, which has a half-life of ∼ 2.3 days [24], dissipate before vascular endothelial growth factor, which mediates the

(a)

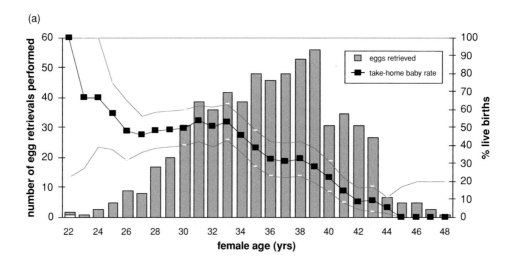

(b)

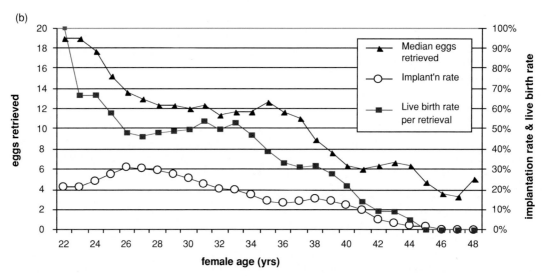

Figure 7.1 Double jeopardy. (a) Take-home baby rates (95% confidence limits) from one unselected egg retrieval at Sydney IVF in 1998, followed by embryo transfers at day 3, including subsequent transfers of cryostored day 3 embryos until a term birth was achieved or no suitable embryos remained for transfer [1]. Data smoothed over a rolling 3-year interval incorporating previous and subsequent year. (b) Take-home baby rates for maternal age are compared with the implantation rate per embryo (gestational sacs/embryos transferred) and the median number of eggs retrieved. The double jeopardy of age is revealed by a quantitative fall in retrieved eggs to fewer than 10 after age 37 years and by a qualitative fall in ability of eggs and embryos to result in a baby evident after age 34 years, a phenomenon of physiological sterility that can be permanent in more than 50% of women by age 40 (see text) and which has been referred to as the "oopause."

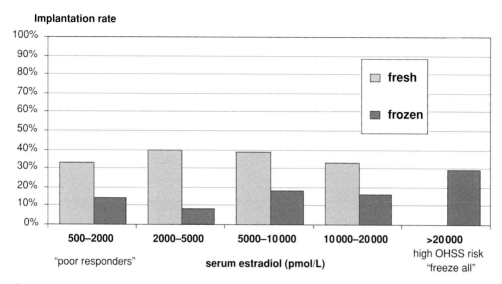

Figure 7.2 Embryo implantation rates (gestational sacs/embryos transferred) among women < 35 years having a first or second egg retrieval at Sydney IVF in the 1998 cohort depicted in Figure 7.1, according to the final serum estradiol performed before egg retrieval. The highest cryostored embryo implantations occurred where response was accompanied by extremely high estradiol levels, trigger doses of hCG were minimal (see text) and all usable embryos were cryostored to obviate the risk of ovarian hyperstimulation syndrome (OHSS). An hypothesized harmful effect on oocyte or embryo quality caused by high periovulatory steroid levels can be ruled out.

condition [25], ordinarily peaks; (2) extinguishing endogenous LH levels effectively to zero through the luteal phase by discontinuing GnRH agonists at the time of the hCG trigger (LH levels and thus the risk of OHSS risk are greatly reduced by discontinuing GnRH agonists [26] and not by continuing them); and (3) cryostoring all embryos, thus obviating the risk of pregnancy supervening and having endogenous hCG levels potentially precipitating the patient into a full and prolonged OHSS, with effusions and hemoconcentration, and be put at risk of the more serious hazards of stroke or death.

This course of management is, in our clinical experience, safe, but clearly must only be undertaken with a high level of patient understanding and agreement, and considerable experience on the part of the clinician. But if there is PCOS with a major ovulatory disturbance, alternative strategies are often repeatedly unsatisfactory. Normally ovulating young women might do well with natural cycle IVF or, given their typical superabundance of

responsive follicles, with minimal stimulation for the retrieval cycle [8], albeit still involving low ovulating doses of hCG and ready recourse to the practice of cryostoring all embryos.

Direct harmful effects of estrogen on endometrium?

The endometrium is unique in its receptors' responses to estradiol and progesterone, early studies revealing that, apart from a basal level of estrogen receptor alpha activity, estradiol action on the estradiol receptor ERα is required for induction of progesterone receptors as well as for escalating the production of estradiol receptors. Then, and particularly importantly, rising progesterone levels acting on the endometrial glands inhibit not only a major proportion of estradiol receptor expression in the glands, but also inhibit further expression of progesterone receptors of PRA isoform, and, a little more slowly into the secretory phase, of PRB isoform receptors [27, 28], producing a natural resistance within the glands and surface epithelium that is visible morphologically [27–29]; the stroma, on the other hand, is not subject to progesterone-induced progesterone receptor loss and shows persistent expression of PRA [28], so that decidualization of the stroma is satisfactory if exposure to progesterone is maintained.

With standard gonadotropin-based ovarian stimulatory regimens for retrieving multiple eggs, estradiol levels rise sufficiently above normal levels, and for long enough, that a functionally abnormal response is likely in the endometrium. Although measurable on ultrasound if looked for carefully using patients as their own controls [30, 31], this function abnormality will not be recognizable on histology [32, 33], short of the development of overt cystic hyperplasia. The endometrium at the time of follicular maturity following high estrogen exposure will have substantially elevated progesterone receptor levels: it is poised to overrespond to progesterone. Then, as the ovaries' multiple follicles luteinize, progesterone is overproduced [34]. The consequence is an acceleration of progesterone action that advances the window of endometrial receptivity by 1 to 2 days, judged on the morphological criteria of an earlier appearance of stromal edema and of endometrial surface "pinopodes" [35, 36]. The paradoxical but predictable subsequent event has been well known since the early days of IVF: an early termination of progesterone effect in the endometrial glands and surface epithelium as their progesterone receptors are prematurely depleted [37], which is presumed to close the implantation window early as well as being demonstrable as a substantially out-of-phase endometrium if the endometrium is biopsied and dated late in the luteal phase [38, 39]. The effect on the window cannot be detected for clinical management purposes short of performing an endometrial biopsy at about the time of embryo implantation, which obviously is not recommended.

In those cases in which the advanced window of receptivity of the endometrium occurs to a crucial degree, even if it happens to this extent uncommonly, all embryos transferred will have

been wasted. Because these are ordinarily the best embryos, it is preferable that the number of embryos put at risk this way is minimized. In other words, while the endometrial phenomenon of sequential hyperresponse and then hyporesponse is not commonly often serious enough to not transfer an embryo fresh, it is another reason to elect to transfer just one embryo fresh and to not transfer more.

The contribution of blastocyst culture to eSET

At Sydney IVF the opportunity of moving to eSET was born of necessity as the twin pregnancy rate rose with our progression from day 3 to routine day 5–6 embryo culture. With a general policy of DET, the twin rate rose to close to 40% among younger women; triplets were not rare. Broadly, there are two clinically important differences for IVF clinics moving to transferring embryos at the blastocyst stage from 6- to 8-cell cleavage stage culture and transfer (in addition to the doubling of embryo culture capacity in the laboratory that is required).

The first difference is metabolic. Cleavage is largely a catabolic process [40]. The ovulating oocyte becomes responsible for its own ATP production as gap junction-bearing cytoplasmic processes from cumulus cells withdraw. The egg and zygote do not metabolize glucose efficiently, so ATP production is through oxidative phosphorylation, with pyruvate as the principal substrate. Whereas the oocyte cytoplasm brings abundant protein and nucleic acid to the early embryo – enough to provide essential amino acids and, through the nucleic acid salvage pathways, the purines and pyrimidines needed for the limited new DNA needed for the first three cleavage divisions – further cell divisions will place geometrically increasing requirements for additional deoxyribose nucleotides, genomic activation demands new species of RNA, and epigenetic differentiation into inner cell mass and trophectoderm and beyond places fresh demands on methylation pathways.

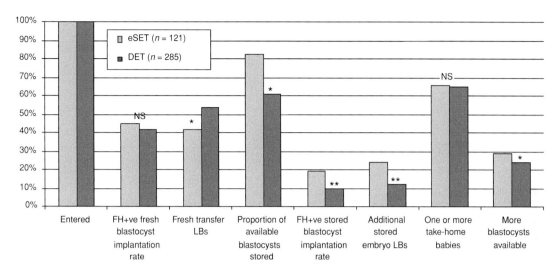

Figure 7.3 When prenatal and neonatal losses are accounted for, eSET can ultimately produce the same chance of at least one "baby-at-home" as women who elect to have DET can achieve [4]. The eSET mothers had more blastocysts remaining for future attempts at pregnancy than did the DET mothers. FH+ve, fetal heart positive pregnancy on ultrasound (slightly fewer than gestational sacs); LB, live birth; NS, not significant; $^*p < 0.05$; $^{**}p < 0.001$.

With successful blastulation, an intensely anabolic metabolic push gets underway, requiring rapid availability of ATP from cytoplasmic glycolysis and a shift in mitochondrial responsibility from catabolism and tricarboxylic acid oxidation (i.e. oxidative phosphorylation) to a number of synthetic pathways, including the crucial electron-transport chain-dependent oxidation of dihydro-orate to enable the formation of pyrimidine precursors for the synthesis of thymidylate. If blastocysts with uncompromised cell numbers are to result then anaerobic metabolism must be encouraged. The mitochondria must enter a state of uncoupled, or "hot", respiration and cease significant oxidative phosphorylation. If oxygen is delivered at room air concentrations, the Pasteur effect will force its uptake and risks production of excessive reactive oxygen species.

Second, it is plain from several studies that the chromosomal complement of the average blastocyst is different from that of the average cleavage stage embryo [41, 42] there being by this stage many fewer surviving monosomies other than 45,X, once calls begin to be made on the embryonic genome

through blastulation and subsequent embryo development. The net result is that blastocysts have almost twice the probability of implanting than cleavage stage embryos will have in all but perhaps the youngest women (although recent data show a similarly high prevalence of abnormal karyotypes in eggs being donated after ovarian stimulation for superovulation in women of college age as those seen among the typically older women having ovarian stimulation for their own IVF [43]). A high implantation rate is an obvious requirement for an effective program of eSET.

From April 2000 to December 2001, women < 38 years at Sydney IVF who had at least three usable blastocysts were increasingly encouraged to have just one embryo transferred fresh (see Figure 7.3); their outcomes were compared with the outcomes for the women who elected to have two embryos transferred fresh [4]. As was the case with the 1998 data that involved the transfer of a median of two day 3 embryos (see earlier), the live birth rates were accumulated by adding pregnancies for as long as it took for a viable birth to take place or until there were no more embryos available. As expected, after

Table 7.1 The cumulative chance of a baby from a median of 1.1 biopsied blastocysts for a variety of indications was 45% (average age 37 years), with a number of patients still trying from cryostored, biopsied embryos, yielding a likely eventual live baby rate after biopsied blastocyst transfer of about 50%, based on known cryostored biopsied embryo pregnancy rates (12 of 28 has been assumed)

	PCR Mutation testing	Aneuploidy screening, reproductive failure	T'locations	Aneuploidy screening, healthy	Overall
Patients with b'cysts to transfer	23	29	11	56	119
Patients with at least one baby	12	11	6	24	53
	52%	38%	55%	43%	45%
Patients not pregnant, still with chance	5	2	2	19	28
					$45 + 5 = 50\%$

PCR = polymerase chain reaction.
Adapted from [5]

just the fresh transfers within the retrieval cycle there were fewer live births in the eSET group. As anticipated, however (see wastage of embryos in fresh cycles due to sporadic endometrial factors, above), the eSET women had more cryostored blastocysts available for further transfers than did the DET women – and, the data show, their embryos were of better average quality. Because women in each arm of the study could elect to have two cryostored blastocysts transferred, the multiple pregnancy rate in the eSET group overall was still 7% (it was 1% from the fresh eSET, this being the sole identified monozygotic twin pregnancy in this group); there were no perinatal deaths in this group. This compares with a 34% multiple pregnancy rate and five neonatal deaths in the DET group. This study was the first to show that, when the pregnancies and deliveries are adjusted for perinatal losses, an eSET group can in time reach a probability of having at least one baby from one egg retrieval which is not different from a DET group.

The impact of embryo biopsy on eSET

General considerations

The study described for Figure 7.3 did not include women having PGD or preimplantation genetic screening (PGS). The effects of embryo biopsy for PGD or PGS on eSET practices are multifaceted. Is the process of embryo biopsy harmful to the chance of implantation? Does limited knowledge of a number of chromosomes in the embryo help or hinder management? Are these effects further dependent on the stage of the embryo studied?

We explored the early effects of moving from day 3 to day 5–6 biopsies contemporaneously with the eSET study described above [2, 5]. In a substantial proportion of cases, embryos at the blastocyst stage were transferred singly, either electively or because there was just one suitable embryo. The implantation rates and pregnancy rates across the different clinical indications are summarized in Table 7.1, with a "take-home" baby rate across the age range of about 50% per retrieval, provided that there is at least one embryo for transfer. The results show a tendency for higher rates for genetic indications than for testing for aneuploidy and there is a relative resistance to the effects of female age (average age for the series was 37 years), perhaps indicative of a selection effect from getting to the stage of having biopsiable blastocysts, this effect operating more strongly among older women, who on average could be expected to have fewer embryos to prove suitable for transfer after testing. Further experience and further analyses have produced firmer conclusions.

Table 7.2 Embryos available for testing for monogenic disease mutations by biopsy for PGD for monogenic diseases on day 3 and on day 5–6. All embryos were developed to blastocysts before transfer on day 5 or 6

	Egg retrievals	Embryos biopsied	Inconclusive test result	Conclusive, favorable test	Embryos transferred fresh	Tested embryos cryostored
d. 3 biopsy d. 5–6 transfer	91	595 av. 6.5 embryos	61* (10.3%)	261 (43.9%)	103	158 (60.5%)
d. 5–6 biopsy d. 5–6 transfer	177	655 av. 3.7 embryos	46* (7.0%)	305 (46.6%)	121	184 (60.3%)

*$p = 0.05$.
Adapted from [6]

Impact of day 5–6 versus day 3 embryo biopsy considerations

If, to begin with, aneuploidy screening cases are removed from consideration and we study the effects of biopsy for a non-fertility-related indication, namely PGD cases performed for detection of embryos carrying a monogenic mutation unrelated to difficulties with conception, we can study the impact of the biopsy on the embryo itself. In a Sydney IVF series [6], we compared biopsies for exclusion of monogenic disease mutation performed on day 3 (cleavage stage) with biopsies performed on day 5 or 6 (blastocyst stage). All embryos were transferred as blastocysts, thus controlling for the variable of an embryo's ability to blastulate. Tables 7.2 and 7.3 imply that, in comparison with the biopsy of blastocysts, day 3 cleavage stage PGD appears to be harmful to at least some embryos.

Table 7.2 shows the technical outcome data for the embryos biopsied (595 for day 3s; 655 for days 5–6), with an average of 6.5 embryos biopsied and tested per retrieval at cleavage, compared with an average of 3.7 embryos biopsied and tested per retrieval when the blastocyst stage was awaited before performing PGD. The proportion of embryos with a conclusive test and with a normal result, thus suitable for transfer, was still approximately 50% in each series, which means that taking the biopsy later in embryo development conferred appreciable efficiency through not having to test embryos whose development was in any case compromised.

The late-biopsied blastocysts had almost twice the chance of implanting than did the blastocysts that had been biopsied on day 3.

Table 7.3 shows the outcomes of the embryo transfer procedures. There was one obvious monozygotic twinning event, involving an embryo biopsied on day 3. In about 60% of cases in each series additional embryos that had tested normally were cryostored for further attempts at pregnancy.

Taking one or two cells for testing on day 3 typically means removing 12.5–25% of the embryo's cells, which, while clearly often tolerated and able to be compensated for by the embryo [44, 45], does not mean that some embryos otherwise capable of implanting and developing are not damaged by the loss. Our study indicates that, on the contrary, random detriment is likely to be present. When biopsy was delayed until after blastulation, the implantation rate per transferred biopsied blastocyst rose from 26.2% to 48.8%. Although the two series within the cohort are sequential rather than contemporaneous, our implantation rates for non-PGD single blastocysts were consistent over the time of the study [3] and our clinical pregnancy results for the day 3 biopsied and day 5–6 transferred embryos (26.2% per retrieval, 34.8% per transfer procedure) is more than comparable with results reported for PGD for monogenic disorders involving day 3 biopsy and transfer, which have been accompanied by implantation rates of about 20% per transfer procedure [44, 45]. Because the two series share the key procedures of zona opening on day 3 and further

Table 7.3. Clinical outcomes following biopsy at the cleavage stage versus biopsy at the stage of blastocyst, each with transfer of embryos fresh on day 5 or 6.

	Embryos transf'd n =	Transfer procedures n =	Pregnancy per retrieval	Implant'n per embryo	Miscarriage	Live birth or ongoing pregnancy	Multiple at confinement		
							sin.	twin	trip.
d. 3 biopsy	1	38	11	11	4	7	7		
d. 5–6 trans.	2	28	12	15	1	10	7	2	
	3	3	1	1	0	1	1		1
$n = 91$ retrievals	all av 1.5	69 (75.8%)*	24/91 (26.4%)	27/103 (26.2%)§	5/91 (5.5%)	18/91 (19.8%)†	15	3 multiples (16.7%)‡	
d. 5–6 biopsy	1	105	54	54	8	46	46		
d. 5–6 trans.	2	8	4	5	1	3	2	1	
	3	0							
$n = 177$ retrievals	all av 1.1	113 (63.8%)*	58/177 (32.8%)	59/121 (48.8%)§	9/58 (15.5%)	49/177 (27.7%)†	48	1 multiple (2%)‡	
		*P = 0.06	n.s.	§P < 0.01	n.s.	†P = 0.2		‡P = 0.04 1-tailed	

n.s., not significant.
Adapted from [6]

hatching through blastulation, this leaves the developmental stage of the embryo at the time of biopsy as the principal and crucial variable in explaining the difference.

As early as 1992, Tarin and colleagues showed that removing one cell for PGD from 4-cell, day 2 embryos retarded cleavage and "strikingly" reduced the size of the inner cell mass and trophectoderm at subsequent blastulation [46]. There appears therefore to be a continuum of increasing damage to cleavage stage embryos the earlier or the more cells are taken, with our study revealing that the damage can begin with just one cell removed from an 8-cell embryo. In conclusion, if PGS is to play a part in selecting embryos for eSET then, on our present evidence, relying on day 3 biopsies for this purpose appears to be inherently compromised. It is also apparent that the ability to blastulate is not itself a sufficient criterion for inferring normal further potential for development. There may be other challenges too.

Is there a role for preimplantation genetic screening in assisting eSET?

Mastenbroek *et al.* have shown recently that biopsy of day 3 (cleavage stage) embryos for limited PGS – screening for aneuploidy of chromosomes 1, 13, 16, 17, 18, 21, X and Y – can reduce the chance of an ongoing pregnancy in women aged 35–41 having IVF [47]. Our considerations above imply that the loss of up to 25% of the cells of a very early embryo might lie behind this detrimental result, but other factors could also be important. These included, for the Mastenbroek study, such straightforward concerns as the time the embryos spent being manipulated in potentially altered culture conditions across the variety of IVF clinics where the biopsies were performed. They also include more complex issues, such as the inadvertent exclusion from transfer of mosaic embryos in which the biopsied cell happened to be the only cell with the trisomy (a situaton that can follow a mitotic non-disjunction event) [48]. Given that the remaining complementarily monosomic cell would usually be rapidly

non-viable, such mosaic embryos might have "self-corrected" if given the opportunity to be transferred and to develop further.

Between August 2004 and November 2006 we studied the impact of screening for aneuploidy in younger infertile women (<38 years, median 33.5 years), employing biopsies of blastocysts [49]. All women were in their first or second attempt at IVF. Agreement to have one embryo transferred (eSET) was a precondition for entry. Patients were withdrawn from the study if there were fewer than eight ovarian follicles over 1 cm diameter at 8–10 days of stimulation, fewer than four embryos with seven or more cells on day 3 of culture, or fewer than three blastocysts for biopsy on day 5 or 6; no women had cycles canceled because of a poor response. The biopsies consisted of two to nine trophectoderm cells and were tested by five-color fluorescent *in situ* hybridization (FISH) for chromosomes 13, 18, 21, X and Y (and in the latter part of the study, also for chromosomes 16 and 22).

We compared outcomes between the screened group (Group A, normal five-color pattern in all the removed trophectoderm cells for the transferred embryo) and the principal control group (Group B, with zona opening but no biopsy); we also made comparisons with the women who were withdrawn from the study before randomization because of suboptimal responses to stimulation (Group C) and with comparable women who were eligible but who elected not to take part in the study (Group D). Table 7.4 gives the results up to the time the trial was suspended. The live birth rates for the two principal groups was high overall (47% of egg retrieval procedures) and is consistent with results we [4, 5] and others [50] have reported previously.

Among the women who underwent biopsy for aneuploidy screening (Group A), the fetal heart positive clinical pregnancy rate at 39.3% compares favourably with the 25% clinical pregnancy rate reported by Mastenbroek *et al.* [47], but was less than among women who were eligible for the trial but did not take part (Group D, 58.7%). Moreover, the embryos subjected to zona opening by infrared laser opening of the zona, a standard

Table 7.4 Live birth rates after preimplantation genetic screening for aneuploidy from biopsy of blastocysts on day 5 or 6 of development using five- or seven-color FISH

Consented $n =$	Entered $n =$	Pregnant $n =$	FH +ve $n =$	no LB $n =$	M/C $n =$	LB $n =$
Group A. Biopsy (Including one patient in who all biopsied were abnormal and not transferred)						
55	55	25	22	35	5*†	20
		45.5%*†	39.3%*†			35.7%*†
Group B. No Biopsy (Control) (intention at time of randomization)						
46	46	28	27	17	1*	27
		60.9%*	58.7%*			58.7%*
Group C. Poor Response, Withdrawn (women with no oocyte retrieval not entered)						
111	106	37	30	79	7	27
		34.9%	28.3%			25.4%
Group D. Eligible, Non-Participant (elective single blastocyst transfer)						
NA	554	325	288	283	54†	271
		58.7%†	52.0%†			48.9%†
		*p = 0.16	*p = 0.07		*† NS	*p = 0.03
		†p = 0.06	†p = 0.12			†p = 0.09

Groups A, B and D are elective single blastocyst transfers; Group C includes poor responders with up to two blastocysts transferred.

LB, live birth; M/C, miscarriage; NA, not applicable; NS, not significant. From [49].

preparatory step for biopsy and performed on day 3–4 [2, 5] (Group B), produced the highest clinical pregnancy rate of the groups (58.7%), a strong trend opposite to that required to disprove the null hypothesis and sufficient to lead to the trial being stopped. Subsequent analysis of live birth rates (Table 7.4) accentuated the difference.

The reason for the strong performance of the embryos in the principal control group, if it is true, is not clear. Assisted hatching by opening of the zona, while advocated from time to time for the embryos of older women to facilitate hatching and implantation has not been shown to be beneficial among women under 40 years of age or with good blastocyst development. More likely, a set of criteria for assumed meiotic non-disjunction that was too strict led to overinterpretation and rejection of otherwise optimally developing blastocysts that would have developed normally if left unscreened. There was a highly significant difference in the proportion of embryos transferred or cryostored (the "uti-

lization rate") between Group A (25%) and Group B (44%). On the other hand, a linear decline in IVF fecundity has been observed from age 33 to 45 years (Figure 7.1a), and when the first of several planned interim examinations of the data was carried out there happened to be a difference in randomization outcome with respect to average female age (Group A, 34.5 years vs. Group B, 32.1 years); correcting for this age discrepancy in fact largely removed the apparent difference between Groups A and B, and at this point the data are still consistent with little or even no clinically important detriment from blastocyst biopsy in women of normal reproductive age, a conclusion that finds support in our PGD series for monogenic disease, as discussed above. However this did not alter the fact that there is little or likely substantial benefit to be realized from presently available PGS techniques in women without specific indications for such screening.

In summary it remains to be shown that routine screening for aneuploidy can be beneficial for young infertile women undergoing IVF. To take this field further, a molecular method is needed that at once can (1) distinguish meiotic non-disjunctions affecting the embryo generally from mitotic non-disjunctions that, in a proportion of cases, develop normally if given the chance, and (2) recognize trisomies in any of the 24 chromosomes, not just the aneuploidies of chromosomes 13, 16, 18, 21, 22, X and Y that produce miscarriage or birth defects, but which will also detect trisomies of the remaining chromosomes that stop embryos more abruptly and thus from the outset compromise the efficacy of eSET.

Conclusions

The following principal conclusions can be drawn from the data and theory discussed in this chapter.

1. Examination of a restricted number of chromosomes using FISH for aneuploidy screening is at best unhelpful in selecting a single embryo to transfer and can be harmful if PGS is performed before blastulation.
2. Blastulation of the embryo is a useful adjunctive milestone but in itself is neither necessary nor sufficient to ensure that the embryo that is transferred is normal. If culture is performed in reliable conditions, blastocysts produce higher fresh clinical pregnancy rates than transfer of day 3 embryos does, and this practice will shorten the average time from egg retrieval to birth. In time, however, the same result might be reached from repeated day 3 transfers of embryos that have been reliably cryostored.
3. The necessary, and for now probably sufficient, requirement for successfully conducting an eSET policy is an effective and affordable embryo cryostorage and transfer program.
4. With follicular phase stimulation when there is deemed to be an excessive response, it is important that follicular development is not compromised in an overzealous attempt to minimize the risk of OHSS. The outcome can be the worst of both worlds, namely that the risk of serious

OHSS remains while the embryos as a cohort have had their development compromised by premature retrieval or subclinical atresia that does not become apparent until many embryos from the cohort have been transferred without success.
5. Abnormal endometrial responses consequent to high estrogen exposure are common but are difficult to quantitate as a cause of implantation failure of competent embryos; but, as an arbitrary and unpredictable phenomenon that renders implantation unlikely for all embryos transferred in an affected retrieval cycle, it constitutes a further argument for the practice of eSET in improving IVF practices.

What do we know?

Blastocysts more commonly have a normal karyotype than cleavage stage embryos do. Second, blastocysts have made a metabolic transition from catabolism and recycling of the oocyte's reserves and resources – processes that fuel the first three days of cleavage – to a state of dependence on the new embryonic genome and activation of a more anabolic mitochondrial metabolic state, both of which are required for successful blastulation and further subsequent development. When electively transferred singly, therefore, a blastocyst *should* be more likely to lead to a viable pregnancy than the transfer of a cleavage stage embryo.

What do we need to know?

Blastocysts appear to be more sensitive to laboratory culture conditions than the morphology of the blastocyst might disclose and often these conditions are in need of improvement. Notwithstanding that all blastocysts are not created karyotypically equal, it is still to be determined to what extent a mosaic karyotype might be a normal feature among embryos and to what extent looking for karyotypic abnormalities by embryo biopsy can help the chance of implantation rather than harm it. It is also still impractical to look at all the chromosomes that can, through their aneuploidy, stand in the way of successful embryonic and fetal development.

What should we do?

If we are correct in assuming that mitotic non-disjunction is common by the stage of the blastocyst and that it is much less ominous than meiotic non-disjunction, then from the perspective of PGS of blastocysts for aneuploidy we must develop methods of analysis that cover all the chromosomes and which can differentiate the triallelic state of meiotically derived aneuploidies from the biallelic state of mitotic aneuploidies.

REFERENCES

1. R. P. S. Jansen, Female age and the chance of a baby from one in-vitro fertilisation treatment. *Med. J. Aust.*, **178** (2003), 258–261.

2. K. A. De Boer, J. W. Catt, R. P. S. Jansen, D. Leigh and S. McArthur, Moving to blastocyst biopsy for preimplantation diagnosis and single embryo transfer at Sydney IVF. *Fert. Steril.*, **82** (2004), 295–298.

3. R. P. S. Jansen, Benefits and challenges brought by improved results from in vitro fertilization. *Intern. Med. J.*, **35** (2005), 108–117.

4. M. Henman, J. W. Catt, K. A.. De Boer *et al.*, Elective transfer of single fresh blastocysts and later transfer of cryostored blastocysts reduces the twin pregnancy rate and can increase the IVF live birth rate in younger women. *Fertil. Steril.*, **84** (2005), 1620–1627.

5. S. J. McArthur, D. Leigh, J. T. Marshall, K. A. De Boer and R. P. S. Jansen, Pregnancies and live births following biopsy and PGD analysis of human embryos at the blastocyst stage. *Fertil. Steril.*, **84** (2005), 1628–1636.

6. S. J. McArthur, D. Leigh, J. T. Marshall *et al.*, Blastocyst trophectoderm biopsy and preimplantation genetic diagnosis for familial monogenic disorders and chromosomal translocations. *Prenat. Diagn.*, **28**(5) (2008), 434–442.

7. H. Foulot, C. Ranoux, J. B. Dubuisson *et al.*, In vitro fertilization without ovarian stimulation: a simplified protocol applied in 80 cycles. *Fertil. Steril.*, **52** (1989), 617–621.

8. E. M. Heijnen, M. J. Eijkemans, C. De Klerk *et al.*, A mild treatment strategy for in-vitro fertilisation: a randomised non-inferiority trial. *Lancet*, **369** (2007), 743–749.

9. M. J. Pelinck, A. Hoek, A. H. Simons and M. J. Heineman, Efficacy of natural cycle IVF: a review of the literature. *Hum. Reprod. Update*, **8** (2002), 129–139.

10. H. Al-Inany and M. Aboulghar, GnRH antagonist in assisted reproduction: a Cochrane review. *Hum. Reprod.*, **17** (2002), 874–885.

11. B. C. Tarlatzis, B. C. Fauser, E. M. Kolibianakis *et al.*, GnRH antagonists in ovarian stimulation for IVF. *Hum. Reprod. Update*, **12** (2006), 333–340.

12. X. Shumin, E. Johannisson, B.-M. Landgren and E. Diczfalusy, Pituitary, ovarian and endometrial effects of progesterone released prematurely during the proliferative phase. *Contraception*, **27** (1983), 177–193.

13. S. J. Baker and N. Spears, The role of intra-ovarian interactions in the regulation of follicle dominance. *Hum. Reprod. Update*, **5** (1999), 153–165.

14. R. P. S. Jansen and K. A. De Boer, The bottleneck: mitochondrial imperatives in oogenesis and ovarian follicular fate. *Mol. Cell. Endocrinol.*, **145** (1998), 81–88.

15. J. Menken, J. Trussell and U. Larsen, Age and infertility. *Science*, **233** (1986), 1389–1394.

16. J. Dor, E. Rudak, S. Mashiach *et al.*, Periovulatory 17 beta-estradiol changes and embryo morphologic features in conception and nonconceptional cycles after human in vitro fertilization. *Fertil. Steril.*, **45** (1986), 63–68.

17. A. Pellicer, D. Valbuena, F. Cano, J. Remohí and C. Simón, Lower implantation rates in high responders: evidence for an altered endocrine milieu during the preimplantation period. *Fertil. Steril.*, **65** (1996), 1190–1195.

18. P. R. Koninckx, W. Heyns, G. Verhoeven *et al.*, Biochemical characterization of peritoneal fluid in women during the menstrual cycle. *J. Clin. Endocrinol. Metab.*, **51** (1980), 1239–1244.

19. M. Arslan, S. Bocca, E. Jones *et al.*, Effect of coasting on the implantation potential of embryos transferred after cryopreservation and thawing. *Fertil. Steril.*, **84** (2005), 867–874.

20. R. F. Williams and G. D. Hodgen, Disparate effects of human chorionic gonadotropin during the late luteal phase in monkeys: normal ovulation, follicular atresia, ovarian acyclicity, and hypersecretion of follicle-stimulating hormone. *Fertil. Steril.*, **33** (1980), 64–68.

21. J. B. Brown, J. H. Evans, F. D. Adey, M. P. Taft and L. Townsend, Factors involved in the induction of fertile ovulation with human gonadotrophins. *J. Obstet. Gynaecol. Br. Commonw.*, **76** (1969), 289–307.

22. D. W. Schmidt, D. B. Maier, J. C. Nulsen and C. A. Benadiva, Reducing the dose of human chorionic gonadotropin in high responders does not affect the outcomes of in vitro fertilization. *Fertil. Steril.,* **82** (2004), 841–846.

23. K. E. Elkind-Hirsch, S. Bello, L. Esparcia *et al.,* Serum human chorionic gonadotropin levels are correlated with body mass index rather than route of administration in women undergoing in vitro fertilization–embryo transfer using human menopausal gonadotropin and intracytoplasmic sperm injection. *Fertil. Steril.,* **75** (2001), 700–704.

24. M. D. Damewood, W. D. Schlaff, W. Shen *et al.,* Disappearance of exogenously administered human chorionic gonadotropin. *Fertil. Steril.,* **52** (1989), 398–400.

25. D. R. Meldrum, Vascular endothelial growth factor, polycystic ovary syndrome, and ovarian hyperstimulation syndrome. *Fertil. Steril.,* **78** (2002), 1170–1171.

26. U. Sungurtekin and R. P. S. Jansen, Profound luteinizing hormone suppression after stopping the gonadotropin-releasing hormone-agonist leuprolide acetate. *Fertil. Steril.,* **63** (1995), 663–665.

27. S. Matsuzaki, T. Fukaya, T. Suzuki *et al.,* Oestrogen receptor alpha and beta mRNA expression in human endometrium throughout the menstrual cycle. *Mol. Hum. Reprod.,* **5** (1999), 559–564.

28. P. A. Mote, R. L. Balleine, E. M. McGowan and C. L. Clarke, Colocalization of progesterone receptors A and B by dual immunofluorescent histochemistry in human endometrium during the menstrual cycle. *J. Clin. Endocrinol. Metab.,* **84** (1999), 2963–2971.

29. L. Chan and B. W. O'Malley, Mechanism of action of the sex steroid hormones. *N. Engl. J. Med.,* **294** (1976), 1322–1372.

30. J. Balasch, F. Miró, I. Burzaco *et al.,* The role of luteinizing hormone in human follicle development and oocyte fertility: evidence from in-vitro fertilization in a woman with long-standing hypogonadotrophic hypogonadism and using recombinant human follicle stimulating hormone. *Hum. Reprod.,* **10** (1995), 1678–1683.

31. G. Fried, J. Harlin, G. Csemiczky and H. Wramsby, Controlled ovarian stimulation using highly purified FSH results in a lower serum oestradiol profile in the follicular phase as compared with HMG. *Hum. Reprod.,* **11** (1996), 474–477.

32. D. Navot, T. L. Anderson, K. Droesch *et al.,* Hormonal manipulation of endometrial maturation. *J. Clin. Endocrinol. Metab.,* **68** (1989), 801–807.

33. J. S. Younis, N. Mordel, A. Lewin *et al.,* Artificial endometrial preparation for oocyte donation: the effect of estrogen stimulation on clinical outcome. *J. Assist. Reprod. Genet.,* **9** (1992), 222–227.

34. R. J. Chetkowski, R. J. Kiltz and W. R. Salyer, In premature luteinization, progesterone induces secretory transformation of the endometrium without impairment of embryo viability. *Fertil. Steril.,* **68** (1997), 292–297.

35. B. A. Kolb, S. Najmabadi and R. J. Paulson, Ultrastructural characteristics of the luteal phase endometrium in patients undergoing controlled ovarian hyperstimulation. *Fertil. Steril.,* **67** (1997), 625–630.

36. G. Nikas, O. H. Develioglu, J. P. Toner and H. W. Jones, Jr., Endometrial pinopodes indicate a shift in the window of receptivity in IVF cycles. *Hum. Reprod.,* **14** (1999), 787–792.

37. R. G. Forman, B. Eychenne, C. Nessmann, R. Frydman and P. Robel, Assessing the early luteal phase in in vitro fertilization cycles: relationships between plasma steroids, endometrial receptors, and endometrial histology. *Fertil. Steril.,* **51** (1989), 310–316.

38. M. J. Graf, J. V. Reyniak, P. Battle-Mutter and N. Laufer, Histologic evaluation of the luteal phase in women following follicle aspiration for oocyte retrieval. *Fertil. Steril.,* **49** (1988), 616–619.

39. A. C. Van Steirteghem, J. Smitz, M. Camus *et al.,* The luteal phase after in-vitro fertilization and related procedures. *Hum. Reprod.,* **3** (1988), 161–164.

40. R. P. S. Jansen and G. J. Burton, Mitochondrial dysfunction in reproduction. *Mitochondrion,* **4** (2004), 577–600.

41. H. J. Clouston, M. Herbert, J. Fenwick, A. P. Murdoch and J. Wolstenholme, Cytogenetic analysis of human blastocysts. *Prenat. Diagn.,* **22** (2002), 1143–1152.

42. S. Ziebe, K. Lundin, A. Loft *et al.,* FISH analysis for chromosomes 13, 16, 18, 21, 22, X and Y in all blastomeres of IVF pre-embryos from 144 randomly selected donated human oocytes and impact on pre-embryo morphology. *Hum. Reprod.,* **18** (2003), 2575–2581.

43. S. Munné, J. Ary, C. Zouves *et al.,* Wide range of chromosome abnormalities in the embryos of young egg donors. *Reprod. Biomed. Online,* **12** (2006), 340–346.

44. P. Braude, S. Pickering, F. Flinter and C. Mackie Ogilvy, Preimplantation genetic diagnosis. *Nat. Rev. Genet.,* **3** (2002), 941–953.

45. K. Sermon, A. Van Steirteghem and I. Liebaers, Preimplantation genetic diagnosis. *Lancet*, **363** (2004), 1633–1641.

46. J. J. Tarin, J. Conaghan, R. M. Winston and A. H. Handyside, Human embryo biopsy on the 2nd day after insemination for preimplantation diagnosis: removal of a quarter of embryo retards cleavage. *Fertil. Steril.*, **58** (1992), 970–976.

47. S. Mastenbroek, M. Twisk, J. van Echten-Arends *et al.*, In vitro fertilization with preimplantation genetic screening. *N. Engl. J. Med.*, **357** (2007), 9–17.

48. A. Kuliev and Y. Verlinsky, Meiotic and mitotic nondisjunction: lessons from preimplantation genetic diagnosis. *Hum. Reprod. Update*, **10** (2004), 401–407.

49. R. P. S. Jansen, M. C. Bowman, K. A. de Boer, D. B. Lierberman and S. J. McArthur, What next for preimplantation genetic screening (PGS)? Experience with blastocyst biopsy and testing for aneuploidy. *Hum. Reprod.*, **23**(7) (2008), 1476–1478.

50. A. A. Milki, M. D. Hinckley, L. M. Westphal and B. Behr, Elective single blastocyst transfer. *Fertil. Steril.*, **81** (2004), 1697–1698.

Sequential embryo selection for single embryo transfer

Lynette Scott

Introduction

Singleton births are the most desired outcome of any pregnancy, be it natural or assisted. Outcome indicators for all twin and certainly triplet pregnancies show increased risk in many areas, including low birth weight, cerebral palsy, prematurity, delayed speech and cognitive functions and increased infant mortality [1]. The risks to the mother can also be large with pre-eclampsia, gestational diabetes and not least post-delivery stress, exhaustion and feelings of isolation. The subject of reducing multiple pregnancies was recently addressed in a symposium [2] where the overall impact of triplets and twins on fetal, child and maternal health was considered. Additionally, the economic cost of multiple pregnancies was also shown to be high, both to families and to society [3].

Within the assisted reproductive technologies (ART) there was a steady rise in the incidence of twin, and greater, gestations through the 1980s and 1990s as methods of stimulation, oocyte retrieval, embryo culture and transfer improved, resulting in higher quality embryos, but with the continued use of too many embryos in transfer. The competitive drive to have better and higher pregnancy rates and the increasing cost of treatment cycles may be the reason there has been a slow reaction to this problem. Finally some countries began to mandate the use of one or two embryos to alleviate this issue

[4]. However, success and the patients' desire to be pregnant at any cost has made for a slow progression to the reduction in numbers of embryos transferred, unless there is a strict mandate [5].

Part of the problem with reducing the numbers of embryos transferred to one is that overall the pregnancy rate will drop, since at present the maximum implantation rate that can be realized is in the order of 60% in young healthy donors, with the general infertile couple having significantly lower rates, even with two and three embryos [6]. When media were improved to allow for the extended development of embryos in vitro, the concept of blastocyst transfer for higher pregnancy rates and reduced embryo numbers was advanced. This strategy is not feasible in countries where extended culture for selection by attrition is banned (Germany, Switzerland, Austria). However, from a large meta-analysis and published reports such as SART (Society for Assisted Reproductive Technology), it is clear that the use of blastocyst transfers only benefits high responders and good prognosis patients, and may not eliminate the use of multiple embryos in transfer [7]. It may also be associated with higher incidences of monozygotic twinning, an outcome that is most undesirable [8]. The concept of selecting the most viable embryos by the tools currently available, microscopy and morphometrics, in a rigorous sequential selection strategy is gaining credence, especially when it is coupled with biology and the

Single Embryo Transfer, ed. J. Gerris, G. D. Adamson, P. De Sutter and C. Racowsky. Published by Cambridge University Press.
© Cambridge University Press 2009.

idea that it is the embryo that is important and not the day of transfer.

Sequential embryo selection (SES) is a systematic documentation of the embryo's development from day to day, using key morphological features that have been shown to correlate with increased implantation so that on the day of transfer multiple criteria can be used for single embryo selection. Beginning with perhaps the gametes, a pedigree for each embryo is developed so that at the stage of transfer embryos that have not met criteria on each day can be eliminated from the selection pool. Sequential embryo selection also becomes important in countries where there are already regulations regarding numbers of fertilized oocytes that can be cultured and where cryopreservation needs to be performed on day 1 (1-cell fertilized oocyte). However, to make SES functional, the most important point to consider is time of scoring, because embryos move rapidly, are dynamic and do not follow rules, and even a 2 hour difference early in development and 4–5 hours difference in later development could affect the data significantly [9]. Using the model of SES, the day of performing the elective single embryo transfer (eSET) is then dictated by the embryo, and is not policy or protocol driven.

Gamete selection

It is recognized that a healthy embryo with full developmental potential is unlikely to develop from a flawed oocyte or sperm with damage to the DNA or mid-piece. Sperm selection is currently performed at a gross level with the use of density gradients to eliminate many of those with abnormal morphologies and perhaps sperm with fragmented DNA. During intracytoplasmic sperm injection (ICSI) there is further selection of sperm, again through morphology and by viability and movement. Some new techniques such as hyaluran binding have been proposed as a means of sperm selection but no real clinical data exist as yet. Ultramicroscopic analysis of sperm head, especially for the presence or absence of vacuoles, has been suggested but insufficient quality data exist to date to generalize this approach [10].

Oocyte selection is rarely performed, with all available material being used in either ICSI or standard insemination, and selection occurring at the embryo level. There are also minimal data on oocyte morphologies that contribute to final outcome although there is evidence that exogenous stimulation does result in oocytes with numerous abnormal morphologies [11]. In countries where limited numbers of oocytes can be used in insemination procedures, the use of oocyte selection becomes important. Light microscopy and morphology have not proven particularly helpful in oocyte selection; however new polarized light microscopy may allow oocyte selection. Visualization of the spindle, its position and shape, by using polarized light microscopy, has been correlated with outcome in both fresh and frozen cycles. However, no definitive controlled prospective trials have been reported where it can be shown that this system augments or supersedes embryo selection for increased delivery results. The spindle is a very dynamic structure and it disassociates as the temperature drops by even 2 degrees from 37 °C. Positioning of the oocyte is also crucial for shape documentation. These factors, oocyte manipulation, sensitive working environment and dedicated equipment, have resulted in a minimal use of this technique for oocyte and embryo selection.

Another emerging use of polarized microscopy of oocytes is documentation of the zona pellucida and abnormalities therein. The zona pellucida is a tri-laminate structure laid down by the oocyte during development and which has an aspect of polarized structure, which allows it to be visualized by polarized light microscopy. Many variations in zona structure and sperm binding have been shown with electron microscopy (invasive) and which may correlate with abnormal embryo development [12–14]. Abnormalities in the zona would imply a functional abnormality in the oocyte. Two different properties of the zona can be seen with polarized light microscopy. The first is the birefringence of the layers, since the outside layer should be polarized, the inner scattered and the middle layer partially polarized. However, although these differences have been documented, there are still not enough clinical data or controlled trials which indicate that this is an effective means of embryo selection. The second aspect of the zona that can be measured with polarized light microscopy is the regularity of the zona [15]. Oocytes in which the zonas display breaks and irregularities in birefringence have lowered post-fertilization potential. Again, this is an emerging technique and it has not been fully validated in a clinical setting and requires the investment and introduction of new technology into the laboratory.

At present the selection of gametes remains at the morphological assessment stage and is primarily to rule out the extreme cases.

Fertilized oocyte scoring

Once fertilization has occurred, the early pronuclear zygote or 1-cell embryo can be scored for certain characteristics. These include the number, position and size of the pronuclei, the number, alignment and size of the visible structures within the pronuclei, the nucleolar precursor bodies (NPBs) and the appearance of the cytoplasm, or "halo" [16, 17].

The male and female pronuclei appear on the periphery of the oocyte early in the fertilization process and rotate into the center by approximately 16–18 hours post-insemination, or 56–58 hours post-human chorionic gonadotropin (hCG). The nuclei should be approximately the same size. If one is much larger than the other, this is abnormal with a large percentage of these oocytes being aneuploid [18]. Within the nuclei the pattern and numbers of NPBs can be scored, pronuclear/zygote (PN/Z) scoring. Two main systems for grouping fertilized oocytes into normal and abnormal exist, but are essentially the same, the Tesarik [19] and Z-Score systems [17, 20] (Figure 8.1). In both systems, equality of alignment of NPBs in the two nuclei is

Normal Forms

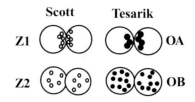

Abnormal Forms

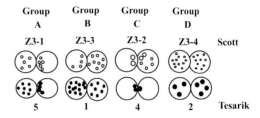

Figure 8.1 Diagrammatic representation of fertilized oocyte scoring: normal groups have equal numbers of NPBs with equal distribution. Abnormal fertilized oocytes have unequal alignment, numbers or sizes of NPBs. Both the Tesarik [19] and Scott [17] scoring systems are represented.

important, with the numbers of NPBs also being correlated with implantation and development. Where there is equality in both alignment and numbers, there is greater blastocyst development and increased implantation. A new finding is that the numbers of NPBs at a set time of scoring is also important, and this should be between 5 and 7 per nucleus [20]. Other authors have used and explored the possibilities and limitations of this methodology in specific circumstances [21–25].

The most crucial aspect of PN/Z scoring is the ability to "see" the oocyte as a three-dimensional ball with two spherical nuclei within it, aligned on a structure that has polarity and direction (the mitotic spindle). Appreciating that the nuclei and NPBs are juxtaposed onto the spindle and that the spindle may lie in any plane between them, and that the chromatin and then chromosomes need to condense onto the spindle, allows an embryologist to mentally rotate the nuclei in order to look at the

NPBs relative to a slice or two-dimensional plane, between the nuclei. In this way, equality and alignment can be easily assigned.

The question is why are NPBs and their number and alignment important? During oocyte development (primordial to mature MII oocyte) nucleoli actively synthesize protein and at the final stages of maturation they disassemble into component parts, only to reform when the embryonic genome is in place and the newly formed embryo is growing. Nucleoli are where all proteins of any cell are constructed and are the site of rRNA production. Some growth factors and developmental regulatory proteins are also produced within the nucleoli [26]. Nucleoli develop on DNA at sites where the genes for ribosomal RNA are located (rDNA), and these sites are the nucleolar organizing regions (NORs) [27].

Another very important aspect of NPB scoring is that the NORs are clustered on the DNA and this is dependent on heterochromatin adjacent to rDNA genes. There are only five NOR-bearing chromosomes: 13, 14, 15, 21 and 22; the heterochromatic chromosomes [28], which are also most likely to be abnormal in any aneuploidy screen.

Nucleoli contain three functional components: the dense fibrillar component (DFC), which is required for transcription, the fibrillar component (FC), which is surrounded by the DFC and which stores inactive transcription factors and is the center of the nucleolus, and the granular or cytoplasmic component (GC) [27, 29]. When the nucleoli disassemble during development the FC region remains and it is this that is scored or seen during pronuclear scoring, the NPBs are the FC region. Since these only reside on the five heterochromatic chromosomes, what is also being indirectly seen is the condensation of chromatin from chromosomes 13, 14, 15, 21 and 22 onto the spindle.

All human cells, including embryos and sperm, have between two and seven nucleoli per cell which dissociate into their component parts during any mitotic cycle, even in the early oocyte at fertilization. When chromatin begins to condense onto the mitotic spindle (in an oocyte at sperm entry), the NPBs will appear to condense onto the spindle. In PN scoring the lack of symmetry in this condensation is seen as unequal alignment of NPBs, unequal numbers of NPBs and different sizes which means delayed or fast condensation in one nucleus. This may indicate abnormal or asynchronous karyo- and cytokinesis, which may result in embryos with little developmental potential.

There is also a correlation between PN score and aneuploidy with the incidence of chromosomally normal embryos being highest with equal-sized nuclei and equal numbers of NPBs that are aligned [22, 30–32].

Early cleavage

Early cleavage, after fertilization on day 1, has been reported as another means of embryo selection for increased implantation [33–36]. One of the main issues with doing early cleavage checks is timing, with reports varying in as much as 4 hours. At the stage of entry into the first mitotic division the fertilized oocyte moves very rapidly with fast breakdown of the nuclear membranes and then cleavage to the 2-cell stage. The timing issue may be why the reports on the use of this parameter vary widely. However, what is also true is that embryos that do undergo early cleavage also tend to be those that score better on day 2 and on day 3 and then also result in higher implantation rates [33]. Using early cleavage when there are very few oocytes and embryos may not be effective and it may just add another time point at which the embryos need to be removed from the incubator. However, if a case presents with many good quality PN scores, the addition of an early cleavage check at approximately 23–24 hours post-insemination [33] could add another point in the SES.

First and second mitotic cleavage

Following sperm entry, pronuclear formation and alignment on the mitotic spindle, the event of

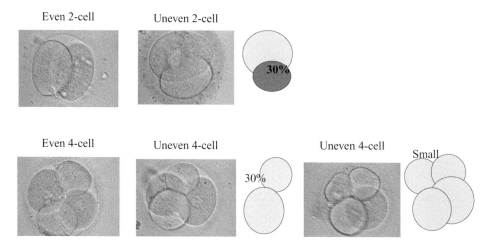

Figure 8.2 Blastomere relative size.

fertilization is completed with the first cleavage division, forming a 2-cell embryo which now has a unique genetic constitution contributed by oocyte and sperm. Fertilization is only complete with the formation of a 2-cell embryo.

The positioning of the meiotic spindle in the oocyte could greatly affect this first cleavage event. If it is off center, the oocyte may cleave down a plane that would result in a 2-cell embryo with greatly different cell sizes. Considering linage in cell divisions, abnormal cytokinesis such as this could lead to blastocysts with allocation of cellular constituents that are very abnormal [20, 37–41]. Even if unequal cleavage was not due to aberrant positioning of the spindle, any cytokinesis that resulted in embryos with two cells of grossly different sizes would suggest abnormal cellular processes and thus an embryo with little developmental potential [42]. The same can be true of the 4-cell embryo, resulting from the second mitotic division. Four-cell embryos that have very uneven cell sizes may arise from a normal second mitotic division after an abnormal/unequal first one or from a normal first division (equal-sized 2-cell) followed by an abnormal second division (unequal 4-cell). Subsequent cell divisions from either or a combination of these unequal cell divisions will result in 8-cell embryos that have very abnormal allocation of cell components to the different cells, which may be translated to the blastocyst.

There is evidence that at the 4-cell stage only one of the blastomeres in the embryo continues to grow into the clone of cells in the blastocyst that produce hCG, which signals to the endometrium that the embryo is ready to implant. If there has been abnormal cytokinesis in the early stages of development, cellular components may be incorrectly allocated to cells resulting in blastocysts that are incapable of producing the necessary signals for implantation [37, 40, 41, 43].

Uneven cell number at a set time (42–44 hours post-insemination) where the cells are of equal size (three, five and greater) correlate with poor outcome. After the first cleavage division, the embryo rapidly transitions to 4-cells, through a 3-cell phase first to form a 4-cell tetrahedron embryo [20, 38, 39, 44]. An embryo with 3 equal-sized cells, or one that does not progress rapidly to a 4-cell, is abnormal. The same can be said of embryos that are at the 5-cell stage and greater at 42–44 hours post-insemination, which means it is progressing too rapidly [45] (Figure 8.2).

Blastomere size after the first and second mitotic divisions is easily scored and even- or equal-sized blastomeres is essential for normal development.

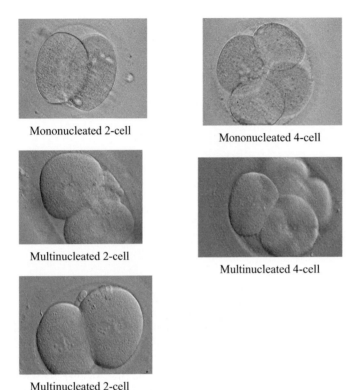

Mononucleated 2-cell

Mononucleated 4-cell

Multinucleated 2-cell

Multinucleated 4-cell

Multinucleated 2-cell

Figure 8.3 Mono- and multinucleation.

After the first two mitotic divisions the state of nucleation of the blastomeres is very easily scored and has been shown to be highly correlated with outcome [46]; [20, 47–51].

Each blastomere should have one clearly defined nucleus (Figure 8.3). Lack of a nucleus may indicate that the cell is in a transition phase, however, at a set point (42–44 hours post-insemination) most embryos should be resting with a visible nucleus in each blastomere. Multi, micro and fragmented nuclei correlate with very poor outcome, even when the embryos keep growing [20, 42, 49, 52, 53]. Two mechanisms are responsible for the multinucleation in the early cleavage divisions: [46] blastomeres proceeding with karyokinesis without cytokinesis, or by errors in chromosome segregation or other mitotic errors. During the first mitotic division the chromosome segregation error and/or

mitotic error is most likely why >70% of embryos displaying multinucleation are aneuploid after fluorescent *in situ* hybridization analysis [52].

Day 2 scoring for cell number, evenness/equality of cell size and state of nucleation is simple and correlates very well with outcome and delivery, and is simple and easy to perform. In SES, the results from day 1 scoring could then be coupled with the results from day 2 scoring, eliminating any embryo that not only did not have a good PN score but also an embryo that passed the first score but did not pass the second.

Day 3 cleaving embryo morphology

After the 4-cell stage each of these cells proceeds through a mitotic event, each halving their volume

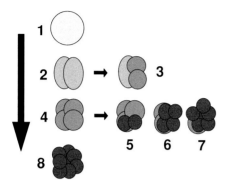

Figure 8.4 Relative cell sizes during mitotic divisions. See color plate section.

since no real growth in the embryo occurs until after the 8-cell stage. During these mitotic events the embryo is very dynamic and moves slightly within the confines of the zona pellucida but it does not rotate. During all early cleavage divisions in human embryos, as seen by time-lapse video images, there is also a vast amount of cellular blebbing and the beginnings of fragments being extruded, most likely due to apoptosis (Figure 8.4).

Scoring of embryos on day 3 must also be by time, since the transition from a 6-cell to an 8-cell embryo can be very fast. The use of a "day 3" score for comparative purposes is meaningless. As with day 2 scoring, it needs to be set according to some definite parameter, generally time of hCG. With most laboratories working on a morning time frame, day 3 scoring is best accomplished at between 64–66 hours post-insemination. Embryos at this stage should be between 6- and 8-cells with little to no fragmentation and with even cell size and without the presence of multinucleation.

A 6- or 7-cell embryo should have two cell sizes. A 6-cell embryo where all the cells are the same size is abnormal, since from the 4-cell stage to the 6-cell stage only 2 of the 4 cells will have completed their next mitotic division (see Figure 8.4).

Thus in SES, the embryo that is an even 6- to 8-cell stage with no fragmentation, and came from a good score on day 2, and a normal PN score, can be chosen for single embryo transfer. These embryos will

have the highest potential for implantation. If only one or two embryos pass gates 1 and 2 then a day 2 transfer can be performed.

If there are sufficient embryos that have passed the gates of SES on day 1, day 2 and day 3, extended culture to the blastocyst stage can be performed, in order to add another selection point to the scoring.

Blastocyst morphology and selection

The relationship between blastocyst development, quality and outcome are no different than that seen with day 1, 2 or 3 development parameters. Morphological criteria also pertain at this stage of development, as not all blastocysts are equal. Retrospective data abound on the relationship between blastocyst morphology and delivery outcome, but there are only a few reports that link early morphological parameters to late ones, or blastocyst development [16, 54]. In all reports, day 1 and day 3 morphology is closely correlated with blastocyst development, the embryos that pass through the early gates are those most likely to result in good quality blastocysts.

High-scoring blastocysts, using one of the many systems available, point to the fact that there is a very high correlation between blastocyst quality and outcome [55, 56], which is no different to early scoring parameters. What is important to remember is that even abnormal day 1, 2 and 3 embryos can develop into morphological *normal appearing* blastocysts. Top morphologically scoring blastocysts result from about 20% of all cultured embryos (40% in high prognosis patients), which means that some patients require more than one blastocyst in embryo transfer [56], which again defeats the concept of eSET. When only low-scoring blastocysts are available (15% of cases) the implantation and pregnancy rates are no different to those obtained with day 3 transfer. Here there are no data on delivery, which is the ultimate proof of successful embryo selection [56].

A good quality blastocyst at 113–116 hours post-insemination should have intact cells; no granular

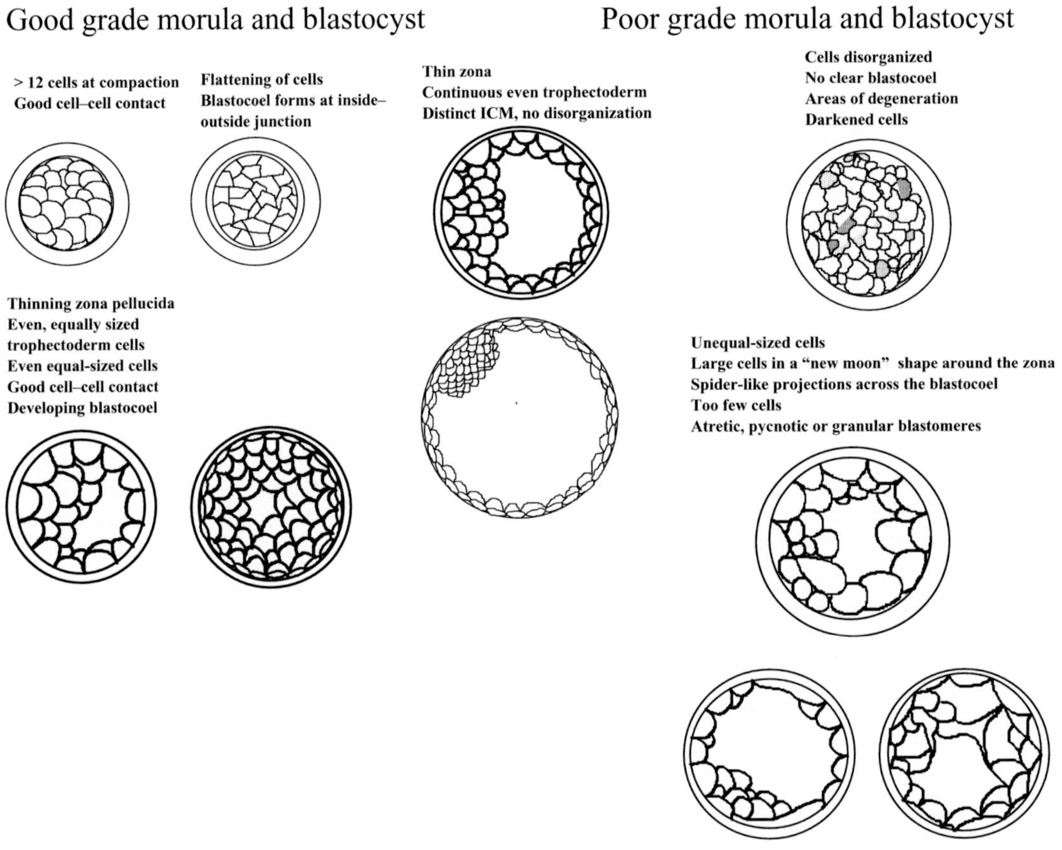

Good grade morula and blastocyst

> 12 cells at compaction
Good cell–cell contact

Flattening of cells
Blastocoel forms at inside–
outside junction

Thin zona
Continuous even trophectoderm
Distinct ICM, no disorganization

Thinning zona pellucida
Even, equally sized
trophectoderm cells
Even equal-sized cells
Good cell–cell contact
Developing blastocoel

Poor grade morula and blastocyst

Cells disorganized
No clear blastocoel
Areas of degeneration
Darkened cells

Unequal-sized cells
Large cells in a "new moon" shape around the zona
Spider-like projections across the blastocoel
Too few cells
Atretic, pycnotic or granular blastomeres

Figure 8.5 Good grade morula and blastocyst. ICM, inner cell mass.

cells; a continuous well-defined outer perimeter of cells with good cell–cell contact; and no long thin cells. Cells in the next layers have clear membranes, good cell–cell contact, clear cytoplasm and an obvious blastocoel. Over the following 2 hours embryos can expand by at least 1/3 of their size, but must have a well-defined inner cell mass, without giant cells; they should have at least 80 cells which could be counted by scanning through the embryo on the inverted microscope. By 5 hours later many will be well-expanded blastocysts. Processes, or finger-like projections, through the blastocoel are also abnormal [57, 58]. A feature of blastocysts in culture is that as they expand they go through cycles of collapsing

and re-expanding. This is a normal process, in vitro, and indicates a healthy blastocyst, which is likely to hatch easily (Figure 8.5).

Poor quality blastocysts present with one or many of: too few cells; granular darkened areas; too few cells in the outer layer resulting in long thin cells expanding over a large portion of the blastocyst; inner cell mass disorganized or with cells of very uneven sizes; spidery cellular projections through the blastocoel cavity; many small fragments localizing to the outside of the embryo.

Thus using SES, blastocysts can be selected based on day 1, 2, 3 and 5 data, which will allow for a very high implantation rate.

REFERENCES

1. C. Bergh, How to promote singletons. Contributions from the Bertarelli Foundation Meeting: "Triplets End Point" (online-only publication). *Reprod. Biomed. Online*, **15**: Suppl. 3 (2007). www.rbmonline.com/Article/2749.

2. Bertarelli Foundation Meeting: "Triplets End Point" (online-only publication). *Reprod. Biomed. Online*, **15**: Suppl. 3 (2007).

3. J. Collins, Global epidemiology of multiple birth. Contributions from the Bertarelli Foundation Meeting: "Triplets End Point" (online-only publication). *Reprod. Biomed. Online*, **15**: Suppl. 3 (2007). www.rbmonline.com/Article/2578.

4. P. Saldeen and P. Sundström, Would legislation imposing single embryo transfer be a feasible way to reduce the rate of multiple pregnancies after IVF treatment? *Hum. Reprod.*, **20** (2005), 4–8.

5. S. de Lacey, M. Davies, G. Homan, N. Briggs and R. Norman, Factors and perceptions that influence women's decisions to have a single embryo transferred, *Reprod. Biomed. Online*, **15** (2007), 526–531.

6. Z. Pandian, S. Bhattacharya, O. Ozturk, G. Serour and A. Templeton, Number of embryos for transfer following in-vitro fertilisation or intra-cytoplasmic sperm injection. *Cochrane Database Syst. Rev.*, **18** (2004), CD003416.

7. A. Styer, D. Wright, A. Wolkovich, C. Veiga and T. Toth, Single-blastocyst transfer decreases twin gestation without affecting pregnancy outcome. *Fertil. Steril.*, **89**(6) (2008), 1702–1708 Epub 2007 Jul 20.

8. V. Wright, L. Schieve, A. Vahratian and M. Reynolds, Monozygotic twinning associated with day 5 embryo transfer in pregnancies conceived after IVF. *Hum. Reprod.*, **19** (2004), 1831–1836.

9. M. Johnson and M. Day, Egg timers: how is developmental time measured in the early vertebrate embryo? *BioEssays*, **22** (2000), 57–63.

10. B. Bartoov, A. Berkovitz, F. Eltes *et al.*, Pregnancy rates are higher with intracytoplasmic morphologically selected sperm injection than with conventional intracytoplasmic injection. *Fertil. Steril.*, **80** (2003), 1413–1419.

11. J. Van Blerkom, Occurrence and developmental consequences of aberrant cellular organization in meiotically mature human oocytes after exogenous ovarian hyperstimulation. *J. Electron Microsc. Tech.*, **16** (1990), 324–346.

12. G. Familiari, M. Relucenti, R. Heyn, G. Micara and S. Correr, Three-dimensional structure of the zona pellucida at ovulation. *Microsc. Res. Tech.*, **69** (2006), 415–426.

13. S. Nottola, S. Makabe, T. Stallone *et al.*, Surface morphology of the zona pellucida surrounding human blastocysts obtained after in vitro fertilization. *Arch. Histol. Cytol.*, **68** (2005), 133–141.

14. P. Schwartz, B. Hinney, P. Nayudu and H. Michelmann, Oocyte-sperm interaction in the course of IVF: a scanning electron microscopy analysis. *Reprod. Biomed. Online*, **7** (2003), 192–198.

15. M. Montag, T. Schimming, M. Köster *et al.*, Oocyte zona birefringence intensity is associated with embryonic implantation potential in ICSI cycles. *Reprod. Biomed. Online*, **16** (2008), 239–244.

16. L. Scott, Pronuclear scoring as a predictor of embryo development. *Reprod. Biomed. Online*, **6** (2003), 57–70.

17. L. Scott, R. Alvero, M. Leondires and B. Miller, The morphology of human pronuclear embryos is positively related to blastocyst development and implantation. *Hum. Reprod.*, **15**(11) (2000), 2394–2403.

18. S. Sadowy, G. Tomkin and S. Munne, Impaired development of zygotes with uneven pronuclear size. *Zygote*, **63** (1998), 137–141.

19. J. Tesarik and E. Greco, The probability of abnormal preimplantation development can be predicted by a single static observation on pronuclear stage morphology. *Hum. Reprod.*, **14**(5) (1999), 1318–1323.

20. L. Scott, A. Finn, T. O'Leary, S. McLellan and J. Hill, Morphologic parameters of early cleavage-stage embryos that correlate with fetal development and delivery: prospective and applied data for increased pregnancy rates. *Hum. Reprod.*, **22** (2007), 230–240.

21. A. Borini, M. Cattoli, E. Sereni, R. Sciajno and C. Flamigni, Predictive factors for embryo implantation potential. *Reprod. Biomed. Online*, **10** (2005), 653–668.

22. S. Kahraman, M. Bahce, H. Samli *et al.*, Healthy births and ongoing pregnancies obtained by preimplantation genetic diagnosis in patients with advanced maternal age and recurrent implantation failure. *Hum. Reprod.*, **15** (2000), 2003–2007.

23. M. Ludwig, B. Schopper, A. Katalinic *et al.*, Clinical use of a pronuclear stage score following intracytoplasmic sperm injection: impact on pregnancy rates under

the conditiions of the German embryo protection law. *Hum. Reprod.*, **15**(2) (2000), 325–329.

24. A. Senn, F. Urner, A. Chanson *et al.*, Morphological scoring of human pronuclear zygotes for prediction of pregnancy outcome. *Hum. Reprod.*, **21** (2006), 234–239.

25. U. Zollner and T. Steck, Pronuclear scoring. Time for international standardization. *J. Reprod. Med.*, **48** (2003), 365–369.

26. T. Pedersen, Growth factors in the nucleolus? *J. Cell Biol.*, **143** (1998), 279–281.

27. G. Goessens, Nucleolar structure. *Int. Rev. Cytol.*, **87** (1984), 107–108.

28. P. Dimitri, N. Corradini, F. Rossi and F. Vernì, The paradox of functional heterochromatin. *BioEssays*, **27** (2005), 29–41.

29. H. Schwarzacher and W. Mosgoeller, Ribosome biogenesis in man: current views on nucleolar structure and function. *Cytogenet. Cell Genet.*, **91** (2000), 243–252.

30. W. Edirisinghe, R. Jemmott, C. Smith and J. Allen, Association of pronuclear Z scores with rates of aneuploidy in in vitro-fertilised embryos. *Reprod. Fertil. Dev.*, **17** (2005), 529–534.

31. P. Gamiz, C. Rubio, M. de los Santos, A. Mercader and C. Simone, The effect of pronuclear morphology on early development and chromosomal abnormalities in cleavage stage embryos. *Hum. Reprod.*, **18** (2003), 2413–2419.

32. L. Gianaroli, M.C. Magli, A.P. Ferraretti, D. Fortini and N. Grieco, Pronuclear morphology and chromosomal abnormalities as scoring criteria for embryo selection. *Fertil. Steril.*, **80**:2 (2003), 341–349.

33. C. Lawler, H. Baker and D. Edgar, Relationships between timing of syngamy, female age and implantation potential in human in vitro-fertilised oocytes. *Reprod. Fertil. Dev.*, **19** (2007), 482–487.

34. K. Lundin, C. Bergh and T. Hardarson, Early embryo cleavage is a strong indicator of embryo quality in human IVF. *Hum. Reprod.*, **16** (2001), 2652–2657.

35. A. Salumets, C. Hydén-Granskog, S. Mäkinen *et al.*, Early cleavage predicts the viability of human embryos in elective single embryo transfer procedures. *Hum. Reprod.*, **18** (2003), 821–825.

36. A. Van Montfoort, J. Dumoulin, A. Kester and J. Evers, Early cleavage is a valuable addition to existing embryo selection parameters: a study using single embryo transfers. *Hum. Reprod.*, **19** (2004), 2103–2106.

37. M. Antczak and J. Van Blerkom, Oocyte influences on early development: the regulatory proteins leptin and STAT3 are polarized in mouse and human oocytes and differentially distributed within the cells of the preimplantation stage embryo. *Mol. Hum. Reprod.*, **3**(12) (1997), 1067–1086.

38. R. Gardner, The early blastocyst is bilaterally symmetrical and its axis of symmetry is aligned with the animal-vegetal axis of the zygote in the mouse. *Development*, **124** (1997), 289–301.

39. R. Gardner and T. Davies, An investigation of the origin and significance of bilateral symmetry of the pronuclear zygote in the mouse. *Hum. Reprod.*, **21** (2006), 492–502.

40. C. Hansis and R. Edwards, Cell differentiation in the preimplantation human embryo. *Reprod. Biomed. Online*, **6** (2003), 215–220.

41. C. Hansis, J. Grifo and L. Krey, Candidate lineage marker genes in human preimplantation embryos. *Reprod. Biomed. Online*, **8** (2004), 577–583.

42. H. Ciray, L. Karagenc, U. Ulug, F. Bener and M. Bahceci, Use of both early cleavage and day 2 mononucleation to predict embryos with high implantation potential in intracytoplasmic sperm injection cycles. *Fertil. Steril.*, **84** (2005), 1411–1416.

43. R. Edwards and C. Hansis, Initial differentiation of blastomeres in 4-cell human embryos and its significance for early embryogenesis and implantation. *Reprod. Biomed. Online*, **11** (2005), 206–218.

44. C. Roux, R. Borodkine, C. Joanne, J. L. Bresson and G. Agnani, Morphological classification of human in-vitro fertilization embryos based on the regularity of the asynchronous division process. *Hum. Reprod. Update*, **1**(5) (1995), 488–496.

45. C. Racowsky, K. Jackson, N. Cekleniak *et al.*, The number of eight-cell embryos is a key determinant for selecting day 3 or day 5 transfer. *Fertil. Steril.*, **73** (2000), 558–564.

46. S. Pickering, A. Taylor, M. Johnson and P. Braude, An analysis of multinucleated blastomere formation in human embryos. *Hum. Reprod.*, **10** (1995), 1912–1922.

47. T. Hardarson, C. Hanson, A. Sjogren and K. Lundin, Human embryos with unevenly sized blastomeres have lower pregnancy and implantation rates: indications for aneuploidy and multinucleation. *Hum. Reprod.*, **16** (2001), 313–318.

48. C. Hnida, I. Agerholm and S. Ziebe, Traditional detection versus computer-controlled multilevel analysis

of nuclear structures from donated human embryos *Hum. Reprod.*, **20** (2004), 665–671.

49. J. Meriano, C. Clarke, K. Cadesky, and C. Laskin, Binucleated and micronucleated blastomeres in embryos derived from human assisted reproduction cycles. *Reprod. Biomed. Online*, **9** (2004), 511–520.

50. T. Moriwaki, N. Suganuma, M. Hayakawa *et al.*, Embryo evaluation by analysing blastomere nuclei. *Hum. Reprod.*, **19**:1 (2004), 152–156.

51. E. Van Royen, K. Mangelschots, D. De Neubourg *et al.*, Calculating the implantation potential of day 3 embryos in women younger than 38 years of age: a new model. *Hum. Reprod.*, **16**:2 (2001), 326–332.

52. I. Kligman, C. Benadiva, M. Alikani and S. Munne, The presence of multinucleated blastomeres in human embryos is correlated with chromosomal abnormalities. *Hum. Reprod.*, **11** (1996), 1492–1498.

53. M. Pelinck, M. De Vos, M. Dekens *et al.*, Embryos cultured in vitro with multinucleated blastomeres have poor implantation potential in human in-vitro fertilization and intracytoplasmic sperm injection. *Hum. Reprod.*, **13** (1998), 960–963.

54. B. Balaban, B. Urman, A. Isklar *et al.*, The effects of pronuclear morphology on embryo quality parameters and blastocyst transfer outcome. *Hum. Reprod.*, **16** (2001), 2357–2361.

55. B. Balaban, B. Urman, A. Sertac *et al.*, Blastocyst quality affects the success of blastocyst-stage embryo transfer. *Fertil. Steril.*, **74** (2000), 282–287.

56. D. Gardner, M. Lane, J. Stevens, T. Schlenker and W. Schoolcraft, Blastocyst score affects implantation and pregnancy outcome: towards a single blastocyst transfer. *Fertil. Steril.*, **73** (2000), 1155–1158.

57. L. Scott, The origin of monozygotic twinning. *Reprod. Biomed. Online*, **5** (2002), 276–284.

58. L. Scott, The biological basis of non-invasive strategies for selection of human oocytes and embryos. *Hum. Reprod. Update*, **9** (2003), 237–249.

Cryo-augmentation after single embryo transfer: the European experience

Aila Tiitinen

Introduction

An optimal standard of success in assisted reproductive technology (ART) should reflect both the risk aspects and the effectiveness of the treatment. The most important parameter for the couple is the ultimate birth rate per started cycle [1]. This means that we should calculate the cumulative delivery rate per stimulated cycle after all embryo transfers, fresh and frozen, have been performed.

A good strategy to avoid multiple pregnancies is elective single embryo transfer (eSET) with freezing of spare embryos [1, 2]. This strategy also highlights the importance of the quality of cryopreservation programs when implementing eSET into daily clinical routine. Actually, the policy of limiting the number of embryos transferred is not possible without a good cryopreservation program. There is a need for an evaluation system not only of the laboratory technology but also for the true augmenting effect of cryopreservation [3]. Only cryopregnancies occurring after an unsuccessful fresh cycle truly reflect the augmentation potential of cryopreservation.

Cryopreservation in European countries

The number of cryopreservation cycles has been quite constant in Europe during the 1990s, but showing some increase during the last years. More than 60 000 frozen embryo transfers (FETs) were performed in 2003, with a mean pregnancy rate of 18.6% and multiple birth rate of 15.1% [4]. The delivery rate per FET – between 11.9% and 33% – varied more than with fresh in vitro fertilization/intracytoplasmic sperm injection (IVF/ICSI), in different European countries. In Finland the number of FETs in relation to fresh transfers seems to be higher than in other countries, because Finland has had a policy with extensive use of cryopreservation [4]. According to Finnish IVF statistics 41.5% of all embryo transfers in 2005 were FETs [5]. In our clinic this number is around 50% (Figure 9A.1). Furthermore 35.7% of ART deliveries in 2005 came from cryopreservation [5] and near to 50% in our clinic (Figure 9A.2). This is a substantial part of all ART children born. Therefore, in order to maximize the efficiency of the IVF/ICSI cycles, more emphasis should be given to effective embryo freezing.

Contribution of cryopreservation in the 1990s

Studies on the cryo-augmented pregnancy rates before the eSET era exist. One of the first studies on the contribution of embryo cryopreservation following IVF/ICSI was reported from Norway [6]. This found a 5.2% increase in the take-home baby rate for women entering the IVF program with cryopreservation and an 11.6% increase in the number of children. It draws our attention to the primary interest

Single Embryo Transfer, ed. J. Gerris, G. D. Adamson, P. De Sutter and C. Racowsky. Published by Cambridge University Press.
© Cambridge University Press 2009.

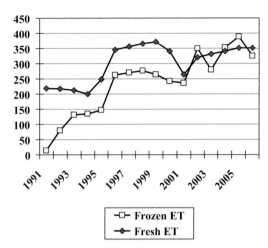

Figure 9A.1 The number of embryo transfers (ET) at Helsinki University Hospital 1991–2006 (Hydén-Granskog, unpublished).

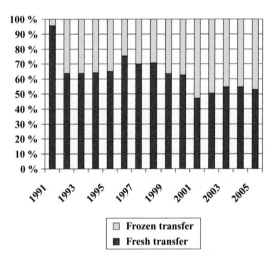

Figure 9A.2 The proportion of children born after fresh or frozen embryo transfer (Hydén-Granskog, unpublished).

of the efficacy of IVF: the proportion of the couples entering an IVF program that obtain a child. Others have reported increases of 11% [7] or even 19% after three completed IVF cycles [8].

The delivery of healthy babies has confirmed at least the short-term safety of the use of the freezing/thawing technique. The cryopreservation process does not adversely affect the growth and health of children during infancy and early childhood [9].

This knowledge has enabled the increase of cryopreservation programs in many clinics. Already 10 years ago the value of cryopreservation in several clinical situations was stated as follows [10]: it allows patients an increased chance of pregnancy by the subsequent transfer of thawed embryos, reduces the risk of multifetal gestation by limiting the number of embryos replaced, decreases the potential risk of ovarian hyperstimulation syndrome in women showing an exaggerated ovarian response to stimulation by the elective embryo cryopreservation of all embryos and it can be used in a donor oocyte program.

The value of cryopreservation in eSET programs

We analyzed in a follow-up study all embryo transfers carried out at our clinic during 1998 and 1999 [11]. Following eSET (127 cases) the pregnancy rate per embryo transfer was 38.6% and after double embryo transfer (DET) 40.0%, respectively. The contribution of embryo cryopreservation in eSET cycles resulted in the cumulative delivery rate of 52.8% per oocyte retrieval after fresh and frozen transfers. After increasing the proportion of eSET cycles yearly we still have deliveries in > 50% of eSET cycles [12]. We have updated our present situation in Figure 9A.3. It is obvious that a significant impact of eSET is an increase in the number and quality of embryos available for cryopreservation. In the Finnish prospective randomized study the cumulative pregnancy rate in the eSET and DET group was 47.3% and 58.6%, respectively [13]. The significance of cryopreservation is important to be considered when the real effectiveness of eSET is evaluated.

A randomized multicenter study performed in Scandinavia showed that in women under 36 years old, transferring one fresh embryo, followed (if there was no live birth) by the transfer of one frozen embryo, dramatically reduced the multiple delivery rate while achieving a rate of live births that is not substantially lower than that which is achievable with one DET [2]. As shown in the study by Thurin

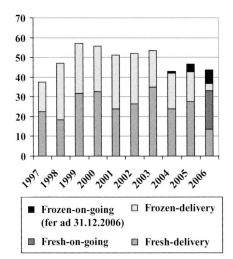

Figure 9A.3 The cumulative delivery rate after fresh and frozen embryo transfer in eSET cycles (Hydén-Granskog, unpublished).

et al. [?] the transfer of frozen-thawed embryos has a significant impact on the safety aspects and final results of ART per oocyte retrieval when eSET is carried out in the fresh cycle.

Similar results have been achieved in other European countries, too. Between June 2002 and December 2004, all patients (first cycle, female age ≤ 38 years) were offered the choice between having one (SET) or two (DET) embryos transferred in a French clinic [14]. Among 493 couples, 428 had at least two good quality embryos and, out of them, 32% opted for SET. The SET and DET populations were not comparable (patients in the SET group were younger and had more oocytes retrieved), and therefore a paired, case-controlled analysis was performed involving 130 SET couples and 130 DET couples, matched according to the female partners' ages and the numbers of embryos available. All the SET patients, and 82% of the DET group, had at least one embryo cryopreserved (3.9 vs. 2.8 embryos). The option of SET was continued for the frozen-thawed embryo transfers. The pregnancy rate following embryo transfer was significantly lower after SET compared to DET for both fresh (27.6% vs. 36.9%) and frozen-thawed (14.5%

vs. 23.4%) embryos. But the cumulative live birth rates following the transfer of fresh and frozen embryos were identical between the two groups (43% vs. 45%), with a high prevalence of twins following DET (34% vs. zero).

SET with cryopreserved embryos in non-optimal patients

The results from Finland demonstrate for the first time that the eSET policy is applicable to women in the age group of 36 to 39 years [15]. In this age group, a clinical pregnancy rate of 33% was achieved after eSET, which was similar to that (30.8–34.5%) found in previous studies on eSET in younger women [13, 16]. In this study, after one or two FET cycles the cumulative pregnancy rate was 54%, with a live birth rate of over 40%. The result in this selected group of older women is very satisfactory, although in younger women we have reported even higher pregnancy rates, up to 60%. In conclusion, the particular study demonstrated that the eSET policy is applicable to women older than 35 years in order to increase the safety of ART and minimize the health risks faced by these women. The results support the view that embryo morphology is a more important determinant of outcome than age, at least until the age of 40.

In the same study, eSET was also performed in a smaller group of subjects with only non top quality embryos [15]. As expected, the pregnancy rate in fresh cycles was rather low (below 20%). However, through several FET cycles, this group reached an acceptable cumulative pregnancy rate of 33%, with a multiple birth rate of 3%. Hence, even if no top quality embryo is available, eSET combined with cryocycles seems to be possible and beneficial to women who are at increased risk of pregnancy complications.

Techniques

Many variables may influence the outcome of embryo cryopreservation and FET. In 1990

Hartshorne *et al.* reported that cryothawed embryos with one or more blastomeres damaged had the same capacity to produce pregnancies as did those with all blastomeres intact [17]. However, several reports indicate that transfer of partially damaged cryothawed embryos results in lower pregnancy and implantation rates compared to transfer of fully intact embryos [18, 19]. In our program we observed an implantation rate of 33.7% for embryos cryopreserved on day 2 as 4-cell and after thawing having all blastomeres intact, fragmentation < 20% and no multinuclear blastomeres [19]. This implantation potential of cryopreserved embryos is supported by the study in which intact cryothawed embryos were shown to have the same implantation potential as fresh embryos of identical quality [18].

The outcome in FET cycles can be improved, and SET in frozen-thawed cycles has to be considered as well. In order to do this, the selection criteria for embryos to be cryopreserved should be optimized and cryopreservation methods further developed. We have shown that SET policy can be adopted into a cryopreservation program [19]. Single embryo transfer may be particularly useful in cycles with frozen-thawed embryos, since the embryos can be frozen and thawed individually, one by one. However, this strategy increases the workload in the laboratory [20]. Others have also supported this recommendation [21]. They suggest that frozen embryos should be thawed individually and if the thawed embryo survives with all its blastomeres intact (and preferably divides after thawing) serious consideration should be given to transferring this embryo alone, saving surplus embryos for future cycles.

Optimal stimulation

Success of ART has long been focused towards technical aspects of treatment: the number of follicle and oocytes harvested, the fertilization and cleavage rate. The most important outcome of interest is, however, whether the treatment will lead to the birth of a healthy baby. In treatment cycles where

ovarian stimulation in conjunction with IVF/ICSI results in a large number of fertilized oocytes, cryopreservation offers the opportunity to select the best embryo for fresh transfer and to freeze the others. This optimizes the clinical use of available good quality embryos. Recent studies have suggested that ovarian stimulation strategies should avoid maximizing oocyte yield, but aim at generating a sufficient number of chromosomally normal embryos by reduced interference with ovarian physiology [22].

The health-economic dimension

It has been concluded that DET is the most expensive strategy, but it is also most effective if performed in a fresh cycle. Elective SET is preferred from a cost-effectiveness point of view when performed in good prognosis patients and when frozen-thawed cycles are included [23]. If frozen-thawed cycles are excluded, the choice between eSET and DET depends on how much society is willing to pay for one extra successful pregnancy. The inclusion of frozen-thawed cycles usually causes relatively more live births for eSET than for DET, because more and better quality embryos are left for freezing after eSET.

Since FET does not involve ovarian stimulation and oocyte retrieval, and is mainly performed in natural cycles requiring no hormonal stimulation, it can be considered less costly and easier for the patients to go through. Frozen embryo transfer also represents less work for the clinic as a whole [20]. No randomized controlled trial on cumulative live births comparing SET with DET and including on fresh and all subsequent frozen cycles has so far been published.

Conclusions

Correct counseling of the couples on the risk of multiple pregnancy is very important. If only one embryo is transferred, it does not mean that the other embryos are discarded; they are only stored for later use. Of course, it has to be remembered that some of the embryos will not survive the freezing-thawing process, and we might lose some pregnancies. It has also been claimed that there are factors which could limit the acceptability of eSET for patients and their physicians [24]. Given the lower success rate inherent in the transfer of one, rather than two fresh embryos, the increased likelihood of having to undergo the subsequent transfer of frozen-thawed embryos entails some inconvenience and stress (although, in many cases, a cycle not requiring ovarian stimulation and the induction of ovulation). This risk can be minimized with improvements in cryopreservation and thawing methods.

Even if the long-term follow-up of the treatment cycles is difficult in practice, we would stress that more emphasis should be given to embryo freezing, in order to maximize the efficiency of the IVF/ICSI cycles. It should be remembered that it is important to take into account the effect of all embryos achieved during one single oocyte pick-up [25]. In Finland the implementation of single embryo transfer has been possible with good cryopreservation programs. After the establishment of reliable embryo selection criteria, eSET, combined with an effective cryopreservation program, has been shown to result in a high cumulative pregnancy rate of at least 50% per oocyte retrieval. The cumulative pregnancy rate achieved after FETs is the best indicator of the efficacy of ART.

What do we know?
We know that cryopreservation gives further opportunities to increase cumulative pregnancy rate per oocyte pick-up.

What do we need to know?
We do not know what is the magnitude of this cryo-augmentation and how cryopreservation protocols affect the final outcome.

What should we do?
We should perform long-term follow-up studies after eSET, including all frozen transfers with a single embryo. We should further improve our cryopreservation techniques.

REFERENCES

1. A. Tiitinen, C. Hydén-Granskog and M. Gissler, What is the most relevant standard of success in assisted reproduction? The value of cryopreservation on cumulative pregnancy rates per single oocyte retrieval should not be forgotten. *Hum. Reprod.*, **19** (2004), 2439–2441.

2. A. Thurin, J. Hausken, T. Hillensjö *et al.*, Elective single-embryo transfer versus double-embryo transfer in in vitro fertilization. *N. Engl. J. Med.*, **351** (2004), 2392–2402.

3. J. Gerris, D. De Neubourg, P. De Sutter *et al.*, Cryopreservation as a tool to reduce multiple birth. *Reprod. Biomed. Online*, **7** (2003), 286–294.

4. A. N. Andersen, V. Goossens, L. Gianaroli *et al.*, Assisted reproductive technology in Europe, 2003. Results generated from European registers by ESHRE. *Hum. Reprod.*, **22** (2007), 1513–1525.

5. STAKES. Finnish IVF statistics 2005 and preliminary data for 2006. National Research and Development Centre for Welfare and Health, accessible at www.stakes.info/files/pdf/Tilastotiedotteet.

6. J. Kahn, V. von During, A. Sunde *et al.*, The efficacy and efficiency of an in-vitro fertilization program including embryo cryopreservation: a cohort study. *Hum. Reprod.*, **8** (1993), 247–252.

7. X. J. Wang, W. Ledger, D. Payne, R. Jeffrey and C. D. Matthews, The contribution of embryo cryopreservation to in-vitro fertilization/gamete intrafallopian transfer: 8 years experience. *Hum. Reprod.*, **9** (1994), 103–109.

8. C. Bergh, B. Josefson, L. Nilsson and L. Hamberger, The success rate in a Swedish in-vitro-fertilization unit: a cohort study. *Acta Obstet. Gynecol. Scand.*, **74** (1995), 446–450.

9. U.-B. Wennerström, K. Albertsson-Wikland, C. Bergh *et al.*, Postnatal growth and health in children born after cryopreservation as embryos. *Lancet*, **351** (1998), 1085–1090.

10. G. Horne, J. D. Critchlow, M. C. Newman *et al.*, A prospective evaluation of cryopreservation strategies in a two-embryo-transfer program. *Hum. Reprod.*, **12** (1997), 542–547.

11. A. Tiitinen, M. Halttunen, P. Härkki, P. Vuoristo and C. Hydén-Granskog, Elective single embryo transfer. The

value of cryopreservation. *Hum. Reprod.*, **16** (2001), 1140–1144.

12. C. Hydén-Granskog and A. Tiitinen, Single embryo transfer in clinical practice. *Hum. Fertil.* (Camb)., **7** (2004), 175–182.

13. H. Martikainen, A. Tiitinen, C. Tomás *et al.*, One versus two-embryo transfer after IVF and ICSI: a randomized study. *Hum. Reprod.*, **16** (2001), 1900–1903.

14. D. Le Lannou, J. F. Griveau, M. C. Laurent *et al.*, Contribution of embryo cryopreservation to elective single embryo transfer in IVF-ICSI. *Reprod. Biomed. Online*, **13** (2006), 368–375.

15. Z. Veleva, S. Vilska, C. Hydén-Granskog *et al.*, Elective single embryo transfer in women aged 36–39 years. *Hum. Reprod.*, **21** (2006), 2098–2102.

16. A. Tiitinen, L. Unkila-Kallio, M. Halttunen and C. Hyden-Granskog, Impact of elective single embryo transfer on the twin pregnancy rate. *Hum. Reprod.*, **18** (2003), 1449–1453.

17. G. M. Hartshorne, K. Wick, K. Elder and H. Dyson, Effect of cell number at freezing upon survival and viability of cleaving embryos generated from stimulated IVF cycles. *Hum. Reprod.*, **5** (1990), 857–861.

18. D. H. Edgar, H. Bourne, A. L. Speirs and J. C. McBain, A quantative analysis of the impact of cryopreservation on the implantation potential of human early cleavage stage embryos. *Hum. Reprod.*, **15** (2000), 175–179.

19. C. Hydén-Granskog, L. Unkila-Kallio, M. Halttunen and A. Tiitinen, Single embryo transfer is an option in frozen embryo transfer. *Hum. Reprod.*, **20** (2005), 2935–2938.

20. K. Lundin, and C. Bergh, Cumulative impact of adding frozen-thawed cycles to single versus double fresh embryo transfers. *Reprod. Biomed. Online*, **15** (2007), 76–82.

21. R. Tang, J. Catt and D. Howlett, Towards defining parameters for a successful single embryo transfer in frozen cycles. *Hum. Reprod.*, **21** (2006), 1179–1183.

22. E. B. Baart, E. Martini, M. J. Eijkemans *et al.*, Milder ovarian stimulation for in-vitro fertilization reduces aneuploidy in the human preimplantation embryo: a randomized controlled trial. *Hum. Reprod.*, **22** (2007), 980–988.

23. A. A. A. Fiddelers, J. L. Severens, C. D. Dirksen *et al.*, Economic evaluations of single versus double embryo transfer in IVF. *Hum. Reprod. Update*, **13** (2007), 5–13.

24. O. K. Davis, Elective single-embryo transfer – has its time arrived? *N. Engl. J. Med.*, **351** (2004), 2440–2441.

25. A. Pinborg, A. Loft, S. Ziebe and A. Nyboe Andersen, What is the most relevant standard of success in assisted reproduction? Is there a single 'parameter of excellence'? *Hum. Reprod.*, **19** (2004), 1052–1054.

Cryo-augmentation after single embryo transfer: the American experience

Marius Meintjes

Introduction

Even though the first successful birth after in vitro fertilization (IVF) was the result of transferring a single 8-cell embryo [1], the transfer of single embryos is rarely practiced in the United States [2, 3]. In contrast, the transfer of a single, cleavage stage embryo is common in much of Europe, with emphasis on the cumulative fresh-frozen cycle outcome [4].

With fewer options for third-party financial coverage of IVF in the United States, physicians and patients insist on an individualized approach rather than mandated practice patterns to be better able to balance the perceived drawbacks of single embryo transfer (SET) against the risks and costs associated with multiple pregnancies. Many IVF programs can now limit higher-order multiple pregnancies to less than 5% by transferring no more than two embryos. However, it is frequently perceived that risks associated with twinning are manageable and that the increased medical costs of caring for mother and two babies are preferentially covered by insurance companies when compared with the expense of repeat IVF. As a result, some patients even insist on twins to have one pregnancy and two babies for the same financial outlay they would incur for one. Clearly, twin pregnancies may be curtailed only by transferring single embryos. However, it is feared that SET may compromise pregnancy rates, mandate more treatment cycles, delay or deprive the patient of a successful outcome and ultimately lead to higher out-of-pocket treatment expenses [5].

To gain acceptance in the United States, SET clinical outcomes must be justifiable and comparable to outcomes after double embryo transfers. A critical question is, therefore, at which developmental stage should we transfer a single embryo to achieve this goal? The best SET pregnancy rate will be accomplished with embryos associated with the highest implantation rate. To date, the highest published implantation rates resulted from transferring blastocysts [6]. Cleavage stage embryos are essentially a promise of an embryo, cleaving under the direction and support of proteins, nutrients and messenger RNA packed into the oocyte during earlier growth and maturation processes. Experience in the laboratory suggests that, on average, only 20% of IVF embryos will convert to viable implantations due to genetic [7] and metabolic [8] deficiencies. In contrast, a blastocyst with a verifiable inner cell mass (ICM) has demonstrated activation of the embryonic genome and some initial metabolic competency. Therefore, the transfer of one proven blastocyst instead of a single unproven cleavage stage embryo should be much more likely to result in a healthy baby.

Elective single blastocyst transfer (SBT) mandates a complimentary blastocyst cryopreservation program. Blastocyst culture and subsequent SBT have been discouraged, in part, by less than

Table 9B.1 Clinical outcome of blastocyst transfers (two good quality vs. two of any quality) for patients ≤ 34 years of age and patients with donor oocytes

	N	Clinical pregnancies (%)	Implanted (%)	Multiple implantations (%)	Patients with cryo (%)
2 Any quality blastocysts donor	260	196 (75.4)	332 (63.8)	131 (66.8)	120 (46.2)
2 Any quality blastocysts ≤ 34 Years	660	418 (63.3)	675 (51.1)	219 (52.4)	220 (33.3)
Total any quality blastocysts	920	614^a (66.7)	1007^a (54.7)	350^a (57)	340^a (37.0)
2 Good quality blastocysts donor	102	84 (82.4)	154 (75.5)	65 (77.4)	73 (71.6)
2 Good quality blastocysts ≤ 34 Years	194	143 (73.7)	233 (60.1)	86 (60.1)	124 (63.9)
Total 2 quality blastocysts	296	227^b (76.7)	387^b (65.4)	151^b (66.5)	197^b (66.6)

[a,b] Numbers in columns with different superscripts are different. χ^2; $p < 0.008$.

acceptable blastocyst cryopreservation outcomes. Frozen-thawed blastocyst cycles have been plagued by discouraging post-thaw survival [9], a high biochemical pregnancy rate followed by a high incidence of miscarriages [10] and an overall less than anticipated take-home baby rate [11].

For SBT to be a viable option in the United States the following are essential: (1) an optimized blastocyst culture system to support the development of quality blastocysts; (2) clinical outcomes for fresh SBT must be competitive with those of day 3 or multiple blastocyst transfers; (3) clinician and patient reluctance to consider SBT must be overcome; and (4) a reliable blastocyst cryopreservation program with acceptable clinical outcomes must be established. Insurance companies that support the birth of a single term infant rather than a positive pregnancy test, regardless of obstetrical and neonatal complications, may compliment any such efforts towards SBT.

Consequences of transferring two blastocysts

Excellent live birth rates can be realized when transferring two blastocysts obtained in an opti-

mized blastocyst culture system. Optimization may include incubation in physiological sequential culture media, culturing at a reduced oxygen concentration [12], using appropriate equipment at all stages of gamete and embryo manipulation and practicing vigorous quality management.

In an investigation of more than 1000 patients, the clinical and cryopreservation outcomes were compared for patients with two good quality embryos for transfer on day 5 and patients not having at least two good quality embryos [13] (Table 9B.1). Two patient populations were identified as having a high risk for twins: young patients (≤ 34 years) and patients using donor oocytes. The lowest implantation rate (51.1%) was obtained in young patients not having at least two quality blastocysts for transfer and the highest (75.5%) in patients using donor oocytes with at least two quality blastocysts for transfer. Even though these implantation and pregnancy rates were considered excellent, the resulting twin implantation rates between 52% and 77% were unacceptable.

It has been well established that twin pregnancies are not benign, but that it poses significant risks to the mother and babies [14]. Furthermore, multiple births have a significant financial and psychological impact on the prospective parents, their families, the healthcare industry and society in general [15]. With the rate of blastocyst cryopreservation (37% to 67%) observed in this study population, it became clear that the threshold to act should no longer be to contain triplet pregnancies, but to reduce twin pregnancies in this high-risk target population.

Initial experience with single blastocyst transfer

To incorporate SBT into routine clinical practice, one must be convinced and convey to the patients that the benefits of transferring a single blastocyst and the risk of not becoming pregnant outweigh the benefit of transferring two blastocysts and the associated risk of twins. A trial period was initiated to evaluate patient acceptance when recommending SBT and to document the clinical outcomes with or without SBT [16]. Single blastocyst transfer was offered to patients ≤ 37 years of age and to patients using donor oocytes. A SBT was offered only at the time of transfer if at least two quality blastocysts were available for transfer. This resulted in a 100% day 5 cryopreservation rate following the SBT.

A total of 103 patients accepted a SBT; 187 refused and insisted on the transfer of two quality blastocysts. A further 103 patients were identified during this period that qualified for a SBT but were not offered it due to the initial inexperience of the clinical team in presenting this concept to couples. Implantation rates were not different for SBT (73.8%) and two-blastocyst transfers (71.2%). The initial live birth rate for two-blastocyst transfers was higher than that for SBT (79.0% and 70.9%, respectively). However, when accounting for additional frozen-thawed blastocyst transfers, the live birth rate was not different for the two-blastocyst transfer and SBT groups (83.4% and 79.6%, respectively). The twin implantation rate was reduced from 67.8% when transferring two blastocysts to 2.4% (two monozygotic twins) for SBT.

Overall, roughly one third (35.5%) of the patients that were given a choice accepted a SBT. Upon inquiry, it became apparent that the two main rea-

sons for insisting on two blastocysts for transfer were a lack of appreciation for the risk inherent to carrying and delivering twins and an absolute intolerance to incur any additional expense for a subsequent frozen-thawed cycle, should the SBT fail to result in a live born baby.

The effect of a comprehensive incentive program on SBT patient participation

It became evident that a comprehensive educational and financial incentive program would be needed to increase patient participation in SBT, even though we could demonstrate that there was no difference in the cumulative fresh-frozen live birth rate between SBT and two-blastocyst transfers. Consequently, a continuing patient education effort was initiated that would begin as soon as a decision was made to undergo IVF treatment. During this time prior to retrieval, patients were educated on: (1) the risks and potential serious consequences associated with twins; (2) the availability and details regarding the SBT initiative; and (3) the need to make a decision only on the day of blastocyst transfer.

The incentive program included free cryopreservation and storage of frozen blastocysts for SBT patients, regardless of pregnancy outcome. If the SBT did not result in a live birth (~ 30% of patients) the program would perform a subsequent thawed blastocyst transfer at no additional cost. The patient age and blastocyst-quality criteria applied were the same as those described during the initial experience with SBT. When meeting these criteria on the day of transfer, a SBT was offered. The scope and implications of the incentive program was reviewed with the couple after which they were asked to sign an agreement to formally accept or refuse a SBT.

The cumulative fresh-frozen term pregnancy rate was not different for patients accepting or declining a SBT (74.6% and 79.9%, respectively). The multiple pregnancy rate for patients declining a SBT was 78.8% to include one monozygotic triplet pregnancy. After the incentive plan was introduced,

Table 9B.2 Acceptance rate and clinical outcomes before and after implementation of the SBT incentive program

	No incentive program		With incentive program	
	Donor oocytes	Patient oocytes	Donor oocytes	Patient oocytes
Patients offered SBT	56	96	31	80
Patients accepting SBT	15[a]	32[A]	20[b]	47[B]
Acceptance rate	26.8	33.3	64.5	58.8
Ongoing/term pregnancies (%)	11 (73.3)	19 (59.4)	13 (65.0)	32 (68.1)
Twin pregnancies (%)	0	1 (5.2)	0	1 (3.1)

[A,B,a,b] Numbers in rows with different superscripts are different. Fisher's Exact Test, $p < 0.01$.

participation in SBT more than doubled for patients using donor oocytes and almost doubled for patients using their own oocytes (Table 9B.2). This study suggests that with preemptive education and removal of the financial burden of a follow-up thawed blastocyst transfer, on average, two out of three patients will choose a SBT [17].

Optimization of blastocyst cryopreservation

Post-thaw inner cell mass (ICM) survival

High biochemical pregnancy and miscarriage rates are frequent observations when transferring frozen-thawed blastocysts. A biochemical pregnancy is defined as a positive beta-human chorionic gonadotropin result failing to progress to a clinical pregnancy. It has been observed that the ICM is preferentially damaged by cryopreservation and that the resulting clinical outcomes directly relate to ICM quality [18].

When transferring frozen-thawed blastocysts with poor quality ICMs, the biochemical pregnancy, clinical pregnancy and ongoing/live birth rates were 25%, 28% and 18%, respectively. Several healthy-appearing post-thaw trophoblasts with no discernable ICM were transferred which resulted in clinical pregnancies followed by first-trimester miscarriages. In contrast, when frozen-thawed blastocysts with good quality ICMs were transferred during the same time period, the biochemical pregnancy rate was lower (7%), the clinical pregnancy

rate higher (63%) and the ongoing pregnancy/live birth rate higher (57%).

Efforts to improve blastocyst cryopreservation should focus to a significant degree on ICM survival, which may be improved by careful selection of blastocysts for cryopreservation, pre-freeze cytoskeletal stabilization, optimization of cryoprotectant solutions and the application of ultra-rapid vitrification techniques.

A place for assisted hatching of frozen-thawed blastocysts?

It is known that the composition and function of the zona pellucida may change during freezing and thawing. It is tempting to speculate that assisted hatching may improve frozen-thawed blastocyst transfer outcomes. In a randomized prospective study comparing assisted-hatched ($n = 76$) and non-hatched ($n = 76$) frozen-thawed blastocyst transfers, it was observed that the initial implantations were improved with hatching (increased from 38.2% to 46.9%), however, without a lasting effect on the ongoing pregnancy/live birth rate (assisted hatching 47.4%, no assisted hatching 50.0%) [19].

Day 5 and day 6 cryopreserved blastocysts

The exact timing and blastocyst developmental stage at the time of cryopreservation may be imperative to optimal frozen-thawed blastocyst pregnancy outcomes. Embryologists frequently face

Table 9B.3 Live birth outcomes for age-specific frozen-thawed blastocyst transfers

Patient age (Years)	Number of transfers	Blastocysts/ transfer	Live-birth implantation rate	Ongoing/ live-birth rate
≤ 34	199	1.7	44.5^a	58.3^a
35 to 37	105	1.6	34.7^b	46.7^b
38 to 40	71	1.5	35.2^b	45.1^b
> 40	13	1.5	35.0^{ab}	38.5^{ab}
Donor oocytes	63	1.8	40.5^{ab}	57.1^{ab}
Total	451	1.7	40.0	52.8

a,b Numbers in columns with no common superscript are different. χ^2; $p < 0.04$.

decisions in freezing expanding blastocysts with reduced cell numbers on day 5 or freezing the next day with increased cell numbers, but risking ICM degeneration or in vitro hatching. A study observing 301 frozen-thawed blastocyst transfers found that blastocysts frozen late on day 5 resulted in higher implantation (47.0% vs. 36.4%) and ongoing pregnancy/live birth rates (54.6% vs. 43.7%) than blastocysts frozen early on day 6 [18].

Expectations for an optimized blastocyst cryopreservation program

The optimization of a blastocyst cryopreservation program mandates a comprehensive approach. Freezing and thawing protocols/solutions are crucial, however, these represent only a part of the overall cryopreservation scheme.

Even with the limitations of slow-rate blastocyst freezing, live birth rates close to those of fresh blastocyst transfers can be achieved (Table 9B.3). From the table, it is apparent that fewer patients will have blastocysts to cryopreserve with increasing age. Interestingly, it seems that as long as quality blastocysts are frozen, pregnancy rates are not as much affected by the age of the patient than what is observed when transferring fresh blastocysts [20].

Vitrification of embryos is now becoming a viable option and should be considered [21]. Human blastocyst vitrification is not yet proven to be convincingly better than optimized conventional blastocyst cryopreservation [22]. However, vitrification may open the door to the cryopreservation of embryos currently not frozen reliably, such as early blastocysts, hatched blastocysts, borderline ICMs and preimplantation genetic diagnosis embryos, or the refreezing of embryos. In addition, vitrification may be a helpful tool where time and technical resources are a limiting factor.

The impact of cryo-augmentation after SBT

To date, SBT has been offered to 893 patients in our program (Table 9B.4). Blastocyst implantation rates were identical when transferring one or two blastocysts, indicating an absence of embryonic synergism when transferring two blastocysts. However, patients refusing a SBT had $\sim$ 10% higher live birth rate at the expense of a multiple pregnancy rate of > 60%. When accounting for some cryo-augmentation after the initial fresh blastocyst transfer (all frozen blastocysts not yet used), the initial small difference in the fresh live birth rate was absent with cumulative fresh-frozen live birth rates now in excess of 80%, regardless of the number of blastocysts transferred.

Nine (1.8% of pregnancies) patients with two-blastocyst transfers had monozygotic twins resulting in triplet pregnancies. Four (2.4% of pregnancies) of the SBT patients had monozygotic twins. In addition, $\sim$ 40% of patients refusing a SBT did not have any blastocysts cryopreserved. In contrast, 100% of patients electing a SBT had one or more blastocyst cryopreserved. Twin rates for the

Table 9B.4 Live birth and cryopreservation outcomes after offering SBT

	No. of patients	Live-birth rate	Live-birth implantation rate	Multiple pregnancy rate	Patients with cryo rate	Cumulative fresh-frozen live-birth rate
SBT Donor	63	71.4^a	71.4	2.2^a	100^a	84.1
SBT ≤ 37 Years	191	62.3^A	62.3	2.5^a	100^a	80.6
SBT Total	254	64.6	64.6	2.4	100	81.5
Refuse SBT Donor	191	82.7^b	71.5^a	73.4^b	66.5^b	86.7
Refuse SBT ≤ 37 Years	448	75.7^B	60.4^b	59.9^b	58.0^b	80.1
Refuse SBT Total	639	77.8	63.7	64.2	60.6	82.2

^{A,B,a,b} Numbers in columns with different superscripts are different. χ^2; $p < 0.04$.

follow-up thawed transfers were not different for the SBT or two-blastocyst transfer groups (30.2% and 39.3%, respectively).

Conclusions

We now know that even though the initial live births are slightly less for patients with a SBT, identical or better cumulative fresh-frozen live birth rates are possible. All patients electing SBT in this program have a second chance to become pregnant if the reason for not conceiving is suspected to be other than blastocyst quality. In contrast, about 40% of patients electing two blastocysts for transfer will not have cryopreserved embryos and, therefore, no second chance. Twin pregnancies are drastically reduced to < 3% when transferring a single blastocyst. Although SBT is offered to a selected patient population, the average number of embryos transferred to all donor-recipients and for all day 5 transfers, in general, can be reduced to < 2 in a large IVF program.

Using morphological criteria only could not result in a > 70% live birth rate. At least 30% of the best patients with the best embryos still fail to become pregnant. We should consider alternative means of blastocyst evaluation such as non-invasive genetic or metabolic analyses to achieve even higher success rates with SBT or to offer SBT to a broader spectrum of patients.

With the current lack of emphasis on single live births by the American insurance industry, the common patient perception that twin pregnancies are harmless and the personal financial burden associated with IVF in the United States, it is clear that comprehensive education combined with significant financial incentives will be necessary to encourage SBT. Our experience indicates that with such a comprehensive incentive program in place, two out of three patients may elect a SBT.

Frozen-thawed blastocyst live birth rates comparable to those obtained with fresh blastocysts for patients of all ages should now improve the feasibility of offering routine SBT to selected patients. Even though cryo-augmentation can be implemented successfully, refinements to current protocols and investigation of alternative techniques such as vitrification will be prudent to further improve ICM survival after thawing. Live births should no longer be compromised when transferring single blastocysts to selected patients. On the contrary, the success rate for delivering healthy infants may be improved. Results obtained from SBT with cryo-augmentation strongly suggest that we not only should, but have an obligation to offer patients the opportunity to avoid twin pregnancies without having to compromise the ultimate outcome they have sought.

ACKNOWLEDGEMENTS

The author wishes to recognize Vitrolife Inc., EMD Serono Inc. and Presbyterian Healthcare System for continued support to make an efficient SET program a reality in the United States. The participating physicians Drs Brian Barnett, David Bookout, Samuel Chantilis, James Douglas, Jerald Goldstein, Reza Guerami, Robert Kaufmann, Karen Lee, James Madden and Alfred Rodriguez and the embryologists Hannalie Adriaanse, Tonya Davidson, Carlos Guerrero, Hetal Mistry, Oscar Perez and David Ward are acknowledged for their dedication and willingness to allow our patients the choice to transfer a single blastocyst.

REFERENCES

1. R. Edwards and P. Steptoe, *A Matter of Life. The Story of a Medical Breakthrough.* (New York: William Morrow & Company Inc., 1980), p. 150.
2. A. Criniti, A. Thyer, G. Chow *et al.*, Elective single blastocyst transfer reduces twin rates without compromising pregnancy rates. *Fertil. Steril.*, **84** (2005), 1613–1619.
3. D. K. Gardner, E. Surrey, D. Minjarez *et al.*, Single blastocyst transfer: a prospective randomized trial. *Fertil Steril.*, **81** (2004), 551–555.
4. A. Thurin, J. Hausken, T. Hillensjö *et al.*, Elective single embryo transfer versus double-embryo transfer in in vitro fertilization. *N. Engl. J. Med.*, **351** (2004), 2392–2402.
5. N. Gleicher and D. Barad, The relative myth of elective single embryo transfer. *Hum. Reprod.*, **21** (2006), 1337–1344.
6. D. K. Gardner, and M. Lane, Towards a single embryo transfer. *Reprod. Biomed. Online*, **6** (2003), 470–481.
7. A. Kuliev, J. Cieslak, Y. Ilkevitch and Y. Verlinsky, Chromosomal abnormalities in a series of 6733 human oocytes in preimplantation diagnosis for age-related aneuploidies. *Reprod. Biomed. Online*, **6** (2003), 54–59.
8. D. K. Gardner, M. Lane, J. Stevens and W. B. Schoolcraft, Noninvasive assessment of human embryo nutrient consumption as a measure of developmental potential. *Fertil. Steril.*, **76** (2001), 1175–1180.
9. E. Van Den Abbeel, M. Camus, G. Verheyen *et al.*, Slow controlled-rate freezing of sequentially cultured human blastocysts: an evaluation of two freezing strategies. *Hum. Reprod.*, **20** (2005), 2939–2945.
10. T. S. Kosasa, P. I. McNamee, C. Morton and T. T. Huang, Pregnancy rates after transfer of cryopreserved blas-

tocysts cultured in a sequential media. *Am. J. Obstet. Gynecol.*, **192** (2005), 2035–2039.
11. N. Desai and J. Goldfarb, Examination of frozen cycles with replacement of a single thawed blastocyst. *Reprod. Biomed. Online*, **11** (2005), 349–354.
12. M. Meintjes, K. Hill, S. Johnston *et al.*, The effect of lowered incubator oxygen tension on implantation-, pregnancy- and cryopreservation rates in a predominantly day-5 embryo transfer program. *Fertil. Steril.*, **74**: 3 Suppl. 1 (2000), S256.
13. M. Meintjes, K. Hill, S. J. Chantilis *et al.*, Selective quality blastocyst transfer and blastocyst cryopreservation eliminate twin pregnancies without compromising pregnancy rates. *Fertil. Steril.*, **78**: 3 Suppl. 1 (2002), S244.
14. E. R. Norwitz, V. Edusa and J. S. Park, Maternal physiology and complications of multiple pregnancy. *Semin. Perinatol.*, **29** (2005), 338–348.
15. T. L. Callahan, J. E. Hall, S. L. Ettner *et al.*, The economic impact of multiple-gestation pregnancies and the contribution of assisted-reproduction techniques to their incidence. *N. Engl. J. Med.*, **331** (1994), 244–249.
16. M. Meintjes, D. M. Bookout, S. J. Chantilis *et al.*, Towards single blastocyst transfers – preliminary experience. *Fertil. Steril.*, **82**: Suppl 2 (2004), S35.
17. D. Marek, J. Madden, S. Chantilis *et al.*, The effect of a comprehensive incentive program on patient participation in elective single blastocyst transfers. *Fertil. Steril.*, **84**: Suppl 1 (2005), S85–S86.
18. J. Rodriguez, J. Douglas, D. Bookout *et al.*, The effect of post-thaw blastocyst quality and the day of freeze on the clinical outcome of a blastocyst cryopreservation program. *Hum. Reprod.*, **17** (2002), 21.
19. H. Adriaanse, O. Perez, B. D. Barnett *et al.*, Assisted hatching of frozen-thawed blastocysts. Does it make a difference? *Fertil. Steril.*, **82**: Suppl 2 (2004), S117.
20. D. Ward, S. Chantilis, J. Madden *et al.*, Expectations for blastocyst cryopreservation and frozen-thawed blastocyst transfer outcomes. *Fertil. Steril.*, **84**: Suppl 1 (2005), S184.
21. K. Takahashi, T. Mukaida, T. Goto and C. Oka, Perinatal outcome of blastocyst transfer with vitrification using cryoloop: a 4-year follow-up study. *Fertil. Steril.*, **84**: 1 (2005), 88–92.
22. M. Kuwayama, G. Vajta, S. Ieda and O. Kato, Comparison of open and closed methods for vitrification of human embryos and the elimination of potential contamination. *Reprod. Biomed. Online.*, **11** (2005), 608–614.

Single embryo transfer in recipients of donated oocytes

Viveca Söderström-Anttila

Introduction

For more than two decades oocyte donation (OD) has successfully been used to treat infertility in women who lack healthy or viable oocytes. According to recently published statistics from European registers by the European Society of Human Reproduction and Embryology (ESHRE) > 7000 embryo transfers from donated oocytes were carried out in 2003 [1]. In the United States, > 13 000 embryo transfers, which is 15% of all in vitro fertilization (IVF) transfer cycles performed in 2004, involved egg donation [2].

Transfer of one embryo at a time in recipients of donated oocytes is, thus far, uncommon. There are, however, several reasons why elective single embryo transfer (SET) should increasingly be implemented in this group of patients. This chapter focuses on factors influencing the embryo transfer strategy in oocyte recipients and presents experiences from OD-SET.

Pregnancy outcome

In general, pregnancy outcome after OD treatment is good with clinical implantation and pregnancy rates (PRs) comparable to or higher than those achieved in conventional IVF [3]. The cumulative live birth rate reaches almost 90% after four OD cycles [4]. During recent years, improvements

in treatment outcome have been demonstrated in spite of a decreasing number of embryos being replaced [5]. Still, in most OD programs at least two or three embryos are routinely transferred at a time. As the implantation rate in oocyte recipients is high, the rate of multiple pregnancies has remained high, usually 30–45% [1, 5–7]. According to the last statistics from the United States, 55% of all OD infants born in 2004 originated from multiple pregnancies [2]. As repeatedly stated in this book, the multiple pregnancies will cause increased health risks both for the mother and the children.

Why SET in oocyte recipients?

Why is it essential to avoid multiples in oocyte recipients? The following background factors all support a clinical practice towards consideration of elective SET in these patients.

1. The excellent outcome in OD is due to the usage of good quality oocytes retrieved from young healthy donors, and is not dependent on the age of the recipient up to the age of at least 45 years [6, 8]. This also means that if we have a young donor, older age of the recipient will not reduce the risk of multiple pregnancies, as in conventional IVF [9].

2. Oocyte recipients include patients with special health conditions that merit attention, for example women with Turner syndrome, women over

Single Embryo Transfer, ed. J. Gerris, G. D. Adamson, P. De Sutter and C. Racowsky. Published by Cambridge University Press.

the age of 40, cancer survivors and women with autoimmune disorders. Caution should be taken with Turner women, as they are at risk of several chronic diseases, such as thyroid dysfunction, hypertension and cardiac complications. During pregnancy their risk of rupture or dissection of the aorta is estimated to be 2% or higher [10].

3. In general, there seem to be more obstetric complications, for example pregnancy-induced hypertension, even in singleton OD pregnancies, compared with standard IVF pregnancies [11–13]. The increased risk of adverse obstetric outcome does not occur merely in older but also in young recipients of donated oocytes [11]. Multiple pregnancies further increase these risks.

Outcome after SET in oocyte recipients

Worldwide, introduction of SET in OD programs has been slow. Clinics in many countries are now actively working towards the reduction of the number of embryos transferred from three to two. A recent study compared the outcome after transfer of two or three embryos and found similar PRs but significantly reduced incidence of twins and triplets following transfer of two embryos [14].

Two observational studies from the Väestöliitto Fertility Clinic in Helsinki, Finland have been published about SET in OD [15, 16]. For the past seven years at our clinic, elective SET has been recommended to all recipients of donated oocytes, if they had one good quality embryo available for transfer. A good quality embryo was defined as an embryo in the 4- to 5-cell stage on day 2 and at the 6- to 8-cell stage on day 3, with mononuclear blastomeres and fragmentation less than 20%. If there was a medical contraindication for twin pregnancy, for example diabetes, Turner syndrome, previous hysterotomy, or uterine malformation, SET was performed regardless of the quality of the embryos [15]. During 2000–4, 77% of all transfers were SET and the PR was 43.2% and delivery rate 31.1% [16]. The delivery rate

after SET was 30.4% with no twins and after double embryo transfer (DET) it was 33.3% with 40% twins. The pregnancy and delivery rates did not differ from those achieved in the late 1990s when DET was performed in the majority of regular IVF cases. However, the twin rate in the OD programme went down from 29% to 10% [15, 16]. The PR after transfer of a fresh good quality cleavage stage embryo was 55%, which was statistically significantly better than with a suboptimal quality embryo (27%; $p < 0.01$). In 2000–6, 79% of all frozen-thawed embryo transfers were SET and the clinical PR was 28%. By an active embryo freezing policy, the combination of a transfer of one embryo at a time in fresh and subsequent frozen cycles, a PR of at least 57% can be reached per recipient treatment cycle [16].

Blastocyst transfer has been shown to increase the efficiency of egg donation [7]. Prolonged culture and single blastocyst transfer could be one option for the future, for example in Turner patients and other recipients with medical contraindications for multiple pregnancy. Selection criteria for the one good embryo on day 2, 3 and 5 have been constantly refined and with accumulating knowledge more precise selection of the embryo to be transferred should be possible [17].

Counseling

Patients seeking OD treatment have often experienced disappointments in their conventional IVF cycles and they might have difficulties in accepting a cautious embryo transfer strategy [16]. These recipients need information about differences in standard IVF and OD, and why fewer OD embryos can be replaced. Risks of obstetric complications, health problems of the children and the burden of multiples for family life should also be thoroughly and objectively discussed with the couple well before the day of embryo transfer. The parents-to-be need time to consider their wishes regarding embryo transfer strategy, before the final decision is taken.

Conclusions

Today too many OD children in the world originate from multiple pregnancies, exposing them to increased risk of neonatal and long-term problems in life. Transfer of fewer embryos and increased application of SET is the obvious solution to the problem. The first step is to convince the IVF doctors that the birth of one baby at a time is really the ideal goal and that SET functions well. If the quality of the embryos is good, and supernumerary embryos can be frozen, elective SET is strongly recommended in oocyte recipients.

What do we know?

We know from observational studies that elective SET gives good pregnancy and delivery rates in oocyte recipients, if the oocyte donor is young. If more than one embryo is transferred at a time, the multiple PR is high, usually 30–40%.

What do we need to know?

We need more precise data about early embryo development to be able to select the best embryo for transfer.

What should we do?

We should recommend SET to oocyte recipients, if there is a good quality embryo available for transfer. A prospective randomized controlled study between SET and DET in oocyte recipients would help to get more exact data about SET outcome and to convince doctors and patients of a cautious embryo transfer strategy.

REFERENCES

1. A. N. Andersen, V. Goossens, L. Gianaroli *et al.*, Assisted reproductive technology in Europe, 2003. Results generated from European registers by ESHRE. *Hum. Reprod.*, **22** (2007), 1513–1525.
2. V. C. Wright, J. Chang, G. Jeng, M. Chen and M. Macaluso, Assisted reproductive technology surveillance – United States 2004. *MMWR Surveill. Summ.*, **56** (SS06) (2007), 1–22.
3. M. Sauer and S. Kavic, Ethics, social, legal, counseling. Oocyte and embryo donation 2006: reviewing two decades of innovation and controversy. *Reprod. Biomed. Online*, **12** (2006), 153–162.
4. J. Remohi, B. Gartner, E. Gallardo *et al.*, Pregnancy and birth rates after oocyte donation. *Fertil. Steril.*, **67** (1997), 717–723.
5. E. Budak, N. Garrido, S. R. Soares *et al.*, Improvements achieved in an oocyte donation program over a 10-year period: sequential increase in implantation and pregnancy rates and decrease in high-order multiple pregnancies. *Fertil. Steril.*, **88** (2007), 342–349.
6. J. P. Toner, D. A. Grainger and L. M. Frazier, Clinical outcomes among recipients of donated eggs: an analysis of the U.S. national experience, 1996–1998. *Fertil. Steril.*, **78** (2002), 1038–1045.
7. W. B. Schoolcraft and D. K. Gardner, Blastocyst culture and transfer increases the efficiency of oocyte donation. *Fertil. Steril.*, **74** (2000), 482–486.
8. M. A. Cohen, S. R. Lindheim and M. V. Sauer, Donor age is paramount to success in oocyte donation. *Hum. Reprod.*, **14** (1999), 2755–2758.
9. M. A. Reynolds, L. A. Schieve, G. Jeng *et al.*, Risk of multiple birth associated with *in vitro* fertilization using donor eggs. *Am. J. Epidemiol.*, **154** (2001), 1043–1050.
10. M. F. Karnis, A. E. Zimon, S. I. Lalwani *et al.*, Risk of death in pregnancy achieved through oocyte donation in patients with Turner syndrome: a national survey. *Fertil. Steril.*, **80** (2003), 498–501.
11. V. Söderström-Anttila, A. Tiitinen, T. Foudila and O. Hovatta, Obstetric and perinatal outcome after oocyte donation – comparison with *in vitro* fertilization pregnancies. *Hum. Reprod.*, **13** (1998), 483–490.
12. O. Salha, V. Sharma, T. Dada *et al.*, The influence of donated gametes on the incidence of hypertensive disorders of pregnancy. *Hum. Reprod.*, **14** (1999), 2268–2273.
13. D. Bodri, V. Vernaeve, F. Figueras *et al.*, Oocyte donation in patients with Turner's syndrome: a successful technique but with an accompanying high risk of hypertensive disorders during pregnancy. *Hum. Reprod.*, **21** (2006), 829–832.
14. D. Dowling-Lacey, E. Jones, J. Mayer *et al.*, Elective transfer of two embryos: reduction of multiple gestations while maintaining high pregnancy rates. *J. Assist. Reprod. Genet.*, **24** (2007), 11–15.
15. V. Söderström-Anttila, S. Vilska, S. Mäkinen, T. Foudila and A. M. Suikkari, Elective single embryo transfer

yields good delivery rates in oocyte donation. *Hum. Reprod.*, **18** (2003), 1858–1863.

16. V. Söderström-Anttila and S. Vilska, Five years of single embryo transfer with anonymous and non-anonymous oocyte donation. *Reprod. Biomed. Online*, **15** (2007), 428–433.

17. L. Scott, A. Finn, T. O'Leary, S. McLellan and J. Hill, Morphologic parameters of early cleavage-stage embryos that correlate with fetal development and delivery: prospective and applied data for increased pregnancy rates. *Hum. Reprod.*, **22** (2007), 230–240.

The impact of single embryo transfer on embryo donation

Jeffrey A. Keenan and Reginald Finger

Embryo donation (ED) is the transfer of an embryo originally created for a couple's own use, to an unrelated woman recipient as a treatment for that woman's infertility. This practice has gained widespread acceptance by the infertility community and the public for two reasons. First, ED is an excellent option to help resolve the disposition of some of the thousands of embryos that are no longer wanted by the couples who created them. Second, it is generally a less expensive and sometimes a more effective way to achieve pregnancy than autologous or donor egg in vitro fertilization (IVF). We recently documented excellent pregnancy and live birth rates seen in embryo donation in seven programs [1]. Generally, ED programs have transferred more than one embryo at a time. In fact, in our study the average number of embryos transferred was 3.05.

However, in recognition of the medical consequences of multiple pregnancy [2–4] and the resulting case for single embryo transfer (SET) that is described elsewhere in this book, it is necessary to recognize SET as a legitimate trend. Therefore we must make two assessments: first, as SET becomes more widely used in IVF generally, what is the impact of that trend on ED? Second, is there any place for the use of SET within ED itself?

No studies have yet been performed that directly assess the impact of SET on ED. Therefore, we must analyze the findings that have been published on SET to estimate what that impact might be.

If there is an impact, it would be expected to come either in the form of an increase or a decrease of cryopreserved embryos available for donation to other couples, or perhaps in a change in the viability of those embryos. It is reasonable to assume that a couple's choice to donate any remaining embryos that they may have is independent of whether they have chosen SET or double embryo transfer (DET) for themselves.

The first and most obvious factor in SET that could lead to availability of more embryos for donation is simply that it might take the couple fewer embryos to achieve pregnancy. Then they might cryopreserve, and perhaps donate, the rest.

In the simplest case scenario (scenario A), a couple has just two embryos and intend to achieve just one pregnancy. If they choose DET they will have no embryos left to donate, regardless of the outcome. If they choose SET and the first transfer is successful, they will have one embryo to donate. If not, they would have a second transfer procedure, thus having none left to donate. In this scenario, the number of additional embryos for donation resulting from SET is (the implantation rate of the first embryo) × (the number of couples choosing SET).

A couple with more embryos at the start would come up with essentially the same result, though the

Single Embryo Transfer, ed. J. Gerris, G. D. Adamson, P. De Sutter and C. Racowsky. Published by Cambridge University Press.
© Cambridge University Press 2009.

calculation would be more complicated – so long as each couple foregoes additional transfers once a pregnancy has been fully established.

Data from Europe, however, show that couples choosing SET have an average of 1.1 more embryos cryopreserved [5, 6] but also undergo an average of 1.1 more frozen transfer cycles [6] than those choosing DET. In other words, they are not following the pattern of scenario A but are, for the most part, going ahead and transferring the additional frozen embryo themselves rather than stopping after a successful fresh SET (scenario B).

We do not know whether the experience in the USA would come closer to scenario A or to scenario B. In 2005, the average number of embryos transferred per cycle in the USA in women under age 35 was 2.4 [7], so it is likely that changing to SET would create about one more embryo cryopreserved per cycle, just as in Europe. However, because most couples in the USA have to pay for their own treatment, and cycles are expensive, the number of additional frozen transfer cycles in the USA might average less than one. That is, more couples might follow scenario A than in Europe. Our experience tells us that there are couples pursuing IVF who want just one child, and so who at least in theory would be potential candidates to donate embryos after successful SET.

To assess this possibility further, it would help to know how many IVF-conceived children the average couple has when they cease infertility treatments. We do not, however, have findings on this item to cite.

One factor in SET that could lead to fewer embryos available is that with SET couples have very few twins. They might experience less stress, having one baby at a time, and thus might continue with IVF efforts as long as they have embryos available.

Recently, blastocyst stage transfer has become more widely used by programs practicing SET [8]. The impact of switching to blastocyst stage transfer on the number of embryos available for donation might also be either positive or negative.

Blastocyst transfer could result in more embryos available for donation because implantation rates with blastocysts are generally higher [8, 9] than those documented in IVF transfers performed at the cleavage stage [7]. Higher success rate on the first (fresh) cycle could mean more embryos available for donation.

However, a possible impact in the opposite direction is that blastocyst stage transfer results in *fewer embryos available* for the fresh transfer [8]. Even though one would suspect that an embryo that died before reaching the blastocyst stage would have a poor implantation potential, evidence exists that some of them might have survived in utero [10] and so possibly in cryostorage as well. Certainly, as culture systems continue to improve, one would expect this potential negative consequence to decrease or be eliminated.

Overall, however, we believe it is likely that implementation of SET would slightly increase the number of embryos available for donation in the USA.

The other major issue to consider is whether SET has a place in donated frozen embryo transfer itself ("elective single frozen embryo transfer", or eSFET). Hydén-Granskog *et al.* in Finland showed pregnancy rates for eSFET equal to those for double frozen embryo transfer (DFET) [11]. Le Lannou *et al.*, by contrast, showed a lower rate for SET than for DET in cryopreserved embryos (14.4% vs. 23.5%) [6]. In ED practice, many couples may decline eSFET because of the low pregnancy rate, especially because cycles are expensive and they may not be able to afford additional cycles if they do not succeed the first time. However, when all the options are explained, some ED couples might choose SET because of the medical complications of twins.

At the National Embryo Donation Center, the current policy is to allow couples a maximum of three cycles to achieve pregnancy. In consideration of a probable lower pregnancy rate with eSFET, this policy might have to be modified for couples choosing eSFET.

Another barrier to be overcome is that most embryos come to our center frozen in units of two to three. If not all embryos thawed are then transferred, some would have to be refrozen. Refreezing compromises the embryo's survival chances enough that if one's goal is to give the embryo the best chance at survival, most would choose to go ahead and transfer all viable embryos from the thaw and take the risk of a multiple birth.

In summary, eSET is an expanding practice that could potentially have a significant impact on ED and adoption. It seems likely that it could increase the number of embryos available for donation to other infertile couples, thus improving the access to this treatment option. However, there are many variables which cannot yet be estimated, and so the final outcome remains uncertain. Finally, eSFET is a viable option that should be discussed with ED recipients, but one that would probably be chosen by a minority of them.

We look forward to the publication of more research directed at both of these policy questions.

REFERENCES

1. J. Keenan, R. Finger, J. H. Check *et al.*, Favorable pregnancy, delivery, and implantation rates experienced in embryo donation programs in the United States. *Fertil. Steril.*, Epub ahead of print.
2. O. Kor-anantakul, C. Suwanrath, T. Suntharasaj, C. Getpook and R. Leetanaporn, Outcomes of multifetal pregnancies. *J. Obstet. Gynaecol. Res.*, **33** (2007), 49–55.
3. W. F. Powers and J. L. Kiely, The risks confronting twins: a national perspective. *Am. J. Obstet. Gynecol.*, **170** (1994), 456–461.
4. B. Blondel, M. D. Kogan, G. Alexander *et al.*, The impact of the increasing number of multiple births on the rates of preterm birth and low birthweight: an international study. *Am. J. Public Health*, **92** (2002), 1323–1330.
5. D. De Neubourg and J. Gerris, Single embryo transfer – state of the art. *Reprod. Biomed. Online*, **7** (2003), 615–622.
6. D. Le Lannou, J.-F. Griveau, M.-C. Laurent *et al.*, Contribution of embryo cryopreservation to elective single embryo transfer in IVF-ICSI. *Reprod. Biomed. Online*, **13** (2006), 368–375.
7. www.sart.org.
8. D. K. Gardner, E. Surrey, D. Minjarez *et al.*, Single blastocyst transfer: a prospective randomized trial. *Fertil. Steril.*, **81** (2004), 551–555.
9. L. L. Veeck, R. Bodine, R. N. Clarke *et al.*, High pregnancy rates can be achieved after freezing and thawing human blastocysts. *Fertil. Steril.*, **82** (2004), 1418–1427.
10. S. Coskun, J. Hollanders, S. Al-Hassan *et al.*, Day 5 versus day 3 embryo transfer: a controlled randomized trial. *Hum. Reprod.*, **15** (2000), 1947–1952.
11. C. Hydén-Granskog, L. Unkila-Kallio, M. Halttunen and A. Tiitinen, Single embryo transfer is an option in frozen embryo transfer. *Hum. Reprod.*, **20** (2005), 2935–2938.

SET in unique clinical situations: single women, lesbians

Karen J. Purcell

Legal aspects

Single women and lesbian couples requesting medical intervention to create a family have been met with varied responses from society and the medical profession [1–3]. Only some countries permit single women to undergo assisted reproductive technology (ART) including Australia, Belgium, Brazil, Canada, Chile, Hungary, India, Israel, Latvia, Netherlands, New Zealand, Peru, Russia, South Africa, United Kingdom, United States and Vietnam. Even fewer countries permit ART use by lesbian couples, including Belgium, Canada, Israel, Netherlands, New Zealand, United Kingdom, Australia, Brazil, South Africa and the United States.

However, even in countries that permit such treatment, there may be laws or regulations regarding the use of donor sperm [3]. In countries such as the Netherlands, Norway, Sweden and the United Kingdom, only known donor sperm may be used whereas in Singapore, Slovenia and Vietnam, only anonymous sperm donors may be used. Alternatively, there may be no legal barriers to providing ART for single women or lesbian couples but access to care in certain regions of the country may be limited given the social climate of the surrounding population or the personal judgment of the physician or clinical staff. Such inconsistencies have led patients to travel to other countries or to other regions within the same country in order to obtain care, a phenomenon commonly termed "reproductive tourism."

Medical aspects

Single women and lesbian couples are expected to have similar fertility risks as their married or heterosexual counterparts, although this may not be correct. The largest difference with this group of patients is the duration of infertility, as they have not had repetitive exposure to sperm in attempts to conceive. As a result, single women and lesbian couples may have fertility more similar to the general population, not the infertile population who may not have conceived even after standard fertility treatment and/or ART. Therefore, single women and lesbians can usually be considered a favorable population for single embryo transfer (SET). However, it is still important to assess their fertility status carefully by taking a comprehensive history regarding infertility factors and possible past exposure to pregnancy through heterosexual sexual relationships, donor sperm insemination or prior ART treatments. Assuming patients have the similar risk factors to the general population, evaluation prior to treatment is often dictated by patient age.

For heterosexual couples, complete evaluation is recommended after 1 year of ovulatory cycles if the patient is less than 35 years old [4]. As age is an important predictor of fertility, a shorter time

Single Embryo Transfer, ed. J. Gerris, G. D. Adamson, P. De Sutter and C. Racowsky. Published by Cambridge University Press.
© Cambridge University Press 2009.

frame is appropriate for older women. Studies have shown that in married women using no contraception, 85% of women eventually achieved pregnancy if less than 35 years old, while only 70% had a child if between ages 35 and 39, and only 64% at age 40 or older [5]. Additionally, most conceptions using donor inseminations occur within the first three to six cycles and therefore patients utilizing donor sperm are often counseled to assess pelvic and hormonal factors at that point even if history would not warrant it. However, given the expense and logistics involved with donor sperm, an appropriately thorough evaluation prior to any attempted conception with donor sperm is also reasonable.

Treatment of single women and lesbian couples has traditionally been approached in a stepwise manner similar to heterosexual couples with complete male factor infertility. Inseminations of donor sperm are performed first. If the woman is young and there are no pelvic or ovulatory factors involved, natural cycles timed for appropriate insemination are performed and if unsuccessful after a certain duration, ovarian stimulation with either clomiphene citrate or gonadotropin injections will be added in an effort to increase the pregnancy rate. If the patient is older, ovarian stimulation with insemination is often considered first, rather than unstimulated cycles. Treatments with insemination have been shown to have an average cycle fecundity of 10.6% [6], with significant differences seen according to the age of the female. For patients less than 35 years old, one study had a pregnancy rate per cycle of 18.5%, if between 35 and 40 years old of 11.9% and if the female was over 40 as low as 5.4%. The cumulative pregnancy rate after eight cycles was 86%, 51% and 32% respectively.

If treatment with insemination has not produced a child after 3 to 12 cycles, only then are women counseled to proceed to in vitro fertilization (IVF), unless the age of the woman is over 40, when direct progression to IVF is recommended [5]. This traditional stepwise approach requires minimal intervention and overall less cost compared with proceeding with ART. However, IVF may be considered initially or after a short duration of attempts with insemination, for several reasons. Given the low cycle fecundity rates with insemination, physicians and patients will often consider treatment with IVF either directly or after only three cycles of inseminations, especially in women with advancing age. Engmann [7] showed that the cumulative pregnancy rate after three cycles of IVF was 57.8% in women over 40.

For single women, proceeding to IVF instead of stimulated insemination cycles has an additional attraction. The option to perform elective SET (eSET) would decrease the risk of multiples, which was found to be approximately one in five in single women undergoing insemination [8].

For lesbian couples, proceeding with ART and eSET also decreases the risk of multiples. However, utilizing the oocytes of one partner to create an embryo which is transferred to the other partner allows both partners to have a link to the child: one as the genetic mother and the other as the biological or birth mother. Within the United States, there are states, such as California, which recognize homosexual partnerships as legal entities having the same rights as heterosexual married couples. In this situation, both partners retain the legal rights of parenting. In other states or in other countries, the partner "donating" her oocyte has no legal parenting rights and only the birth mother maintains those rights. This legislation also contributes to reproductive tourism.

REFERENCES

1. H. Jones, J. Cohen, I. Cooke and R. Kempers, IFFS surveillance 07: marital status. *Fertil. Steril.*, **87** (2007), S17–S18.
2. H. Jones, J. Cohen, I. Cooke and R. Kempers, IFFS surveillance 07: legislation and guidelines. *Fertil. Steril.*, **87** (2007), S8–S13.
3. H. Jones, J. Cohen, I. Cooke and R. Kempers, IFFS surveillance 07: donation. *Fertil. Steril.*, **87** (2007), S28–S32.
4. The Practice Committee of the American Society of Reproductive Medicine. Optimal evaluation of the infertile female. *Fertil. Steril.*, **86** (2006), S264–S267.
5. The Practice Committee of the American Society of Reproductive Medicine. Aging and infertility in women. *Fertil. Steril.*, **86** (2006), S248–S251.

6. I. Ferrara, R. Balet and J. Grudzinskas, Intrauterine insemination with frozen donor sperm. Pregnancy outcome in relation to age and ovarian stimulation regime. *Hum. Reprod.*, **17** (2002), 2320–2324.

7. L. Engmann, N. Maconochie, J. Bekir, H. Jacobs and S. Tan, Cumulative probability of clinical pregnancy and live birth after a multiple cycle IVF package: a more realistic assessment of overall and age-specific success rates? *Br. J. Obstet. Gynaecol.*, **106** (1999), 165–170.

8. R. Weissenberg, R. Landau and I. Madgar, Older single mothers assisted by sperm donation and their children. *Hum. Reprod.*, **22** (2007), 2784–2791.

Preimplantation genetic diagnosis and single embryo transfer

Willem Verpoest

Introduction

Preimplantation genetic diagnosis (PGD) offers couples affected by a genetic disorder an alternative to prenatal diagnosis by chorion villus sampling (CVS) or amniocentesis. Preimplantation genetic aneuploidy screening (PGS) allows ploidy analysis of embryos prior to embryo transfer, thereby reducing the risk of numerical chromosomal abnormalities. Ever since the first application of PGD in the early 1990s [1, 2], it is now well established as a technique, in spite of an ongoing debate about its diagnostic accuracy and clinical relevance [3, 4]. The issues that will be discussed are (1) the implications of single embryo transfer (SET) on clinical reproductive outcome of PGD and (2) the potential benefit of PGS in improving clinical reproductive outcome of SET.

Clinical application of PGD

Preimplantation genetic diagnosis uses polymerase chain reaction (PCR) or fluorescent *in situ* hybridization (FISH), and is applied for over 100 indications ranging from single gene disorders, including late-onset disorders with genetic predisposition, to structural chromosomal abnormalities including reciprocal and Robertsonian translocations [5, 6] (Table 10D.1). In spite of a lack of randomized studies of the clinical efficiency of PGD, there is little controversy about its usefulness [7].

Preimplantation genetic aneuploidy screening is a technique allowing chromosomal aneuploidy analysis by FISH in pre-transfer embryos following in vitro fertilization (IVF) or intracytoplasmic sperm injection (ICSI), and can be considered as an early form of prenatal screening for numerical chromosomal abnormalities (Figure 10D.1). Many studies have argued a potential benefit of PGS in couples at high risk of chromosomally abnormal embryos, including in cases of advanced maternal age [8–11], recurrent miscarriage [12–16] and recurrent implantation failure [17, 18], whereas other authors have not been able to find an unequivocal benefit [19, 20] or have found restrictions to the clinical benefit when a low number of embryos is available for analysis [10, 11]. The clinical benefit of PGS in improving live birth rate may therefore be under scrutiny, but this technique may appear to be useful in improving selection of euploid embryos, thereby reducing implantation failure and miscarriage rates (for review see [21]).

PGD and SET

Preimplantation genetic diagnosis is performed either on a polar body, sequential polar bodies, blastomeres, or trophectoderm cells from an embryo.

Single Embryo Transfer, ed. J. Gerris, G. D. Adamson, P. De Sutter and C. Racowsky. Published by Cambridge University Press. © Cambridge University Press 2009.

Table 10D.1 Most commonly used indications for PGD or PGS

PGD	
1. Autosomal recessive	cystic fibrosis
	beta-thalassemia
	spinal muscular atrophy
	sickle-cell anemia
2. Autosomal dominant	epidermolysis bullosa
	myotonic dystrophy type 1
	Huntington's disease
	amyloid polyneuropathy
	Charcot-Marie-Tooth disease
	achondroplasia
	Marfan's syndrome
3. Specific sex-linked	Duchenne muscular dystrophy
	fragile-X syndrome
	hemophilia
4. Structural chromosomal abnormalities	Robertsonian translocations
	reciprocal translocations
	sex chromosome aneuploidy

PGS	
1. Advanced maternal age	
2. Recurrent implantation failure	
3. Recurrent miscarriage	
4. Severe male factor infertility	

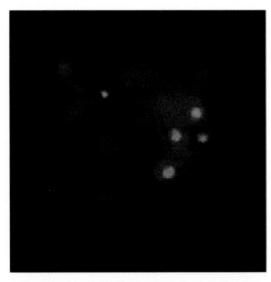

Figure 10D.1 Trisomic blastomere. See color plate section.

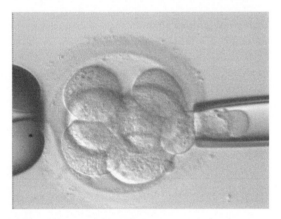

Figure 10D.2 Blastomere biopsy.

All biopsy techniques have in common that an opening is made in the zona pellucida, prior to removal of the organelle, usually by means of laser, by means of needles (polar body biopsy) or by an acidic solution such as Tyrode's (blastomere biopsy) (Figures 10D.2 and 10D.3). There is no in vivo [22] or in vitro [23] evidence that this breech of the zona pellucida significantly impairs further embryo development. More-recent data show that even multiple micromanipulations for PGD do not affect embryo development to the blastocyst stage [24]. In spite of technical progress in embryo biopsy and sequential culture techniques, and despite reports that SET at blastocyst stage gives a significantly better outcome than at cleavage stage [25], there is still considerable apprehension about embryo quality following PGD, not in the least because cryopreservation results remain disappointing in comparison to cleavage stage cryopreservation results [26–28].

Data on PGD and SET is rare. Given the genetic background of the patients, the cost and often the relative inaccessibility of the treatment, PGD clinic protocols often suggest higher-order embryo transfer. However, a retrospective study [29] comparing reproductive outcome in PGD treatment cycles prior to and after the legal implementation of SET in women under 36 years did not show the delivery

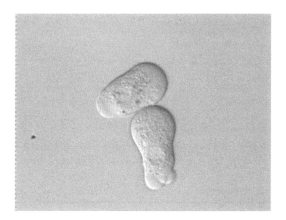

Figure 10D.3 Biopsied blastomeres.

rate to be affected, in spite of a trend towards a lower delivery rate in SET. Further prospective research is required to improve on statistical power and document the implications of SET in patients undergoing PGD for structural chromosomal abnormalities, a group particularly affected by a high abnormality rate at PGD.

PGS and SET

Knowing that even in young patients, the rate of numerical chromosomal abnormalities in embryos is remarkably high following ovarian stimulation for IVF/ICSI [30, 31], some authors argue that PGS may be as useful for this group of patients as for patients at higher risk of developing aneuploid embryos [30], not in the least if a restriction in number of embryos for transfer is introduced. However, in contrast to what one would expect in terms of increased pregnancy rates when SET is combined with PGS, this was not observed in the only prospectively randomized data set presented so far by Staessen *et al.* [32]. The observed euploid embryo rate in this study was 61.6%, in a population of 91 patients with a mean age of 29.9 years. Compared to a control group of 84 couples with an identical mean age, where no PGS was performed, the ongoing pregnancy rate per SET was not significantly different in spite of PGS (47.4% with PGS vs. 42.8% without PGS) [32].

Conclusion and scope

Single embryo transfer does not seem to affect reproductive outcome in PGD, but larger prospective series are needed to assess cumulative reproductive outcome including frozen-thawed embryo transfer, as well as to analyze different (prognostically poor) subgroups. Further development of biopsy techniques and cryopreservation techniques should produce cumulative success rates similar to those of regular IVF/ICSI. Selection of blastocysts with a normal chromosomal complement by single cell PGS does not appear to improve ongoing pregnancy rate or implantation rate in SET.

REFERENCES

1. A. H. Handyside, E. H. Kontogianni, K. Hardy and R. M. L. Winston, Pregnancies from biopsied human preimplantation embryos sexed by Y-specific DNA amplification. *Nature*, **344** (1990), 768–770.
2. Y. Verlinsky, N. Ginsberg, A. Lifchez and C. Strom, Analysis of the first polar body: preconception genetic diagnosis. *Hum. Reprod.*, **5** (1990), 826–829.
3. L. K. Shahine and M. I. Cedars, Preimplantation genetic diagnosis does not increase pregnancy rates in patients at risk for aneuploidy. *Fertil. Steril.* **85** (2006), 51–56.
4. M. Twisk, S. Mastenbroek, M. van Wely *et al.*, Preimplantation genetic screening for abnormal number of chromosomes (aneuploidies) in in vitro fertilisation or intracytoplasmic sperm injection. *Cochrane Database Syst. Rev.*, **1** (2006), CD005291.
5. A. Kuliev and Y. Verlinsky, Place of preimplantation diagnosis in genetic practice. *Am. J. Med. Genet.*, **134A** (2005), 105–110.
6. J. C. Harper, C. de Die-Smulders, V. Goossens *et al.*, ESHRE PGD consortium data collection VII: cycles from January to December 2004 with pregnancy following to October 2005. *Hum. Reprod.*, **23** (2008), 741–755.
7. J. A. Collins, Preimplantation genetic screening in older mothers. *N. Engl. J. Med.*, **357** (2007), 61–63.
8. L. Gianaroli, M. C. Magli, A. P. Ferraretti and S. Munné, Preimplantation genetic diagnosis for aneuploidies in patients undergoing in vitro fertilization with a poor prognosis: identification of the categories for which it should be proposed. *Fertil. Steril.*, **72** (1999), 837–844.

9. A. Kuliev and Y. Verlinsky, The role of preimplantation genetic diagnosis in women of advanced reproductive age. *Curr. Opin. Obstet. Gynecol.*, **15** (2003), 233–238.

10. S. Munné, E. M. Sandalinas, T. Escudero *et al.*, Improved implantation after genetic diagnosis of aneuploidy. *Reprod. Biomed. Online*, **7** (2003), 91–97.

11. P. Platteau, C. Staessen, A. Michiels *et al.*, Preimplantation genetic diagnosis for aneuploidy screening in women older than 37 years. *Fertil. Steril.*, **84** (2005a), 319–324.

12. A. Pellicer, C. Rubio, F. Vidal *et al.*, In vitro fertilisation plus preimplantation genetic diagnosis in patients with recurrent miscarriage: an analysis of chromosome abnormalities in human preimplantation embryos. *Fertil. Steril.*, **71** (1999), 1033–1039.

13. C. Rubio, T. Pehlivan, L. Rodrigo *et al.*, Embryo aneuploidy screening for unexplained recurrent miscarriage: a mini-review. *Am. J. Reprod. Immunol.*, **53** (2005), 159–165.

14. L. Gianaroli, C. Magli, A. Ferraretti *et al.*, Beneficial effects of PGD for aneuploidy support extensive clinical application. *Reprod. Biomed. Online*, **10** (2005), 633–640.

15. S. Munné, S. Chen, J. Fischer *et al.*, Preimplantation genetic diagnosis reduces pregnancy loss in women aged 35 years and older with a history of recurrent miscarriages. *Fertil. Steril.*, **84** (2005), 331–335.

16. P. Platteau, C. Staessen, A. Michiels *et al.*, Preimplantation genetic diagnosis for aneuploidy screening in patients with unexplained recurrent miscarriages. *Fertil. Steril.*, **83** (2005b), 393–397.

17. T. Pehlivan, C. Rubio, L. Rodrigo *et al.*, Impact of preimplantation genetic diagnosis on IVF outcome in implantation failure patients. *Reprod. Biomed. Online*, **6** (2003), 232–237.

18. M. Wilding, R. Forman, G. Hogewind *et al.*, Preimplantation genetic diagnosis for the treatment of failed in vitro fertilisation-embryo transfer and habitual abortion. *Fertil. Steril.*, **81** (2004), 1302–1304.

19. C. Staessen, P. Platteau, E. Van Assche *et al.*, Comparison of blastocyst transfer with or without preimplantation genetic diagnosis for aneuploidy screening in couples with advanced maternal age: a prospective randomized controlled trial. *Hum. Reprod.*, **19** (2004), 2849–2858.

20. S. Mastenbroek, M. Twisk, J. van Echten-Arends, In vitro fertilization with preimplantation genetic screening. *N. Engl. J. Med.*, **357** (2007), 61–63.

21. P. Donoso, C. Staessen, B. Fauser and P. Devroey, Current value of preimplantation genetic aneuploidy screening in IVF. *Hum. Reprod. Update*, **13** (2007a), 15–25.

22. L. Gianaroli, M. C. Magli, A. P. Ferraretti *et al.*, Preimplantation genetic diagnosis increases the implantation rate in human in vitro fertilization by avoiding the transfer of chromosomally aneuploid embryos. *Fertil. Steril.*, **68** (1997), 1128–1131.

23. K. Hardy, K. L. Martin, H. J. Leese, R. M. Winston and A. H. Handyside, Human preimplantation development in vitro is not affected by biopsy at the 8-cell stage. *Hum. Reprod.*, **5** (1990), 708–714.

24. J. Cieslak-Janzen, I. Tur-Kapsa, Y. Ilkevitch *et al.*, Multiple micromanipulations for preimplantation genetic diagnosis do not affect embryo development to the blastocyst stage. *Fertil. Steril.*, **85** (2006), 1826–1829.

25. E. G. Papanikolaou, M. Camus, E. M. Kolibianakis *et al.*, In vitro fertilization with single blastocyst-stage versus single cleavage-stage embryos. *N. Engl. J. Med.*, **354** (2006), 1139–1146.

26. H. Joris, E. Van den Abbeel, A. De Vos and A. Van Steirteghem, Reduced survival after human embryo biopsy and subsequent cryopreservation. *Hum. Reprod.*, **14** (1999), 2833–2837.

27. M. C. Magli, L. Gianaroli, D. Fortini, A. P. Ferraretti and S. Munné, Impact of blastomere biopsy and cryopreservation techniques on human embryo viability. *Hum. Reprod.*, **14** (1999), 770–773.

28. W. Verpoest, M. Bonduelle, E. Van den Abbeel *et al.*, The reproductive outcome of cryopreservation and thawing of blastocysts after biopsy for preimplantation genetic diagnosis. *Hum. Reprod.*, **22** (2007), 208.

29. P. Donoso, W. Verpoest, E. G. Papanikolau *et al.*, Single embryo transfer in preimplantation genetic diagnosis cycles for women < 36 years does not reduce delivery rate. *Hum. Reprod.*, **22** (2007b), 1021–1025.

30. S. Munné, M. Sandalinas, C. Magh *et al.*, Increased rate of aneuploid embryos in young women with previous aneuploid conceptions. *Prenat. Diagn.*, **24** (2004), 638–643.

31. E. B. Baart, E. Martini, I. van den Berg *et al.*, Preimplantation genetic screening reveals a high incidence of aneuploidy and mosaicism in embryos from young women undergoing IVF. *Hum. Reprod.*, **21** (2006), 223–233.

32. C. Staessen, A. Michiels, W. Verpoest *et al.*, Does PGS improve pregnancy rates in young patients with single-embryo transfer? *Hum. Reprod.*, **22**: suppl 1 (2007), i32.

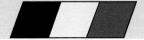

Figure 3.1 The Belgian funding system if IVF/ICSI.

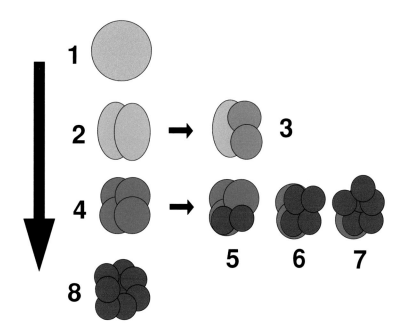

Figure 8.4 Relative cell sizes during mitotic divisions.

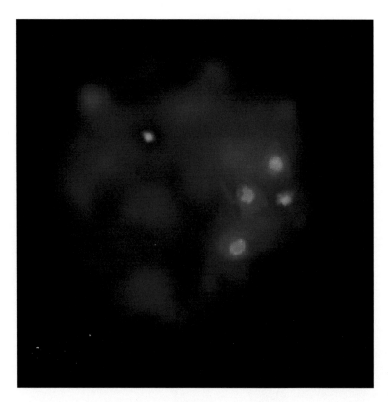

Figure 10D.1 Trisomic blastomere.

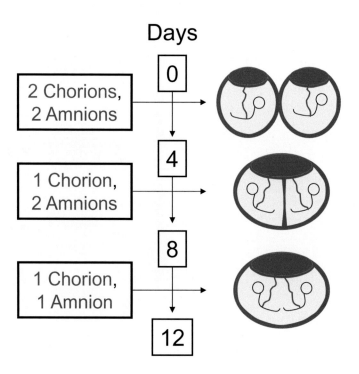

Figure 17.1 Time-sensitive placental development in monozygotic twins.

Counseling patients for single embryo transfer

Sharon N. Covington

Introduction

Technological advances in reproductive medicine in the last quarter-century have offered couples options for parenthood previously beyond most people's imagination. Retrieval of oocytes, fertilization occurring outside the womb and a woman carrying a child that is not biologically related to her are but a few examples of the mind-boggling methods couples may be exposed to in their quest for a baby. Assisted reproductive technology (ART) has given couples more choices in the pursuit of parenthood, while at the same time creating more challenges in the families that are formed by ART. Multiple pregnancies have increased dramatically across the globe and the associated complications, both medically and psychosocially, have become an even greater concern. However, the concern seems more often carried by medical professionals than by infertile couples – in fact, many patients prefer multiples to a singleton [1, 2].

When couples are willing to go to such lengths to have a child, how do we as caregivers provide them assistance in making the best decision, not just for their immediate desires but for the long-term health of their family? Counseling on the medical and psychosocial aspects of multiple pregnancy is the foundation for patient decision-making on elective single embryo transfer (eSET). This chapter will describe the psychological context for patients

considering eSET, factors affecting the choice they make, the role of counseling and approaches to use to assist in decision-making.

The psychological context of eSET

Procreation is fundamental to existence and is defined by social, cultural, legal, psychological and religious norms. The ability to reproduce affects an individual's sense of self, relationship with others, status within the community and position in society. When one's ability to reproduce is thwarted, a psychosocial crisis ensues involving grief and loss that have been well documented in the literature. The losses are multifaceted and numerous, yet personal and unique, involving health, well-being, life-goals, prestige, current and future relationships, and on and on. These losses precipitate a grief response with feelings of shock, disbelief, anger, sadness, shame, blame and guilt. Because of the extended nature of treatment and since the losses of infertility are often invisible to others (i.e., no baby, looking healthy to others, etc.), it is difficult to "mourn" in the traditional sense and couples may find themselves suffering alone. Over time, repeated failure to become pregnant or successfully gestate creates feelings of loss of control, diminished self-esteem, anxiety, depression and chronic bereavement that may persist, with the potential to continue

Single Embryo Transfer, ed. J. Gerris, G. D. Adamson, P. De Sutter and C. Racowsky. Published by Cambridge University Press.
© Cambridge University Press 2009.

throughout treatment and beyond. Thus, infertility can be a painful, psychologically traumatic and life-altering phenomenon that is both isolating and stigmatizing [3].

The distress of infertility creates powerful mood states for many patients or may exacerbate pre-existing psychological conditions in others. Some studies have shown that many women identify infertility as the most distressing event in their lives, more distressing than the loss of a loved one or divorce [4, 5]. Men also report significant emotional distress associated with the diagnosis and treatment of infertility [6, 7] and increased emotional distress over time for both sexes has been shown, due to repeated treatment failures [7, 8]. Symptoms of depression and anxiety are common with infertile patients [9] and may be correlated to the length of treatment [10]. One study found that symptoms of depression and anxiety in infertile women were as prevalent as in patients with other serious, chronic health conditions, such as cancer and hypertension [11]. It should be pointed out that the prevalence of symptoms of depression and anxiety in women undergoing infertility treatment is an international finding, which has been documented in multiple cultures, including Japan, China, Taiwan, Korea, Kuwait and many European countries [12].

Most couples entering an ART program see in vitro fertilization (IVF) as their last, best option for having a child. They usually enter treatment after many months or sometimes years of treatment failure, often at tremendous emotional, physical and financial cost. They may be burdened with grief and disappointment from infertility, acting depressed, angry, tired, dependent and anxious. Although emotionally depleted, couples are attracted to a technology that offers hope and may find themselves drawn into new emotional turbulence of contrasting feelings of hope and despair, which is generated in part by the experience of the technology itself [13].

The intensity and high-tech nature of ART create a stressful atmosphere, where the stakes are high and the chance of success may be relatively low. Assisted reproductive technology is perceived as a gamble, and, like gamblers, patients may have unrealistically high expectations of success [14–16] or feel compelled to try "just one more time" finding it difficult to end treatment without success. Of all infertility treatments, IVF is considered the most stressful [17, 18] with 80% of patients ranking it as extremely or moderately stressful [19].

In order to cope with the psychological trauma of infertility, certain psychological defense mechanisms may be activated. Defense mechanisms are an intra-psychic process used to provide relief from emotional distress, conflict and pain. They are usually unconscious, that is the person is not aware he or she is using it, and seek to protect the psyche of the individual from anxiety, guilt, or loss of self-esteem. Defense mechanisms serve many purposes, reducing emotional conflict, alleviating the effects of traumatic experiences, softening failure or disappointment and, in general, help the individual maintain a sense of adequacy and personal worth. Defense mechanisms, such as avoidance or withdrawal, may be helpful to infertility patients in the short-run to assist in getting through difficult situations (e.g., being invited to a baby shower), but become problematic when they become the primary means of coping. When needing to make important treatment decisions, infertility patients commonly may use denial (the refusal to accept the reality of certain things), repression (the refusal to think about certain things), detachment (distancing emotionally) and minimization (accepting a reality but "watering it down") that distort information being given. Caregivers need to understand the function of these defenses to the individual being counseled (i.e., fear of failure) to find ways to help him or her take in the reality.

Factors affecting attitude and choice of eSET

Patients undergoing IVF may be influenced by varying factors while making a decision about the number of embryos to transfer and the possibility of multiple pregnancies. It is well documented in the literature that infertility patients tend to underestimate the risks associated with multiple births as they weigh the prospect of pregnancy itself during ART treatment. A number of studies have shown that, when given the choice, a significant number of patients prefer the possibility of a multiple birth to a singleton [1, 20, 21] and their desire is, most understandably, related to two factors: a long-standing history of infertility and no previous children. Thus, the longer patients have been trying to become pregnant without success, the more likely they are to want to achieve their dream family quickly. In addition, a prior history of IVF treatment was found to be a significant variable in one study [22] yet not a factor in another [23].

The age of a woman undergoing treatment may, also, be a factor in choice of eSET. Newton and colleagues found that older women were more likely to prefer transfer of three or four embryos as they believed it would increase their chance of pregnancy and limit involvement with treatment, as opposed to desiring a twin pregnancy [23]. On the opposite spectrum, Ryan and associates found a significant correlation between a patient's younger age and the desire for a multiple birth, speculating that younger women may underestimate the physical and economic resources need to raise multiple children [1]. Further, financial concerns may factor into decision-making, since patients with lower income or limited insurance benefits may want to try and maximize their chance for pregnancy in the least number of treatment cycles [1, 24].

A patient's risk-taking attitude may be another factor in choice, with the willingness to take or not take risks based on knowledge about multiple pregnancy and chance of achieving pregnancy with eSET. Couples undergoing infertility treatment may not be aware of risks of perinatal complication associated with multiple gestations. However, a number of studies have demonstrated that when they are given appropriate medical information, patients are risk sensitive and likely to change their desires based on their perception of overall risk [22, 23, 25–27]. A patient's attitude towards risk, whether they are normally cautious or less cautious, will need to be taken into consideration and information adapted to ensure informed consent.

Mood and emotional state may, also, influence decision-making and lead patients to be less risk averse. Strong mood states have been shown to affect risk taking in other situations, such as gambling, but have not been looked at with regards to decision-making during IVF. In an intriguing new study, Newton and associates investigated the role of mood, infertility stress and risk-taking behavior in decision-making regarding embryo transfer. One hundred and twenty-nine female infertility patients answered a standardized questionnaire measuring moods such as anxiety, depression, anger and fatigue, and were given a total score of overall emotional distress. They also filled out a form assessing infertility-specific stress, and then rated their desirability for a multiple birth versus a singleton pregnancy as well as perception of risk. The authors found a strong correlation between negative mood state and multiple embryo transfer, with women estimating the likelihood of having a multiple pregnancy lower when they were experiencing negative moods. In addition, they found that infertility stress was associated with a preference for a multiple pregnancy, but not with the perceptions of risk. The authors surmised that negative moods lead women to be less risk averse and knowingly make more risky choices [28].

In summary, many factors influence choices patients make regarding embryo transfer and their attitudes towards multiple birth. Factors such as patient age, how long they have been undergoing infertility treatment, prior ART treatment failure, income, insurance and emotional state should be taken into consideration when counseling patients. Efforts should be made to tailor information to each patient, understanding that a "one size fits all" approach will be least effective in working towards the goal of eSET with appropriate patients.

Role of counseling

There is growing evidence that counseling and education is the single most important variable in patient decision-making regarding the number of embryos to transfer. What information is communicated, how it is presented, when and by whom has a profound effect in how it is received by a patient. The role of counseling is fundamental in patient care, providing the opportunity for understanding, changing of attitudes and beliefs, and ensuring that patients are in the best place possible to make true informed consent. Counseling is collaboration between patient and healthcare provider, involving sharing of information, listening and giving advice, which allows decisions to be made and change to take place.

Counseling is a communication process of offering and receiving ideas, thoughts and feelings and, as such, must take place along a continuum of care. It also involves a relationship between doctor and patient that is built upon trust, honesty and safety. Communication and education regarding the rational behind eSET and the risk of multiples must start at the beginning of ART treatment, not at the time of embryo transfer or after learning of a multiple pregnancy. In addition, counseling must be individualized and include a discussion about the patient's understanding about treatment, as well as hopes and expectations regarding outcome – is it for one baby or more than one? If it is for twins (or more), why does the patient feel that way? One patient might want to put treatment behind by having several babies at once, while another may be a twin herself and always dreamed of having a family like the one she grew up in. Each patient's knowledge and experience is different so that no assumptions should be made as to what or why s/he thinks a certain way. With a better understanding of where a patient is coming from and their hopes about treatment, the physician can begin the process of providing suitable information and advice.

The counseling role extends beyond the doctor–patient relationship to the broader community. Physicians must take the lead in the counseling process, beginning with educating themselves, their staff and the public about what is "success" in IVF as well as the maternal, neonatal and pediatric risks of multiple gestations [1]. The discussion needs to extend further to legislators and insurance companies with physicians advocating the medical and financial benefits to these groups and their constituents of covering the cost of IVF to reduce multiple births [29]. Decision-making is not made in a vacuum between doctor and patient, and is influenced by family members, friends, social values, norms, finances, etc, so that counseling must go beyond this relationship.

While physicians may have the lead role in the counseling, patient autonomy must be respected. Patient autonomy is considered a fundamental principal in bioethics and patient care. In a free society, reproductive rights, including the right to choose the transfer of more than one embryo, must be considered in treatment decisions. However, as Grobman and associates point out, "true autonomy is achieved only when patients are able to formulate their desires in the context of a thorough understanding of the risks and benefits." [25]. Counseling and treatment must be individualized with the focus, not on limiting reproductive choices, but on avoiding adverse outcome [24].

The role of counseling in eSET is education that allows for decision-making with the shared goal of a healthy baby. These decisions involve uncertainty and risk that must be addressed in the course of counseling. Over the years, there has been a shift away from paternalism in medicine, where the doctor makes treatment decisions regarding care, to a shared decision-making (SDM) model [30]. In SDM there is collaboration between patient and physician, not only in sharing information and ideas, but also in the making of decisions. Today, SDM is thought to be the model of choice for complex medical decisions involving more than one reasonable treatment option [31]. The characteristics of SDM include that: (1) at least two participants (patient and physician) be involved; (2) both parties share information; (3) both parties take steps to build a consensus about preferred treatment; and (4) an agreement is reached on the treatment to implement [32]. A SDM model provides a useful framework for counseling regarding the complex issues surrounding eSET, and achieving the goal of decreasing multiple gestations (with associated complications) and increasing the birth of healthy singletons.

Counseling approaches for decision-making

The ability to communicate effectively in counseling depends on the way something is said (i.e., the choice of words, tone of voice, etc.), timing of discussions, where the interaction takes place and who is involved. Whatever information is being given (whether verbal or written), it must be communicated at a level the patient can understand, in terms that are simple, clear, direct and without technical jargon. Also, it is better not to make assumptions about a patient's knowledge of the subject at hand based on their profession or educational background (i.e., another physician or nurse) and keep consistency with information shared with all ART patients. If possible, it is important to choose surroundings that provide safety and confidentiality for discussions where patient and doctor are "eye-to-eye," such as in an office setting rather than during a physical examination. For many patients, office visits to the doctor are fraught with anxiety and feeling overwhelmed so that only a small amount of what is being communicated will be retained. Thus, it can be helpful on a subsequent visit to ask a patient about their understanding of what was discussed previously (i.e., "Tell me what you remember about our talk last week…") and repeat or go over information again as needed. Using consistent, simple statements, such as "more is not better" and "quality not quantity," may help to drive the message home.

The messenger and the message have a great deal of authority when given with compassion, clarity and purpose. As Alper notes, "Let's face it: Patients tend to listen to us on the basis of how we deliver the message." [33]. The way the message is delivered should go beyond talk, and involve a "multi-media" approach including visual aids, written materials, brochures, hand-outs and web-based information. All verbal discussions should include easy to understand, written materials that patients take with them to review. Classes, web-based educational informa-

Figure 11.1 Example of a visual aid on eSET vs. two-blastocyst embryo transfer (2-blastocyst ET).

	IVF using own eggs		IVF using donor eggs	
	Blast eSET	2-Blast ET	Blast eSET	2-Blast ET
# Cycles	180	698	68	160
% Pregn / ET	68%	61%	67%	67%
% Multiples	1.6%	50%	0.0%	63%

Infant complications from multiple pregnancy births

	Singleton	Twin	Triplet
Ave. Week @ birth	39 wks	36 wks	32 wks
% Very premature	1.7%	14%	41%
Ave. birth weight	3357 gms	2390 gms	1735 gms
% Severe handicap	1.9%	3.4%	5.7%
% Infant mortality	1.1%	6.6%	19 %

Figure 11.2 Example of a visual aid on complications from multiple pregnancy births.

tion placed on a clinic's website, or a listing of internet informational sites provide more materials on eSET and the risks associated with multiple births. "A picture is often worth a thousand words" and visual aids, such as laminates with statistics on a clinic's pregnancy success rates with eSET versus two-blastocyst embryo transfer or complications from multiple births, can be powerful tools during counseling (Figures 11.1 and 11.2.)

Communicating statistics regarding the risks associated with multiple gestations may be difficult for patients to absorb and so it may be important to find ways to have it "hit home." As mentioned, a patient's normal defenses to deal with the emotional trauma of infertility such as denial, detachment and minimization may be activated when hearing about eSET. Compelling statistics, such as "twins are ten times as likely to be damaged by cerebral palsy and three times more likely to die than a single baby," may have more meaning if a couple has known someone who has had problems with a twin pregnancy [34]. Educational booklets detailing the statistics and advantages of single embryo transfer in comparison to the risks and complications associated with double embryo transfer have also been shown to have an influential effect on patient choice [26, 27].

Cryopreservation of supernumerary embryos is another aspect of eSET that should be included in counseling. Patients may fear that if they do not use all embryos created in the cycle, they will be lost forever. However, freezing of excess embryos provides an option for future cycles, minimizes the motivation to transfer more than one and optimizes the potential of pregnancy with the one best embryo. "Cryocounseling" involves informing patients about some of the challenges of cryopreservation: embryos lost in the thaw; decisions regarding which is the best thawed embryo(s) to transfer in a subsequent cycle; lower pregnancy rates; what to do if, later on, patients do not need or want the frozen embryos; and the cost of storage. Nonetheless, knowing that extra embryos can be saved for use at a later time may lessen anxiety for many patients and fortify a willingness to consider eSET.

Counseling regarding the medical risks associated with multiple gestation and birth are substantial and documented throughout this text. What is less well understood, and yet must be addressed in counseling, are the significant psychosocial risks to families of multiples. There is considerable evidence that parenting twins or more negatively affects the emotional well-being of mothers, with a greater incidence of emotional distress and depression as much as 4 years after birth [35–37]. Stress and distress in these families results from short- and long-range concerns around children's health and development; sleep deprivation; financial concerns due

to loss of an income and/or increased expenses; and decrease in marital satisfaction. In addition, parenting multiple children has significant impact on quality of life in a family especially as it relates to parents feeling stigmatized by others' moral judgments of their family as well as compounded losses associated with the pregnancy and birth (i.e., premature birth, miscarriage, selective reduction and neonatal death) [36, 37]. Patients must be counseled about the psychosocial risks for multiple birth families, and how it impacts the short- and long-term functioning of the family, to increase informed decision-making.

An additional psychosocial risk is selective reduction. There is nothing so difficult or painful for a couple that has been longing for a baby and gone through Herculean efforts to achieve a pregnancy, to then face the decision of multifetal reduction. Even when they have made a decision to transfer more than one embryo, or if a single embryo has split and they learn they are carrying twins or more, patients are often shocked and distressed to learn the news. Despite being counseled, they may assume "it will never happen to us" and when faced with the reality of risks associated with a multiple pregnancy must consider the unthinkable – choosing to terminate much desired fetuses. Since the reduction is an active decision (not a miscarriage where there is no choice involved), feelings of guilt, shame, sadness, anguish and grief are overwhelming. One couple described, "It is like the Normandy invasion (during World War II) – you know a lot of people will get killed but you have to do it anyway so others may live." Often the decision to reduce must be made quickly and patients experience the events surrounding the reduction as stressful, chaotic and emotionally disturbing. Counseling and support during this traumatic period are essential for a good final outcome and, as with other losses, couples need the opportunity to grieve for emotional healing to take place [38].

In conclusion, counseling is the vehicle for disseminating information necessary to help patients make an informed decision regarding eSET. The road traveled towards this goal should be filled with signs that are obviously marked and give patients clear direction towards a shared destination – a healthy baby. We, as caregivers, are here to help them navigate the journey, while realizing that patients are in the driver's seat.

What do we know?

Counseling is crucial in helping patients understand and decide to do eSET. Patients often desire twins or more, and typically underestimate the medical and psychosocial risks associated with multiple births. However, counseling has been shown to change patients perspective and affect decision-making. Counseling must start at the very beginning of treatment, with an ongoing process of discussion regarding the risks associated with multiple births and the comparible success rates of eSET versus transfer of multiple embryos.

What do we need to know?

We need to do more research to understand what affects treatment choices and develop evidence-based counseling strategies for eSET.

What should we do?

Counseling should be a fundamental part of ART treatment. We need to consider requiring patients to go through counseling and education on multiple pregnancy as well as provide support for the psychological consequences of protracted infertility treatment (i.e., depression, anxiety, etc.) which can affect transfer choices. The entire treatment team needs to be well versed in the risks of multiple pregnancy and benefits of eSET to provide consistency in patient care.

REFERENCES

1. G. L. Ryan, S. H. Zhang, A. Dorkras, C. H. Syrop, and B. J. Van Voohis, The desire of infertile patients for multiple births. *Fertil. Steril.*, **81** (2004), 500–504.
2. M. D'Alton, Infertility and the desire for multiple births. *Fertil. Steril.*, **81** (2004), 523–525.
3. L. H. Burns and S. N. Covington, Psychology of infertility. In S. N. Covington and L. H. Burns, eds., *Infertil-ity Counseling: a Comprehensive Handbook for Clinicians*, 2nd edn. (New York: Cambridge University Press, 2006), pp. 1–19.
4. E. W. Freeman, A. S. Boxer, K. Rickels *et al.*, Psychological evaluation and support in a program of in vitro fertilization and embryo transfer. *Fertil. Steril.*, **43** (1985), 48–53.
5. P. P. Mahlstedt, S. Macduff and J. Bernstein, Emotional factors and the in vitro fertilization and embryo transfer process. *J. In Vitro Fert. Embryo Transf.*, **4** (1987), 232–236.
6. C. R. Newton, M. T. Hearn and A. A. Yuzpe, Psychological assessment and follow-up after in vitro fertilization: assessing the impact of failure. *Fertil. Steril.*, **54** (1990), 879–886.
7. D. Baram, E. Tourtelot, E. Muechler *et al.*, Psychological adjustment following unsuccessful in vitro fertilization. *J. Psychosom. Obstet. Gynaecol.*, **6** (1987), 165–178.
8. J. Boivin, J. Takefman, T. Tulandi *et al.*, Reactions to infertility based on extent of treatment failure. *Fertil. Steril.*, **63** (1995), 801–807.
9. M. Beutel, J. Kupfer, P. Kirchmeyer *et al.*, Treatment-related stresses and depression in couples undergoing assisted reproductive treatment by IVF or ICSI. *Andrologie*, **31** (1999), 27–35.
10. A. D. Domar, A. Broome, P. C. Zuttermeister *et al.*, The prevalence and predictability of depression in infertile women. *Fertil. Steril.*, **58** (1992), 1158–1163.
11. A. D. Domar, P. C. Zuttermeister and R. Friedman, The psychological impact of infertility: a comparison with patients with other medical conditions. *J. Psychosom. Obstet. Gynaecol.*, **14**, 45–52.
12. K. E. Williams and L. N. Zappert, Psychopathology and psychopharmacology in the infertile patient. In S. N. Covington and L. H. Burns, eds., *Infertility Counseling: a Comprehensive Handbook for Clinicians*, 2nd edn. (New York: Cambridge University Press, 2006), pp. 97–116.
13. S. N. Covington, Patient support in the ART program. In D. K. Gardner, A. Weissman, C. M. Howles and Z. Shoham, eds., *Textbook of Assisted Reproductive Techniques: Laboratory and Clinical Perspectives*, 2nd edn. (London: Taylor & Francis, 2004), pp. 901–910.
14. M. Johnston, R. Shaw and D. Bird, "Test-tube baby" procedures: stress and judgments under uncertainty. *Psychol. Health*, **1** (1987), 25–38.

15. A. E. Reading, Decision making and in vitro fertilization: the influence of emotional state. *J. Psychosom. Obstet. Gynaecol.*, **10** (1989), 107–112.

16. A. Visser, G. Haan, H. Zalmstra *et al.*, Psychosocial aspects of in vitro fertilisation. *J. Psychosom. Obstet. Gynaecol.*, **15** (1994), 35–45.

17. E. J. Kopitzke, B. J. Berg, J. F. Wilson and D. Owen, Physical and emotional stress associated with components of the infertility investigation: professional and patient perspectives. *Fertil. Steril.*, **55** (1991), 1137–1143.

18. J. Boivin and J. Takefman, The impact of the in vitro fertilization–embryo transfer (IVF–ET) process on emotional, physical, and relational variables. *Hum. Reprod.*, **11** (1996), 903–907.

19. K. J. Connolly, R. J. Edelmann, H. Bartlett *et al.*, An evaluation of counselling for couples undergoing treatment for in vitro fertilization. *Hum. Reprod.*, **8** (1993), 1332–1338.

20. N. Gleicher, D. P. Campbell, C. L. Chan *et al.*, The desire for multiple birth in couples with infertility problems contradicts present practice patterns. *Hum. Reprod.*, **10** (1995), 1079–1084.

21. S. Murray, A. Shetty, A. Rattray, V. Taylor and S. Bhattacharya, A randomized comparison of alternative methods of information provision on the acceptability of elective single embryo transfer. *Hum. Reprod.*, **19** (2004), 911–916.

22. T. J. Child, A. M. Henderson and S. L. Tan, The desire for multiple pregnancy in male and female infertility patients. *Hum. Reprod.*, **19** (2004), 558–561.

23. C. R. Newton, J. McBride, V. Feyles, F. Tekpetey and S. Power, Factors affecting patients' attitudes toward single- and multiple-embryo transfer. *Fertil. Steril.*, **87** (2007), 269–278.

24. D. Adamson and V. Baker, Multiple births from assisted reproductive technologies: a challenge that must be met. *Fertil. Steril.*, **81** (2004), 517–522.

25. W. A. Grobman, M. Milad, J. Stout and S. C. Klock, Patient perceptions of multiple gestations: an assessment of knowledge and risk aversion. *Am. J. Obstet. Gynecol.*, **185** (2001), 920–924.

26. J. D. Hutton, Acceptance of single-embryo transfer by patients. *Fertil. Steril.*, **87** (2007), 207–209.

27. G. L. Ryan, A. E. T. Sparks, C. S. Sipe *et al.*, A mandatory single blastocyst transfer policy with educational campaign in a United States IVF program reduces multiple gestation rates without sacrificing pregnancy rates. *Fertil. Steril.*, **88** (2007), 354–360.

28. C. R. Newton, V. Feyles, F. Tekpetey and S. Power, The influence of mood, infertility stress and risk taking behavior on patient decisions about embryo transfer. ESHRE 23rd Annual Meeting, Lyons, France, 2007.

29. R. J. Stillman, A 47-year-old woman with fertility problems who desires a multiple pregnancy. *JAMA*, **297** (2007), 858–867.

30. L. Fraenkel and S. McGraw, What are the essential elements to enable patient participation in medical decision making? *J. Gen. Intern. Med.*, **22** (2007), 614–619.

31. S. N. Whitney, A. L. McGuire and L. B. McCullough, A typology of shared decision making, informed consent, and simple consent. *Ann. Internal Med.*, **140** (2003), 54–59.

32. C. Charles, A. Gafni and T. Whelan, Shared decision-making in the medical encounter: what does it mean? (or it takes at least two to tango). *Soc. Sci. Med.*, **44** (1997), 681–692.

33. M. M. Alper, In vitro fertilization outcomes: why doesn't anyone get it? *Fertil. Steril.*, **81** (2004), 514–516.

34. D. Healy, Damaged babies from assisted reproductive technologies: focus on the BESST (birth emphasizing a successful singleton at term) outcome. *Fertil. Steril.*, **81** (2004), 512–513.

35. C. Glazebrook, C. Sheard, S. Cox, M. Oates and G. Ndukwe, Parenting stress in first-time mothers of twins and triplets conceived after in vitro fertilization. *Fertil. Steril.*, **81** (2004), 505–511.

36. M. A. Ellison and J. E. Hall, Social stigma and compounded losses: quality-of-life issues for multiple-birth families. *Fertil. Steril.*, **80** (2003), 405–414.

37. M. A. Ellison, S. Hotamisligil, H. Lee *et al.*, Psychosocial risks associated with multiple births resulting from assisted reproduction. *Fertil. Steril.*, **83** (2005), 1422–1428.

38. C. Bergh, A. Moller, L. Nilsson and M. Wikland, Obstetric outcome and psychological follow-up of pregnancies after embryo reduction. *Hum. Reprod.*, **14** (1999), 2170–2175.

Stress-reduction techniques to reduce patient dropout rates during elective single embryo transfer

Janetti Marotta

Introduction

Since the first successful in vitro fertilization (IVF) in 1978 more than two million children have been born through assisted reproductive technology (ART). While the benefits of establishing a pregnancy for couples otherwise unable to conceive are significant, the risks are also significant. The most important negative impacts of ART include the elevated twin pregnancy rate and the high treatment dropout rate.

Elective single embryo transfer (eSET) is seen as the only way to reduce twin pregnancy in ART [1]. However, high treatment dropout during eSET remains problematic. Of all the reasons for IVF dropout, the stress of treatment appears to rank highest. Fortunately, studies have found that stress-reduction techniques can improve IVF cycle factors and outcomes, and thus may reduce treatment dropout.

The specific stress-reduction techniques that may reduce the patient dropout rate for eSET have yet to be identified. However, this review of the substantial research on eSET, IVF treatment dropout, IVF-related stress and psychosocial interventions for infertility can make some recommendations for the implementation of clinic-based stress-management programs and suggest directions for future research.

Overview of eSET

Since the 1990s, the success of IVF has led to increases in the multiple pregnancy rate > 30% on average [2]. Assisted reproductive technology has been associated with a 20-fold increase in the rate of multiple pregnancies compared with spontaneous twin pregnancies [3]. Data reveal that half of the children born after ART in Europe originated from multiple pregnancies; these numbers are even higher for the USA [4].

It has been estimated that the excess costs of twin births due to IVF per 10 000 births is roughly $26 million [5]. Prematurity and its associated complications occur five to ten times more often in multiple pregnancies than in singleton pregnancies. Multiple pregnancies lead to obstetrical risks, compromised neonatal outcomes and difficult psychosocial and economic outcomes. From a health-economic point of view, ART twins constitute a major burden on society, since the long-term health problems of surviving twins are often severe [6].

Health-economic analyses that factor in treatment, maternal, delivery and neonatal costs have evaluated eSET versus DET (double embryo transfer) [6, 7]. De Sutter and colleagues calculated the increased risk of obstetrical and neonatal complications of twin pregnancies, taking into account IVF, pregnancy and neonatal-related costs. The authors

Single Embryo Transfer, ed. J. Gerris, G. D. Adamson, P. De Sutter and C. Racowsky. Published by Cambridge University Press.
© Cambridge University Press 2009.

conclude that the cost per child born after eSET
and DET is the same. Though more IVF cycles are
needed to obtain the same number of live births
with eSET, eSET avoids the very high long-term costs
resulting from the increased morbidity after twin
pregnancy. De Sutter *et al.* [8] suggest: "the ultimate aim of each IVF center should be to provide
one healthy child (at a time) to the infertile couple instead of striving to obtain the highest possible pregnancy rates, at the risk of multiple pregnancies." Prospective, large-scale randomized clinical
and health-economic impact studies that compare
eSET and DET are reportedly on their way.

Patients < 34 years of age during their first or second IVF cycles constitute the population responsible for > 80% of all twins, and are the main target
group for twin prevention by eSET [2]. There is a significant body of research to indicate that eSET may
substantially eliminate multiple pregnancies without compromising the cumulative live birth rate per
couple [9, 10]. In a 5-year appraisal study in Belgium
comparing eSET with DET, while the ongoing pregnancy and implantation rates were the same, the
twin rate was significantly different [8].

In both prospective and retrospective studies,
eSET yields an acceptable pregnancy rate while
decreasing the multiple pregnancy rate [9, 10]. If
performed in good prognosis patients, eSET yields
approximately a 40% pregnancy rate per transfer,
which is comparable to DET [11]. The eSET literature highlights the importance of both patient
selection and embryo quality as factors in achieving pregnancy [12]. The key to a successful eSET is
reported to be a woman < 38 years of age, in her first
or second IVF cycle, and with a high implantation
potential embryo [13].

If eSET can eliminate multiple pregnancies without compromising the cumulative live birth rate,
why is it not part of routine practice?

1. Many IVF centers are reluctant to introduce
   eSET for fear that the overall pregnancy rates
   will decrease. Few patients are eligible for eSET.
   Only good prognosis patients with high quality embryos are appropriate. Those centers that
   serve a population with less chance of success,
   i.e. older patients, with a higher incidence of previously failed cycles, find eSET less desirable. The
   success of eSET also depends on identifying the
   embryo(s) with a very high implantation potential, which is not always possible. Not all IVF
   centers have high quality IVF laboratories with
   steady results and good pregnancy rates. Finally,
   though the existing data on eSET are compelling,
   testing on a large scale has not been done, and
   the existing research is not sufficiently convincing to the majority of the IVF community.
2. Physicians are pressured by clinic competition
   for high pregnancy rates; government requirements to report success rates per IVF cycle; insurance companies who determine which clinics
   to include in their network; and patients' need
   for quick success. In those countries that subsi-
   dize the majority of costs (e.g., Europe), physicians tend to agree on a more careful approach,
   whereas in countries where patients pay out of
   pocket (e.g., USA), physicians tend to agree to
   riskier methods.
3. Patients are pressured by economic, emotional
   and physical factors. While patient stress is partially determined by whether costs are subsidized
   or paid out of pocket, it is even more heavily
   determined by emotional and physical factors.
   While the cumulative pregnancy rate for eSET is
   comparable to DET, more transfers may be necessary to achieve pregnancy, intensifying patient
   distress.

A debate has been initiated about how to rede-
fine ART outcome, taking safety as well as efficacy
into account; this in turn would be the most relevant qualifier of IVF performance [14]. An ESHRE
(European Society of Human Reproduction and
Embryology) consensus meeting report stated that
the essential aim of IVF is the birth of one single
healthy child, with a twin pregnancy being regarded
as a complication [15].

Infertility and IVF treatment are extremely distressing for patients. It is not surprising that patients
desire to end infertility as soon as possible. As
a result, it is the attitudes of the patients themselves that significantly contribute to keeping eSET

from routine practice. Patient dropout rates for IVF are already high, even when treatment is financially subsidized, and the necessity of extending treatment for single embryo transfers would likely increase IVF dropout.

To begin to address the issue of reducing patient dropout rates during eSET with stress-reduction techniques, we begin by examining the following questions: who drops out of treatment, when is dropout most likely to occur and what factors are related to dropout?

IVF dropout

Research now demonstrates that the IVF clinic dropout rate is surprisingly high, ranging from 23% to 65%. The patient populations studied have ranged from 144 to 8362. Given the research, it should not be surprising to expect a 50% dropout rate in a typical IVF clinic.

The reasons for IVF treatment dropout are not well understood. While active censoring, discontinued treatment due to poor response or prognosis, financial burden, or achieving pregnancy should be primary factors, they are not [16]. In several studies, only a fraction of the dropout rate was due to active censoring, and poor treatment prognosis did not seem to play an important role [17]. When finances are not a factor, in European or Australian studies that offer three to six IVF cycles without charge, dropout is likewise reported to be high [17, 18]. More than half of US insurance-covered IVF patients are reported to drop out of treatment before using up their entitled benefits [16]. Overall, it is generally recognized that reasonable prognosis, benefits that cover costs and achieving pregnancy are not the major contributors to IVF dropout.

The majority of studies investigating IVF dropout point to psychological factors as primary [16]. Studies describe psychological stress in the following ways: physical and emotional burden; emotional and physical cost/inability to cope with more treatment; stress and frustration; depression and state anxiety; a way out of emotional stress; and fear of failure [17, 19–21].

In a UK study aimed to identify major factors that influence IVF treatment dropout, psychological stress accounted for 36% and lack of success 23% – two factors that are strongly associated. Lack of personal funding and/or National Health Service funding accounted for 23%, changes in personal circumstances accounted for 30% and general discomfort or advice from medical staff accounted for < 10% of dropout [22].

In a qualitative study designed to explore women's decision-making at the end of IVF treatment, Peddie *et al.* [21] found that women were distressed by accepting that their infertility would remain unresolved; had the belief that they began treatment with unrealistic expectations of success; and felt vulnerable to the pressures of media and society. The decision to drop out of treatment offered "a way out of the emotional distress" while simultaneously creating a "confrontation" with the issues previously avoided [21].

Terminating after only one cycle is reported more likely in women found to be more anxious and depressed before beginning IVF treatment [17]. As treatment is extended, emotional distress is reported to increase. Schröder *et al.* found dropout increased from 30.9% after the first IVF cycle to 62.2% after the fourth cycle. The researchers suggest that dropout rate should be used as an important marker of quality control [20]. Other recent studies also indicate that acute stress increases the dropout rates from treatment [22, 23].

Penzias questions his conclusion that couples would rather avoid treatment and "protect their fragile dreams of genetic offspring" and asks: "Is this a normal psychological reaction in an abnormal situation? Do we as physicians fail these patients?" [19]. He argues that it is important to believe that intervention will lead to retention of patients, and that it would be a disservice to patients and IVF centers alike to believe otherwise. What has yet to be determined is what the intervention should be and when it should be applied. Do we agree with Schröder's suggestion that the dropout rate be used as an important marker of quality control?

To address the potential issues of eSET treatment dropout, it is helpful to understand the psychological impact of IVF and its effect on treatment outcome, and then investigate the literature on psychological interventions.

The psychological impact of IVF and its effect on treatment outcomes

The psychological impact of infertility has been well documented [24, 25]. Infertile women have been found to have depression and anxiety levels equivalent to those of women with heart disease, cancer, HIV or chronic pain [26]. Chen *et al.* found 40.2% of infertile women met criteria for a psychiatric disorder, as compared to an average prevalence of 3%. The most common diagnoses were anxiety disorder (23.2%) and major depressive disorder (17%) [27].

In a review of the literature on psychological aspects of IVF, Eugster and Vingerhoets conclude that, beyond a doubt, the IVF procedure is physically and emotionally stressful for both women and their partners, and that anxiety and depression are the most common reactions to treatment. The authors reviewed psychological states before, during and after IVF treatment [28]. These authors cite studies that conclude that stress reactions change with the duration of infertility. In the short term, depression, anxiety, lowered self-esteem and marital problems continue past treatment. The third year of trying to conceive is associated with the highest rates of depression; scores peak during the third year and then slowly fall to levels in the normal range after the sixth year. After repeated failed IVFs, childlessness is more common, because patients show increased vulnerability to developing clinically elevated depression.

The review includes studies on coping strategies. The coping strategies most frequently used by couples when entering IVF treatment were direct action and problem-focused coping. Problem-focused coping was found to be associated with high levels of well-being after a failed IVF. However, women who entered treatment believing that they had

opportunities for control showed lower scores on psychological measures following IVF than women who felt out of control. Because the IVF procedure has elements that are both controllable and outside couples' control, it may be that coping styles need to be multidimensional.

The role of stress and IVF treatment outcome is a topic of current research. A review of the literature on infertility and the mind–body connection by Domar concludes that increased levels of distress are reported in infertile women. Consequently, this may contribute to their infertility. Domar identified 21 studies in the literature on the relationship between distress and IVF outcome. She determined that 15 studies found a positive correlation between stress and pregnancy outcome, two found a trend, three found no relationship and one study lacked the data to support their conclusion [25].

Domar specifically highlights two studies by the same author [29, 30]. Results in the 2001 study indicated that acute and chronic stress prior to IVF affected procedural outcomes or "biologic end points" (i.e., number of oocytes retrieved and fertilized), pregnancy, live birth delivery, birth weight and multiple gestations. Stress from the procedure only influenced biological end points, but the level of stress was significantly related to the biological end points, pregnancy, live birth rate and birth weight. Less distressed women were 93% more likely to give birth than more distressed women.

In the 2004 study, they explored the relationship between biological end points and concerns specific to IVF (i.e., side effects, surgery, anesthesia, not enough information, pain recovery, finances, missing work and live birth delivery) using the Concerns During Assisted Reproductive Technologies (CART) inventory. At baseline, women concerned about the medical aspects of the IVF procedure reduced their percentage of oocytes retrieved by 20% and oocytes fertilized by 19%. A reduction of 30% fewer oocytes fertilized was found in women who were very concerned about missing work. A very high risk of not delivering a live birth was found in women who were extremely concerned about finances associated with IVF.

In Boivin and Takefman's prospective study, results showed that more distress during IVF was reported for women who did not become pregnant than for women who did become pregnant. These women also had poorer biological end point responses in terms of estradiol levels, oocytes retrieved and embryos transferred [31]. However, in another prospective study, no significant differences were found in depression, chronic or acute (trait or state) anxiety at any time during treatment between women who conceived and women who did not conceive. In fact, during the phase of oocyte retrieval, women who conceived scored higher on state anxiety than the women who did not conceive [32].

Smeenk *et al.* established that, after controlling for other factors, a significant relationship exists between both psychological variables and the probability of becoming pregnant after IVF. State anxiety had a slightly stronger correlation with treatment outcome than depression, but both mood states related to persistent or chronic "trait" stress [33]. Koryntova *et al.* found women from the pregnant group had significantly lower scores for trait anxiety than women from the non-pregnant group. The authors concluded that those women reacted in IVF treatment with higher stress, and that this stress response decreased their chance of conception [34].

Bringhenti *et al.* found that, even though women beginning IVF treatment exhibited no signs of psychological maladjustment, they did exhibit elevated levels of state anxiety. The authors suggested this may be an emotional response to their situation [35]. The type of stress response in women during IVF was examined in two studies. Lindheim *et al.* showed that infertile women had a "blunted response" to the stress of IVF [36] whereas Facchinetti *et al.* concluded that infertile women had an elevated response to stress [37]. Harlow *et al.* showed that state anxiety rose during IVF, and also prolactin and cortisol. However, treatment outcome did not appear to be affected by anxiety scores [38].

Csemiczky *et al.* found more suspicion, guilt and hostility in the personality profiles of infertile women as compared to their fertile control, possibly due to their response to infertility. They also found higher stress levels, as measured by circulating prolactin and cortisol levels, in infertile women as compared to their fertile control. The authors concluded that treatment outcome may be related to psychological stress, since the women who did not achieve pregnancy were slightly higher in state anxiety levels than those who did achieve pregnancy [39].

Not all studies found that stress negatively impacted treatment outcome, thus controversy persists. Because of this, it has been suggested that these dimensions be analyzed more carefully, and that standardized instruments and well-defined measures of hormonal stress markers for women in IVF treatment be used. Nevertheless, with the existing data, identifying interventions that will not only decrease psychological distress and treatment dropout, but perhaps also increase chances for success would be of tremendous value.

The effect of psychological interventions on pregnancy

Several studies present promising results of psychological interventions leading to higher pregnancy rates. Some authors reviewed the literature on psychological aspects of infertility to assess the effect of psychological interventions on pregnancy achieved either naturally or from IVF [25, 28]. Boivin's review of the literature focused exclusively on psychosocial interventions and the effects on pregnancy [40], and Campagne's review focused on stress management and reduction in fertility treatment [41].

Eugster and Vingerhoets [28] cite studies that demonstrated a positive relationship between psychosocial treatment and pregnancy outcome. Women in the relaxation training groups, who had unexplained infertility or intended to participate in IVF, had higher pregnancy rates than women in control groups [42]. Women with unexplained infertility who had drug intervention to reduce anxiety also had higher pregnancy rates than the control groups who received a placebo.

Eugster and Vingerhoets [28] conclude that, until there are methodologically well-structured prospective studies that track couples over a longer time period, it cannot be established that psychological factors can predict infertility and outcome. The design would include sample sizes determined on the basis of mean pregnancy chances when undergoing infertility treatment, and psychobiological variables indicating whether distress is experienced.

In an earlier study, Domar *et al.* measured the psychological symptoms and pregnancy rates for infertile women in a behavioral medicine program. Results indicated that not only were psychological symptoms of depression, anxiety and anger reduced in the treatment program, but also 32% of women conceived within six months after completing the program [43].

Domar's subsequent review [25] revealed only one randomized, controlled, prospective study on the effect of a psychological intervention specific to IVF patients [44]. Sixty couples were randomized into a counseling service model provided by a nurse practitioner, or routine infertility care. Counseling was composed of detailed information on IVF, daily telephone contact, personal support during retrieval and transfer, and five discrete counseling sessions. Not only were anxiety and depression scores significantly lower and life satisfaction scores significantly higher in the counseling group versus the control group, but also 43% of the counseling group achieved a clinical pregnancy (fetal heartbeat present), compared with 17% of the control group.

Domar examined mind–body studies that report increased pregnancy rate as a result of psychological interventions. In general, these programs included relaxation training, stress management, coping skills and group support. Programs ranged from five to ten sessions and were conducted by a mental health professional and/or nurse. Not only were psychological and physical symptoms reduced (i.e., depression, anxiety, headaches, insomnia), but also approximately 45% of patients in the intervention groups conceived within 6 months of program completion.

In a randomized, controlled, prospective study of infertile women undergoing mind–body intervention, participants were randomized into a ten-session mind–body group, a ten-session support group, or a routine care control group. While the mind–body group reported significant improvement in psychological symptoms, the support group reported no change, and the control group reported an increase in psychological symptoms. Furthermore, the mind–body group had a 55% birth rate; the support group a 54% birth rate; while the control group had a 20% birth rate [45].

A Japanese prospectively randomized study of 74 women included a five-session mind–body group or routine care control group to assess psychological stress and natural killer cell activity. Both psychological stress and natural killer cell activity decreased significantly in the mind–body group, while there was no change in the control group. Additionally, in the mind–body group, 38% conceived within the year, versus 13.5% for the control group [46].

Domar concludes that emotional symptoms are reduced and pregnancy rates increased through psychological interventions. In particular, mind–body interventions demonstrate greatest promise in improving symptoms and raising pregnancy rates.

The aim of Boivin's review was to examine the outcome studies that exist with the intent of providing directions for future research on the evaluation of effective psychosocial interventions [40]. In all, Boivin found 15 studies that investigated pregnancy outcome that met criteria. Fourteen of these studies sampled women currently involved in fertility treatment, introducing the possibility that medical treatment as opposed to psychosocial intervention accounted for the pregnancies. Therefore, only better quality studies assessing the impact on pregnancy, using a control group ($n = 8$ of 11), were examined. While three studies demonstrated a positive intervention effect on cumulative pregnancy rate (30% to 60% with an average of 48.3%), five studies demonstated no intervention effect (15% to 40% with an average of 24.7%). It was also reported that pregnancy occurred sooner in behavioral skills groups than in the control groups.

Boivin concludes that, on the basis of the evidence examined, one cannot confidently argue that psychosocial interventions increased pregnancy rates among participating couples. She suggests that more research be devoted to the systematic evaluation of pregnancy effects before psychosocial interventions can be recommended as a way of helping couples increase their chances of success.

Campagne entitled his article: *Should fertilization treatment start with reducing stress?* [41]. In his review of stress management and reduction in fertility treatment, he reports that psychological interventions to reduce stress in IVF have demonstrated effectiveness in a number of studies, and that a recent meta-analysis showed that psychotherapy accompanying IVF is also effective. This author observes that it is often the stress from fertility treatment that psychological interventions address; however, more and earlier attention should be paid to chronic stress, as it has an important influence on treatment outcome. It is also reported that the influence of psychological interventions on pregnancy rates varies considerably from one study to another, depending on size, selection criteria, female/male factor and, in particular, study design, concluding that more research is needed. Nevertheless, he believes there is ample preliminary evidence that psychological distress impacts fertility, and thus the outcome of IVF, and that both chronic and acute (trait and state) stress levels be treated before commencing treatment. This, he suggests, could lessen necessary treatment cycles, prepare the couple for an initial failed IVF, or make more-invasive techniques unwarranted.

Are some psychosocial interventions more effective than others?

Boivin's review of psychosocial interventions for infertility asks if some interventions are more effective than others. She grouped interventions into counseling, which emphasized emotional expression and support and/or discussion about thoughts and feelings related to infertility, versus educational, which emphasized knowledge and skills training (i.e., relaxation training) within a supportive group environment. She found seven counseling and ten educational studies that met criteria for review [40].

Results indicated that, across a range of outcomes, educational group interventions were significantly more effective (70% vs. 30% positive intervention effect) in producing positive change. This included changes in interpersonal functioning, negative affect, pregnancy and other specific areas related to infertility. The more successful interventions lasted between 6 and 12 weeks with a follow-up period of at least 6 months. The most important interventions included the acquisition of medical knowledge, stress management and coping techniques. Women and men appeared to benefit equally from psychosocial interventions. To support this conclusion, Boivin cites numerous studies that determined participants' opportunity to increase medical knowledge. Skills training that focused on how to cope with infertility was found to be of particular value.

Boivin interprets the value of the group format as enabling participants to be with others having similar problems. This increased the sense that their reactions were normal and justified. Several studies attest to the importance of sharing and exchange among participants about common experiences of infertility. A common coping strategy among infertile people appeared to be "downward comparison," in which people made themselves feel better by seeing their problem as being more treatable or their distress as being lower than others with the same condition. Infertility then felt less threatening.

It is interesting to note that Boivin's review found participation in educational versus counseling interventions was determined to be significantly different. Even though participants' counseling sessions were theoretically unlimited, they generally enlisted in less than five sessions. In fact, even when the interventions lasted six or eight months, participation rates in educational interventions were more than 70%.

Boivin suggests that future research evaluate interventions with these specific components and identify subgroups that would most highly benefit (i.e., by level of distress). She adds that more rigorous experimental methods to evaluate effectiveness of interventions are imperative: "The aim of future research should now be to answer the 'who', 'what', and 'when' questions – who benefits from interventions, using what kinds of interventions, and delivered when?"

What do we do now?

We need to utilize the pertinent literature on dropout and psychosocial interventions and apply it to the eSET population to investigate those techniques that may enable patients to remain in eSET treatment longer. We need to identify what subgroups would most benefit from interventions; determine when interventions are most indicated; and propose more robust research models to accurately measure the effectiveness of treatment.

Patients' "short-sighted" need to define success as achieving pregnancy rather than a healthy child is not only related to a wish to end infertility as soon as possible, but also to a lack of adequate information on the risks and complications of a twin pregnancy. Indeed, when couples were presented with scenarios of differing pregnancy-associated risk magnitudes between single and multiple pregnancies, their desire for twin pregnancy decreased [47]. As Tiitinen *et al.* recommends: "good counseling should include realistic information, not only on the risks of twin gestation but also on later burdens with multiple births" [48]. It is important to explore whether early interventions that begin with a thorough discussion and written information on both IVF and the advantages and disadvantages of eSET are effective, as this could help establish realistic expectations, and increase couples' ability to cope with stress and invest in a longer course of treatment.

Effectively run IVF programs decrease patients' stress. Studies to understand clinic strategies that decrease emotional distress based on common patient complaints are recommended. Such operational interventions may include: improving the ease in contacting the center or staff; having a contact person if different doctors are seen during the same treatment; prescheduling a follow-up consultation after a failed IVF; and having emotional support resources readily available. Improving the existing system of consultation and support include increasing opportunities for patients to discuss their thoughts and feelings in order to facilitate the decision-making process to reengage or discontinue treatment. Exploring the relationship between eSET dropout rate and program quality also requires more study. It would be interesting to determine if staff training in the mind–body approach facilitates patients' participation in psychological intervention programs; increases patients' satisfaction and ease during treatment; and decreases dropout.

Because depression and anxiety have been found to decrease pregnancy rates during IVF, and also increase treatment dropout, it is important to be more proactive in identifying those patients in the pretreatment phase most at risk of dropping out. It is important to note that the most distressed patients do not seek out psychological support [49]. Targeted patients would include those who are significantly delaying treatment, experiencing treatment failure, significantly distressed with little support, suffering infertility at or near three years duration, with personality-dependent stress responses and low resilience.

Smeenk *et al.* concludes that pretreatment levels of depression predict IVF dropout [17]. The pretreatment clinically depressed group could benefit most from psychological interventions from both a prognostic and a supportive point of view. Proactive interventions during the initial medical workup to establish chronic and acute stress levels through the use of validated questionnaires and/or a structured personal interview with a trained mental health professional should be explored. Campagne recommends that if validated questionnaires are over thresholds, intensive stress reduction techniques be applied for three months. Furthermore, he concludes that: "closer monitoring of stress and stress-induced negative changes, together with early intervention aimed at reducing the influence of stress on fertility and fertility treatment success rates, is where fertilization treatment should start" [41].

Penzias recommends that intervention be multidisciplinary, including improved treatments, simpler protocols, more effective teaching and increased psychological support. Medical and emotional treatment would go hand in hand from the beginning [19].

Psychological support through stress reduction interventions in a mind–body group is reported to be of particular benefit. Investigation for eSET patients is recommended on research-based effective group interventions available to women and men, lasting from 5 to 12 weeks with a follow-up of at least 6 months, led by a psychotherapist and/or nurse, and focusing on relaxation training, stress management, coping skills, medical knowledge and group support. Studies of interventions for eSET patients may also include additional support in combination with group counseling, i.e. receiving detailed information on IVF and eSET, daily telephone contact, personal support during retrieval, transfer and pregnancy outcome along with group counseling sessions and drug interventions to decrease anxiety and depression.

Psychological interventions after an unsuccessful treatment outcome to treat such factors as depression, anxiety, low self-esteem, marital problems and concern about what others say or think need to be studied in the eSET population. Because of the different coping styles required during IVF (taking control vs. relinquishing control), it is important to compare interventions that take a direct action approach or are problem-focused with interventions that are not oriented around taking control, i.e. mindfulness.

Research design recommendations from reviewers, most notably Boivin, suggest higher quality studies analyzing dimensions of interest more carefully, using controlled methodology, standardized instruments, well-defined measures of hormonal markers of stress, biological markers for male and female fertility, ample sample size and randomized groups (when possible). Replication studies and a more cautious approach to recommendations are also advised [40].

Stress-reduction techniques to reduce patient dropout rates during treatment will be an important part of the eventual success of eSET. Although psychological interventions have been hampered by methodological problems, results are promising. Well-controlled studies to evaluate the "who, what, and when" of interventions on the eSET population can be based on the relevant literature to date. Valuable strategies to help patients stay the course of treatment and make a decision based not on ending infertility as soon as possible, but on having a healthy child, deserve important consideration. Complete medical care for eSET would combine medical and emotional treatment from the beginning through to completion.

What do we know?

While eSET is the most effective way to reduce twin pregnancies during ART, the stress of treatment leads to a high rate of dropout. Fortunately, studies have found that stress-reduction techniques can improve IVF outcomes, and thus may reduce eSET treatment dropout.

What do we need to know?

We need to know which stress-reduction techniques will reduce patient dropout rates during eSET. We need to utilize the pertinent literature on dropout and psychosocial interventions and apply it to the eSET population to identify those strategies that will help patients to remain in treatment longer. For the most part, the mind–body group approach (information, emotional support, stress-management, coping skills) appears to be the most effective to reduce symptoms and increase pregnancy rates. We need controlled studies to clarify population needs, intervention parameters and treatment effectiveness.

What should we do?

We should design strategies to help patients stay the course of treatment. We should teach patients how to change focus and make decisions based on having a healthy child, rather than ending infertility treatment as soon as possible. Complete patient care during eSET should combine medical and emotional treatment from the beginning.

ACKNOWLEDGEMENTS

The author would like to thank FPNC staff Heather Rone for research assistance and Leslie Woodward for her invaluable help with manuscript preparation.

REFERENCES

1. Prevention of twin pregnancies after IVF/ICSI by single embryo transfer. ESHRE Campus Course Report. *Hum. Reprod.*, **16** (2001), 790–800.
2. J. Gerris and E. Van Royen, Avoiding multiple pregnancies in ART: a plea for single embryo transfer. *Hum. Reprod.*, **15** (2000), 1884–1888.
3. O. Ozturk, S. Bhattacharya and A. Templeton, Avoiding multiple pregnancies in ART: evaluation and implementation of new strategies. *Hum. Reprod.*, **16** (2001), 1319–1321.
4. J. P. Toner, Progress we can be proud of: U.S. trends in assisted reproduction over the first 20 years. *Fertil. Steril.*, **78** (2002), 943–950.
5. J. Collins, An international survey of health economics of IVF and ICSI. *Hum. Reprod. Update*, **8** (2002), 265–277.
6. P. Wølner-Hanssen and H. Rydhstroem, Cost-effectiveness analysis of in-vitro fertilization: estimated costs per successful pregnancy after transfer of one or two embryos. *Hum. Reprod.*, **13** (1998), 88–94.
7. P. De Sutter, J. Gerris and M. Dhont, A health-economic decision-analytic model comparing double with single embryo transfer in IVF/ICSI. *Hum. Reprod.*, **17** (2002), 2891–2896.
8. P. De Sutter, J. Van der Elst, T. Coetsier and M. Dhont, Single embryo transfer and multiple pregnancy rate reduction in IVF/ICSI: a 5-year appraisal. *Reprod. Biomed. Online*, **6** (2003), 464–469.
9. S. Vilska, A. Tiitinen, C. Hydén-Granskog and O. Hovatta, Elective transfer of one embryo results in an acceptable pregnancy rate and eliminates the risk of multiple birth. *Hum. Reprod.*, **14** (1999), 2392–2395.
10. J. Gerris, D. De Neubourg, K. Mangelschots *et al.*, Prevention of twin pregnancy after in-vitro fertilization or intracytoplasmic sperm injection based on strict criteria: a prospective randomized clinical trial. *Hum. Reprod.*, **14** (1999), 2581–2587.
11. P. De Sutter, T. Coetsier, J. Van Der Elst and M. Dhont, Elective single embryo transfer in IVF/ICSI: an analysis of 126 cases. 16th Annual Meeting of the European Society of Human Reproduction and Embryology. *Hum. Reprod.*, **15**: Abs. Bk1 (2000), 0–157, p. 63.
12. E. Van Royen, K. Mangelschots, D. De Neubourg *et al.*, Calculating the implantation potential of day 3 embryos in women younger than 38 years of age: a new model. *Hum. Reprod.*, **16** (2001), 326–332.
13. D. De Neubourg and J. Gerris, Single embryo transfer – state of the art. *Reprod. Biomed. Online*, **7** (2005), 615–622.
14. J. A. Land and J. L. Evers, What is the most relevant standard of success in assisted reproduction? Defining outcome in ART: a Gordian knot of safety, efficacy and quality. *Hum. Reprod.*, **19** (2004), 1046–1048.
15. G. Griesinger, K. Dafopoulos, A. Schultze-Mosgau, R. Felberbaum and K. Diedrich, What is the most relevant standard of success in assisted reproduction? Is BESST (birth emphasizing a successful singleton at term) truly the best? *Hum. Reprod.*, **19** (2004), 1239–1241.
16. A. D. Domar, Impact of psychological factors on dropout rates in insured infertility patients. *Fertil. Steril*, **81** (2004), 271–273.
17. J. Smeenk, C. M. Verhaak, A. M. Stolwijk, J. A. Kremer and D. D. Braat, Reasons for dropout in an in vitro fertilization/intracytoplasmic sperm injection program. *Fertil. Steril.*, **81** (2004), 262–268.
18. K. Olivius, B. Friden, K. Lundin and C. Bergh, Cumulative probability of live birth after three in vitro fertilization/intracytoplasmic sperm injection cycles. *Fertil. Steril.*, **77** (2002), 505–510.
19. A. S. Penzias, When and why does the dream die? Or does it? *Fertil. Steril.*, **81** (2004), 274–275.
20. A. K. Schröder, A. Katalinic, K. Diedrich and M. Ludwig, Cumulative pregnancy rates and drop-out rates in a German IVF programme: 4102 cycles in 2130 patients. *Reprod. Biomed. Online*, **8** (2004), 600–606.
21. V. L. Peddie, E. van Teijlingen and S. Bhattacharya, A qualitative study of women's decision-making at the end of IVF treatment. *Hum. Reprod.*, **20** (2005), 1944–1951.
22. M. Rajkhowa, A. McConnell and G. E. Thomas, Reasons for discontinuation of IVF treatment: a questionnaire study. *Hum. Reprod.*, **21** (2006), 358–363.
23. C. Olivius, B. Friden, G. Borg and C. Bergh, Psychological aspects of discontinuation of in vitro fertilization treatment. *Fertil. Steril.*, **81** (2004), 276.

24. T. M. Cousineau and A. Domar, Psychological impact of infertility. *Best Pract. Res. Clin. Obstet. Gynaecol.*, **21** (2007), 293–308.

25. A. Domar, Infertility and the mind/body connection. *Female Patient*, **30** (2005), 1–5.

26. A. D. Domar, P. D. Zuttermeister and R. Friedman, The psychological impact of infertility: a comparison with patients with other medical conditions. *J. Psychosom. Obstet. Gynaecol.*, **14** (1993), 45–52.

27. T. H. Chen, S. P. Chang, C. F. Tsal and K. D. Juang, Prevalence of depressive and anxiety disorders in an assisted reproductive technique clinic. *Hum. Reprod.*, **19** (2004), 2313–2318.

28. A. Eugster and A. J. Vingerhoets, Psychological aspects of in vitro fertilization: a review. *Soc. Sci. Med.*, **48** (1999), 575–589.

29. H. Klonoff-Cohen, E. Chu, L. Natarajan and W. Sieber, A prospective study of stress among women undergoing in vitro fertilization or gamete intrafallopian transfer. *Fertil. Steril.*, **76** (2001), 675–687.

30. H. Klonoff-Cohen and L. Natarajan, The concerns during assisted reproductive technologies (CART) scale and pregnancy outcomes. *Fertil. Steril.*, **81** (2004), 982–988.

31. J. Boivin and J. E. Takefman, Stress level across stages of in vitro fertilization in subsequently pregnant and nonpregnant women. *Fertil. Steril.*, **64** (1995), 802–810.

32. D. Merari, D. Feldberg, A. Elizur, J. Goldman and B. Modan, Psychological and hormonal changes in the course of in vitro fertilization. *J. Assist. Reprod. Genet.*, **9** (1992), 161–169.

33. J. M. Smeenk, C. M. Verhaak, A. Eugster *et al.*, The effect of anxiety and depression on the outcome of in-vitro fertilization. *Hum. Reprod.*, **16** (2001), 1420–1423.

34. D. Koryntova, K. Sibrtova, E. Klouckova *et al.*, Effect of psychological factors on success of in vitro fertilization. *Ceska Gynekol.*, **66** (2001), 264–269.

35. F. Bringhenti, F. Martinelli, R. Ardenti and G. La Sala, Psychological adjustment of infertile women entering IVF treatment: differentiating aspect and influencing factors. *Acta Obstet. Gynecol. Scand.*, **76** (1997), 431–437.

36. S. Lindheim, R. Legro, L. Morris *et al.*, Altered responses to stress in women undergoing in vitro fertilization and recipients of oocyte donation. *Hum. Reprod.*, **10** (1995), 320–323.

37. F. Facchinetti, M. L. Matteo, G. P. Artini, A. Volpe, and A. R. Genazzani, An increased vulnerability to stress is associated with a poor outcome of in vitro fertilization-embryo transfer treatment. *Fertil. Steril.*, **67** (1997), 309–314.

38. C. R. Harlow, U. M. Fahy, W. M. Talbot, P. G. Wardle and M. G. R. Hull, Stress and stress-related hormones during in vitro fertilization treatment. *Hum. Reprod.*, **11** (1996), 274–279.

39. G. Csemiczky, B. M. Landgren and A. Collins, The influence of stress and state anxiety on the outcome of IVF-treatment: psychological and endocrinological assessment of Swedish women entering IVF-treatment. *Acta Obstet. Gynecol. Scand.*, **79** (2000), 113–118.

40. J. Boivin, A review of psychosocial interventions in infertility. *Soc. Sci. Med.*, **57** (2003), 2325–2341.

41. D. M. Campagne, Should fertilization treatment start with reducing stress? *Hum. Reprod.*, **21** (2006), 1651–1658.

42. D. Farrar, L. Holbert and R. Drabman, Can behavioral-based preparation counseling increase pregnancy after in vitro fertilization? Paper presented at the Meeting of In Vitro Fertilization Psychologists, 1990 Melbourne, Australia.

43. A. D. Domar, P. C. Zuttermeister, M. Seibel and H. Benson, Psychological improvement in infertile women after behavioral treatment: a replication. *Fertil. Steril.*, **58** (1992), 144–147.

44. F. Terzioglu, Investigation into effectiveness of counseling on assisted reproductive techniques in Turkey. *J. Psychosom. Obstet. Gynaecol.*, **22** (2001), 133–141.

45. A. D. Domar, D. Clapp, E. A. Slawsby *et al.*, Impact of group psychological interventions on pregnancy rates in infertile women. *Fertil. Steril.*, **73** (2000), 805–811.

46. T. Hosaka, T. Matsubayashi, Y. Sugiyama, S. Izumi and T. Makino, Effect of psychiatric group intervention on natural-killer cell activity and pregnancy rate. *Gen. Hosp. Psychiatry*, **24** (2002), 353–356.

47. W. A. Grobman, M. P. Milad, J. Stout and S. C. Klock, Patient perceptions of multiple gestations: an assessment of knowledge and risk aversion. *Am. J. Obstet. Gynecol.*, **185** (2001), 920–924.

48. A. Tiitinen, L. Unkila-Kallio, M. Halttunen and C. Hyden-Granskog, Impact of elective single embryo transfer on the twin pregnancy rate. *Hum. Reprod.*, **18** (2003), 1449–1453.

49. J. Boivin, L. C. Scanlan and S. M. Walker, Why are infertile patients not using psychosocial counselling? *Hum. Reprod.*, **14** (1999), 1384–1391.

13

Barriers for elective single embryo transfer implementation

Arno M. van Peperstraten, Jan A. M. Kremer and Didi D. M. Braat

Introduction

A twin pregnancy after in vitro fertilization (IVF) and intracytoplasmic sperm injection (ICSI) is no longer considered to be a successful outcome [1]. There is extensive evidence on the higher incidence of twin-related complications for both mothers and neonates [2–12] and the related medical costs of these complications have a substantial impact on healthcare budgets [13, 14]. Elective single embryo transfer (eSET) is the key intervention to reduce the twin rate dramatically [15]. When performed in a suitable population, eSET will maintain an acceptable pregnancy rate per cycle [16–21] For this reason, the use of eSET has gained increasing attention and is supported by policymakers and international organizations as the preferred treatment option [1]. However, in Europe the percentage of SET use remains stable around a disappointing 15% in recent years [22]. The majority of countries still have double embryo transfer (DET) as their standard method and some even transfer three embryos or more routinely. This demonstrates that apparently it remains difficult to implement eSET in clinical practice.

The problems with the implementation of eSET are not surprising at all. Difficulties with the implementation of innovations, like eSET, are a common phenomenon in clinical practice [23]. Complete and spontaneous dissemination of a new therapeutic intervention is rare and this could have numerous reasons. For the implementation of eSET we can expect potential barriers at many levels. For instance, the decision for the number of embryos transferred is often taken by multiple people instead of only one. This means that even if you convince the professionals to perform eSET, the couple might decide to perform a transfer with multiple embryos instead. Another potential problem could be that eSET in an unselected or older population might result in a drop in pregnancy rate and therefore policymakers will be very careful with the implementation of eSET for all couples in their clinics. Another example could be that guidelines, reimbursement systems and legislation also have a great impact on eSET use.

Because we can expect many potential barriers for eSET at different levels, it will be necessary to design a thorough, evidence-based strategy to implement eSET successfully in daily practice [24, 25]. Without such a strategy it will be nearly impossible to increase the eSET use. The implementation strategy should be based on the barriers for eSET that exist at all different levels. In this chapter we will describe these potential barriers for eSET, according to theoretical domains of implementation theory and literature on assisted reproductive technology (ART). The theoretical models demonstrate that barriers can exist at four domains [26, 27].

Single Embryo Transfer, ed. J. Gerris, G. D. Adamson, P. De Sutter and C. Racowsky. Published by Cambridge University Press.
© Cambridge University Press 2009.

- Characteristics of the innovation
- Characteristics of the professionals
- Characteristics of the patient
- Characteristics of the context

In this chapter we will follow this structure to describe possible barriers for eSET. It is important to consider that within our description we will assume that no legislation for compelled eSET use exists and that couples and professionals take the decision for the number of embryos transferred through a process of shared decision-making. Furthermore, not all barriers mentioned within the theoretical models were identified through clinical studies. Because of lack of evidence, it was sometimes necessary to describe the barriers through interpretation of implementation theory or through barriers found with other implementation problems. When applicable, we will distinguish clearly within the paragraphs between barriers identified through clinical studies (indicated as "evidence-based" barriers) and barriers found by means of interpretation of implementation theory (indicated as "theory-based" barriers).

The barriers for eSET described in this chapter give an overview of potential barriers for implementation of eSET in daily practice. However, the setting of the IVF/ICSI treatment can vary greatly between countries and even clinics. In every setting other barriers could play an essential role. Therefore, to design a local, national or international implementation strategy, it is important to analyze the barriers according to the local specific setting. Although it is complicated to present a general set of the most important barriers, experiences in some countries do provide us with valuable information on eSET implementation. Consequently, we can end this chapter with a paragraph with suggestions to increase the eSET use in general.

Characteristics of eSET

For optimal implementation, certain aspects of the innovation itself that has to be implemented can impede implementation. Also for eSET, characteristics might act as an extra obstacle for the acceptance of eSET as a standard. The following barriers could be of importance for eSET implementation.

Elective SET could cause a decrease in pregnancy rate per cycle (evidence-based)

The use of eSET can cause a reduction in live birth rate per cycle compared with the transfer of multiple embryos [18], especially in an unselected population [20]. To obtain an equal pregnancy rate compared with a multiple embryo transfer regimen, more cycles may be necessary [17, 19]. For patients lower pregnancy rates are difficult to accept [28], especially since for some patients the number of cycles they can endure is limited [29]. If couples or professionals focus on the change for pregnancy per cycle instead of pregnancy rates per couple or per time period, this fact might act as a barrier for eSET implementation.

Furthermore, when eSET is the standard or even compelled for all patients, couples with an initial lower chance for pregnancy will pay the price for the prevention of twin pregnancies in other couples with better prospects. The concern that some couples are withheld from an acceptable chance for pregnancy is a barrier to using eSET as a standard in clinical practice.

A substantial part of twin pregnancies end up with minor or no complications (evidence-based)

The most important feature of eSET is the prevention of twin pregnancies. Although there is a lot of evidence on complications for mothers and neonates associated with twin pregnancies [30–33], complications only occur in the minority of cases [8, 34]. This could be a barrier for eSET implementation. If the higher risks with twins are not acknowledged as a serious problem, clinicians or couples will probably not be motivated for eSET.

Lack of a sufficient cryopreservation program (evidence-based)

The implementation of eSET is facilitated through a sufficient cryopreservation program. With a successful freezing protocol, the possible reduction in pregnancy rate per fresh cycle, as described above, could be compensated for [19]. Some even state that a good freezing program is a necessity for the general use of eSET and that better cumulative results with frozen-thawed embryos are possible [21]. If no sufficient cryopreservation program exists, or when the success rates of frozen-thawed embryos are disappointing, this is a potential barrier for eSET.

Lack of prognostic models or selection criteria for eSET (evidence-based)

No generally accepted, strict prognostic models are available for the selection of patients eligible for eSET. For couples and professionals it is very important to be able to predict the chance of pregnancy before the choice for the number of embryos to transfer is made. If this chance is considered to be low, the transfer of only one embryo might impede the patient of a reasonable chance of success and DET is probably a better option. The inability to select the right couples for eSET might stimulate couples and professionals to "play it safe" and choose to transfer multiple embryos. Consequently, this could be a barrier for eSET use.

Disadvantages of eSET are easier to recognize for couples and clinicians compared with the advantages (theory-based)

A potential barrier for eSET implementation is that the negative results of the implementation of eSET (lower pregnancy rate per cycle for some couples) become visible immediately and affects the individual couple directly (they fail to become pregnant).

The positive effect of eSET implementation, twin reduction, takes longer to become apparent and for the couple this might not make a very big difference (both a singleton and twin is a pregnancy and therefore a success). For clinicians and policymakers this creates a difficult situation. In the transition phase between multiple embryo transfer and eSET, patients and professionals might focus on the decreasing pregnancy rates per couple, instead of the also decreasing twin rate for the whole population and the unchanged overall success rate.

Characteristics of the IVF professional

In the process of shared decision-making for eSET or multiple embryo transfer between patients and clinicians, the doctor plays an important role. The clinician is often the only one taking part in the decision-making process with a rational instead of emotional involvement. During the counseling process, the professionals' opinion or advice could greatly influence the final decision for the number of embryos to transfer. Therefore, factors related to the clinical professional could impede the use of eSET in practice.

Doubts about the necessity for eSET (evidence-based)

Not all professionals feel the need for the prevention of twin pregnancies and therefore are not stimulated to transfer only one embryo. They are apparently not convinced or willing to define twin pregnancies as a complication of IVF and ICSI [34, 35]. Even though (inter)national organizations classified multiple pregnancies as a negative result instead of a success after IVF/ICSI [1], this did not convince all professionals. A potential reason for this is that fertility specialists often do not see the patient after the pregnancy test has turned positive. The complications of twin pregnancies are regularly dealt with by other clinicians. If fertility clinicians do not feel the need to decrease the twin rate after IVF/ICSI, they will probably advise to transfer multiple embryos to maximize the chance for pregnancy per cycle. This behavior would be a barrier to eSET use.

Insufficient counseling skills (evidence-based)

Good communicating skills are required to be able to discuss all aspects of the choice for one or more embryos in a thorough and unbiased way [36]. Often couples start with IVF and actually desire a twin pregnancy, but change their mind after thorough counseling [28, 30–32]. To discuss the twin-related risks and the pregnancy rates of eSET and multiple embryo transfer, while at the same time ensure the couples' freedom of choice, is an ability that not all clinicians master immediately and probably comes with experience. Without this ability the couples might not be informed correctly and miss out on essential information. This could be a barrier for the use of eSET.

Lack of knowledge of professionals on twin risks and eSET success rates (theory-based)

To make a good decision, patients and their clinicians need the appropriate information. It is primarily the professionals' responsibility to provide the couple with all the necessary facts. Without the essential knowledge on twin-related risks and pregnancy rates related to the number of embryos transferred, it is impossible to make a thorough decision. If professionals do not possess sufficient knowledge this could be a barrier to eSET.

Characteristics of the couples undergoing IVF/ICSI

In most clinical settings, the couples have an important part in the decision for the number of embryos to transfer. Moreover, in a lot of settings the patients make the final decision and the doctor plays an advising role. Therefore, characteristics of couples undergoing IVF/ICSI could impede the general use of eSET in clinical practice.

Female age in the population undergoing IVF/ICSI (evidence-based)

Female age is the most important predictor of success in ART. Younger females achieve higher pregnancy rates compared to couples with an older woman [37–39]. If the IVF/ICSI treatment is applied in a population with relatively older females, this could imply that the pregnancy rates will be lower compared to a population where the females are relatively younger. In such an older population it will be more difficult to perform eSET, because the success rate might fall below an acceptable level. For this reason, a higher female age is an important reason to transfer multiple embryos. The differences in eSET use between countries might be explained by the fact that some countries perform IVF earlier compared with others.

Considering a twin to be a successful outcome (evidence-based)

Patients have difficulty in seeing a twin as a complication instead of a success. Most couples that undergo IVF/ICSI have been trying to conceive for an extensive time period and often already have a history of failed attempts with other therapeutic options like medication or insemination. The patients that finally decide to undergo IVF or ICSI have a strong desire for children and regularly see a twin pregnancy as a success instead of a complication [30, 32, 33, 40]. In addition, patients frequently wish for more than one child to complete their family and in their view a twin pregnancy immediately fulfils this wish [41]. To realize this "ideal" scenario, the transfer of one embryo is not the best option and eSET could only make it take longer before this goal is achieved. When couples simply do not think of twins as a complication, this is a barrier for eSET use. Furthermore, if couples have personal experience with twins and this experience was not negative, this could make it difficult for them to see a twin pregnancy as a complication instead of a success.

Insufficient knowledge of patients on twin risks and eSET success rates (evidence-based)

The possession of accurate information is essential to be able to make a thorough decision about the number of embryos for transfer. If couples do not have the right information, it is impossible for them to make a sufficient consideration [42]. This problem of deficiency of the proper information has three potential causes. First, patients frequently have difficulties with dealing with probabilities and chances. Problems with processing percentages, ratios and statistical numbers are common and could complicate the decision-making process [43, 44]. Second, the individual twin-related risks, when presented to the couple, might not look that impressive. Couples often feel such a strong desire to have children, that during counseling they experience the twin-related risks percentages as less important and unimposing [45]. A third aspect could be the problem that couples might simply not be provided with the information by their IVF professionals. Possibly the professional does not feel responsible, or does not have the knowledge. The lack of information, or the inability to deal with the information, is a potential barrier to eSET. Couples will not be able to see the whole perspective and might just choose for the option that provides them with the maximal chance for pregnancy per cycle.

Couples might dread possible extra necessary cycles with eSET (theory-based)

The potential necessity of extra treatment cycles to maintain similar pregnancy rates compared with multiple embryo transfer regimens [17, 18, 20, 22], is a potential barrier to eSET. In particular patients without experience of IVF or ICSI could be anxious about the burden of hormonal injections and the burden of the uncertainty about success or failure they will have to face with every cycle.

Ethical/religious barriers (theory-based)

If only a limited number of oocytes is fertilized, or when it is impossible to take advantage of cryopreservation, this will reduce the pregnancy rate remarkably [19]. This lower pregnancy rate could be a strong incentive to transfer more than one embryo. Some couples have ethical or religious objections against either fertilizing embryos they might not use, freezing embryos that possibly will not survive or to potentially create supernumerary embryos that might never be transferred. Therefore, this could impede implementation of eSET.

Characteristics of the context in which IVF/ICSI is performed

Besides the characteristics of eSET itself and the people taking the decision for the number of embryos for transfer, the context of the choice for eSET or multiple embryo transfer could have significant impact on eSET implementation as well. If external conditions are not favorable for eSET, this might greatly influence the decision for the number of embryos for transfer.

Legislation for eSET or another form of compelled eSET (evidence-based)

Legislation or rules for compelled eSET are essential factors that have shown immense impact in countries where they were implemented. Evidently, when the use of eSET is compelled, it is not possible for couples or clinicians to choose a multiple embryo transfer regimen. This will increase the eSET rate remarkably [46]. The process of decision-making is presumably non-existent when such legislation or compelled eSET rules are present. In that case, an implementation strategy with a focus on shared decision-making seems unnecessary. However, other identified barriers for eSET implementation are not completely insignificant. Questions on patient autonomy might be raised when couples lose the freedom to choose the number of embryos for transfer [15] and optimal implementation of eSET will only occur if acceptance is achieved at the patient level, even if legislation is present [47].

Legislation could also work the other way around. If legislation forbids the use of cryopreservation techniques or fertilization of possible supernumerary embryos, as is the case in Italy [48], this could actually impede the eSET use.

Reimbursement of IVF/ICSI cycles (evidence-based)

Couples are often billed for their IVF and ICSI treatment per cycle. The average costs per cycle vary greatly between countries, but regularly have a substantial impact on the couples' financial situation. Especially when no reimbursement system exists or when a limited number of cycles are reimbursed, patients might have financial reasons to transfer more embryos to maximize their pregnancy chance per cycle [49].

Lack of clinical guidelines (evidence-based)

National guidelines, developed by societies of peer professionals, could facilitate the quality of care and suggest the appropriate treatment options for clinicians in the field. Unfortunately national subfertility guidelines are not commonly used [50] and, except from a few innovative European countries, no guidelines exist to ensure the use of eSET [48]. If no clinical guidelines are present, clinicians will feel free to decide on the number of embryos according to their own insight. As discussed before, some clinicians might not agree with the need for eSET and therefore use a multiple embryo transfer regimen. The lack of guidelines on the number of embryos for transfer could impede the use of eSET. However, even with existing clinical guidelines, this is no guarantee that they are strictly followed by everyone [51].

Competition between clinics and commercial interest (theory-based)

In modern medicine it is becoming more and more accepted to publish yearly reports of ART results [22, 49]. With the implementation of eSET, clinicians could face a (slight) decrease in pregnancy rate per cycle [18]. This potential decrease may well be commercially unappealing, especially when neighboring clinics did not implement eSET and are able to maintain their success rates per cycle. When the differences in pregnancy rate are published, future patients might decide to go to the other clinic instead. The fear for potential loss of patient supply could be a barrier to eSET.

International differences in eSET use and the possibility to travel abroad (theory-based)

Considerable differences exist between countries in many aspects of subfertility treatment [22, 49]. Apart from technical differences in laboratory interventions, one could also observe different stimulation regimens, variation in oocyte aspiration protocols, availability of donated oocytes and especially the maximal number of embryo for transfer [48]. These differences, combined with possible cultural and ethical variation could stimulate couples to travel abroad and undergo their subfertility treatment elsewhere. This might act as a barrier for eSET use, since it enables couples to escape a national eSET protocol and go for a multiple embryo transfer regimen instead. However, it is difficult to determine the magnitude of this problem, since no exact numbers for this phenomenon are yet demonstrated.

Freedom of choice for the couples; shared decision-making or not? (theory-based)

In some clinics, couples are probably not really counseled or advised about the number of embryos for transfer. Instead, they are simply told how many embryos are going to be transferred. Even if the choice of number of embryos transferred is considered to be a process of shared decision-making, in practice this might turn out with a professional "strongly suggesting" a certain option. If this situation exists, it will be less effective to focus on barriers existing with the couples and more useful to focus on the barriers for eSET at the level of the doctors.

Suggestions to increase eSET use

In the paragraphs above we have demonstrated that many factors can affect the implementation of eSET in daily clinical practice. A summary of the barriers mentioned is shown in Table 13.1. The barriers described can be used for the design of an evidence-based implementation strategy for eSET. However, the list of potential barriers is extensive and until now it is not clear what barriers have the most impact compared with others. Before such a strategy is designed, it will be necessary to assess the own local setting, to be sure that the strategy will be useful for the applicable local, national or international situation. Moreover, other still undiscovered barriers could also play a role. We would therefore strongly recommend further research that focuses on the multifactorial aspects of this implementation problem.

It is important to consider that eSET should not be the option for every subfertile couple [34, 35]. In our opinion optimal use of eSET consists of three domains: maximal twin reduction through the use of eSET, maintaining an acceptable pregnancy rate and a reasonably satisfied couple when the treatment has been finished. Increasing the eSET use regardless of these domains is a bridge too far. For this reason it is important to make sure that the couple is part of the decision-making process. Nevertheless, even when we account for these three domains, we can still report suggestions to increase the eSET use. These suggestions have either shown their influence before or could be expected to result in a higher use of the eSET technique in general.

Legislation or reimbursement system that stimulates eSET

Legislation for a form of compelled eSET use will increase the eSET rate significantly. In Europe there

Table 13.1 Barriers for eSET implementation

- Characteristics of eSET
  - Elective SET could cause a decrease in pregnancy rate per cycle
  - A substantial part of twin pregnancies end up with minor or no complications
  - Lack of a sufficient cryopreservation program
  - Lack of prognostic models or selection criteria for eSET
  - Disadvantages of eSET are easier to recognize for couples and clinicians compared to the advantages
- Characteristics of the IVF professional
  - Doubts about the necessity for eSET
  - Insufficient counseling skills
  - Lack of knowledge of the professionals on twin risks and eSET success rates
- Characteristics of the couples undergoing IVF/ICSI
  - Female age in the population undergoing IVF/ICSI
  - Considering a twin to be a successful outcome
  - Insufficient knowledge of patients on twin risks and eSET success rates
  - Couples might dread possible extra necessary cycles with eSET
  - Ethical/religious barriers
- Characteristics of the context in which IVF/ICSI are performed
  - Legislation for eSET or another form of compelled eSET
  - Reimbursement of IVF/ICSI cycles
  - Lack of clinical guidelines
  - Competition between clinics and commercial interest
  - International differences in eSET use and the possibility to travel abroad
  - Freedom of choice for the couples; shared decision-making or not?

is experience with such a construction in Belgium and Sweden and the eSET use there is remarkably higher compared with other countries [15, 46]. The experiences with the new systems in these two countries are promising. The development of the legislation system does require a lot of input and should be closely supervised by professionals. Obviously, it will take time and effort to convince policymakers to agree with the proposed rules and the development of the rules will involve supervision and extensive evaluation. Therefore we would suggest that, if legislation is considered, this is developed and supervised by IVF professionals or national professional societies.

A reimbursement system that stimulates eSET could also be very important for the implementation of eSET. If couples and professionals do not experience a financial incentive for multiple embryo transfer, this enables them to solely look at the medical aspects of eSET versus multiple embryo transfer. It is important to consider that an eSET regimen with potential extra treatment cycles is actually cost-effective and will reduce costs because of the prevention of the more expensive twin pregnancies [13].

Maintaining higher pregnancy rates per cycle with eSET, through improvement of prognostic models, better embryo selection and enhanced cryopreservation protocols

If the difference in pregnancy rate per cycle between eSET and multiple embryo transfer could be reduced or even diminished, this will be an important facilitator for eSET implementation. The way to achieve this is probably through improvement of the ability to select the right couples for eSET, identifying the best embryos and to obtain better results with frozen-thawed embryos.

If we were able to select the appropriate couples for eSET and DET, we could prevent lower success rates previously reported in an unselected population [20]. New prediction models have recently been published [39, 52], but none of them are generally accepted or have proven their value with eSET especially. The same situation is applicable with embryo selection. Identification of the ultimate "eSET embryo" would enable us to apply eSET only in the applicable population. Big differences between embryo analysis protocols exist and no clear definition of an embryo particularly suitable for eSET could be demonstrated yet. Recent literature did suggest new embryo selection criteria [4],

but it remains uncertain if these criteria can be broadly used.

Good cryopreservation results offer us a "bonus" with every fresh cycle [19]. If we were able to improve the eSET success rates, with a cumulative pregnancy rate comparable with the results of multiple embryo transfer regimens, this will act positively on eSET implementation. The experiences with cryopreservation vary greatly between countries. The Nordic European countries have a tradition of good cryopreservation results, but until now these results could not be repeated in other countries or clinics.

Improvement of information provision

To increase eSET use, couples need to recognize the disadvantages of twin pregnancies and combine this with a realistic view on the pregnancy rates per cycle that come with eSET. It is vital that they are able to recognize that with possible extra cycles they maintain a similar chance for pregnancy compared to a multiple embryo transfer regimen with fewer cycles [17–19]. If couples understand the complications associated with twins, this might result in a change of attitude in favor of eSET [31, 33, 53]. It will not be a simple task to ensure that couples receive the right information in a way they can grasp. Professionals need to invest time and effort in the counseling process and try to ensure their impartiality in the process of decision-making. Furthermore, to make this multifactorial problem understandable and comprehensible, patients will probably require a counseling tool, especially designed for this particular problem [42].

Standardization of presentation of clinical outcomes

Success in IVF and ICSI is not only defined by the live birth rate per cycle but is more a balance between high live birth rates with healthy babies and low numbers of multiple pregnancies with complications. Additionally, the factor time also might play an important role since for couples it is important not only to know if, but also when, they will become pregnant. Therefore, apart from the pregnancy rates per cycle, also total live birth rates, life birth rate per episode, twin rates, complication rates and the use of fetal reduction are very important outcome features. If clinics were to report all these aspects of their treatment results, this could act as a facilitator for eSET implementation. It enables couples and clinicians to base their decisions for eSET and DET on thorough evidence and it could also prevent policymakers from refraining from eSET implementation because of commercial reasons.

In conclusion, in this chapter we have tried to give an overview of possible barriers for eSET implementation in clinical practice. With this overview we hope that clinicians and policymakers will be able to assess their own setting and design their own strategy to implement eSET optimally. Only if this pathway is followed is it likely that we will be able to increase eSET use compared to the current disappointing plateau of 15% [22].

What do we know?

Twin pregnancies are no longer considered to be a successful outcome in IVF and ICSI, and eSET is the most effective intervention to prevent twins. Although this is acknowledged by many professionals and international societies, in Europe the percentage of SET use remains stable around a disappointing 15%. The majority of clinics still have a transfer with multiple embryos as a standard method. Apparently it is very difficult to implement eSET in clinical practice. The question is where barriers exist that cause this implementation difficulty.

What do we need to know?

According to implementation theory, we can expect potential barriers for the implementation of eSET at many levels, such as clinicians, couples or context. Because of all these barriers, it will be necessary to design a thorough, evidence-based strategy to implement eSET successfully in daily practice. The first step for the design of such a strategy is to identify all potential barriers for eSET at all relevant levels.

What should we do?

The barriers described in this chapter can be used for the design of an evidence-based implementation strategy for eSET. However, the list of potential barriers is extensive and until now it is not clear what barriers have the most impact compared with others. Before a strategy is designed, it will be necessary to assess the barriers prevailing in each society. This way, we can assure that the strategy will be useful for the applicable situation. Moreover, other still undiscovered barriers could also play a role. We would therefore strongly recommend further research that focuses on the multifactorial aspects of this implementation problem.

REFERENCES

1. Prevention of twin pregnancies after IVF/ICSI by single embryo transfer. ESHRE Campus Course Report. *Hum. Reprod.*, **16** (2001), 790–800.

2. E. Bryan, The impact of multiple preterm births on the family. *BJOG*, **110**: Suppl. 20 (2003), 24–28.

3. M. Dhont, P. De Sutter, G. Ruyssinck, G. Martens and A. Bekaert, Perinatal outcome of pregnancies after assisted reproduction: a case-control study. *Am. J. Obstet. Gynecol.*, **181** (1999), 688–695.

4. J. M. Gerris, Single embryo transfer and IVF/ICSI outcome: a balanced appraisal. *Hum. Reprod. Update*, **11** (2005), 105–121.

5. F. M. Helmerhorst, D. A. Perquin, D. Donker and M. J. Keirse, Perinatal outcome of singletons and twins after assisted conception: a systematic review of controlled studies. *BMJ*, **328** (2004), 261.

6. A. T. Kjellberg, P. Carlsson and C. Bergh, Randomized single versus double embryo transfer: obstetric and paediatric outcome and a cost-effectiveness analysis. *Hum. Reprod.*, **21** (2006), 210–216.

7. J. Koudstaal, H. W. Bruinse, F. M. Helmerhorst *et al.*, Obstetric outcome of twin pregnancies after in-vitro fertilization: a matched control study in four Dutch university hospitals. *Hum. Reprod.*, **15** (2000), 935–940.

8. A. Pinborg, A. Loft, L. Schmidt, J. Langhoff-Roos and A. N. Andersen, Maternal risks and perinatal outcome in a Danish national cohort of 1005 twin pregnancies: the role of in vitro fertilization. *Acta Obstet. Gynecol. Scand.*, **83** (2004), 75–84.

9. A. Pinborg, IVF/ICSI twin pregnancies: risks and prevention. *Hum. Reprod. Update*, **11** (2005), 575–593.

10. A. Rao, S. Sairam and H. Shehata, Obstetric complications of twin pregnancies. *Best. Pract. Res. Clin. Obstet. Gynaecol.*, **18** (2004), 557–576.

11. C. Sheard, S. Cox, M. Oates, G. Ndukwe and C. Glazebrook, Impact of a multiple, IVF birth on post-partum mental health: a composite analysis. *Hum. Reprod.*, **22** (2007), 2058–2065.

12. H. Verstraelen, S. Goetgeluk, C. Derom *et al.*, Preterm birth in twins after subfertility treatment: population based cohort study. *BMJ*, **331** (2005), 1173.

13. H. G. Lukassen, Y. Schonbeck, E. M. Adang *et al.*, Cost analysis of singleton versus twin pregnancies after in vitro fertilization. *Fertil. Steril.*, **81** (2004), 1240–1246.

14. P. Wolner-Hanssen and H. Rydhstroem., Cost-effectiveness analysis of in-vitro fertilization: estimated costs per successful pregnancy after transfer of one or two embryos. *Hum. Reprod.*, **13** (1998), 88–94.

15. D. De Neubourg, J. Gerris, E. Van Royen, K. Mangelschots and M. Vercruyssen, Impact of a restriction in the number of embryos transferred on the multiple pregnancy rate. *Eur. J. Obstet. Gynecol. Reprod. Biol.*, **124** (2006), 212–215.

16. J. Gerris, D. De. Neubourg, K. Mangelschots *et al.*, Prevention of twin pregnancy after in-vitro fertilization or intracytoplasmic sperm injection based on strict embryo criteria: a prospective randomized clinical trial. *Hum. Reprod.*, **14** (1999), 2581–2587.

17. H. G. Lukassen, D. D. Braat, A. M. Wetzels *et al.*, Two cycles with single embryo transfer versus one cycle with double embryo transfer: a randomized controlled trial. *Hum. Reprod.*, **20** (2005), 702–708.

18. Z. Pandian, A. Templeton, G. Serour and S. Bhattacharya, Number of embryos for transfer after IVF and ICSI: a Cochrane review. *Hum. Reprod.*, **20** (2005), 2681–2687.

19. A. Thurin, J. Hausken, T. Hillensjo *et al.*, Elective single-embryo transfer versus double-embryo transfer in in vitro fertilization. *N. Engl. J. Med.*, **351** (2004), 2392–2402.

20. A. P. van Montfoort, A. A. Fiddelers, J. M. Janssen *et al.*, In unselected patients, elective single embryo transfer prevents all multiples, but results in significantly lower pregnancy rates compared with double embryo transfer: a randomized controlled trial. *Hum. Reprod.*, **21** (2006), 338–343.

21. Z. Veleva, S. Vilska, C. Hydén-Granskog *et al.*, Elective single embryo transfer in women aged 36–39 years. *Hum. Reprod.*, **21** (2006), 2098–2102.

22. A. N. Andersen, V. Goossens, L. Gianaroli *et al.*, Assisted reproductive technology in Europe, 2003. Results generated from European registers by ESHRE. *Hum. Reprod.*, **22** (2007), 1513–1525.

23. R. Grol and J. Grimshaw, From best evidence to best practice: effective implementation of change in patients' care. *Lancet*, **362** (2003), 1225–1230.

24. L. A. Bero, R. Grilli, J. M. Grimshaw *et al.*, Closing the gap between research and practice: an overview of systematic reviews of interventions to promote the implementation of research findings. The Cochrane Effective Practice and Organization of Care Review Group. *BMJ*, **317** (1998), 465–468.

25. R. W. M. E. M. Grol, *Improving Patient Care. The Implementation of Change in Clinical Practice*, 1st edn. (London: Elsevier Butterworth-Heinemann, 2005).

26. M. D. Cabana, C. S. Rand, N. R. Powe *et al.*, Why don't physicians follow clinical practice guidelines? A framework for improvement. *JAMA*, **282** (1999), 1458–1465.

27. M. Peters, M. Harmsen, M. Laurent and M. Wensing, Ruimte voor verandering? (in Dutch) Centre for Quality Care Research (wok), Radboud University Medical Centre, Nijmegen (2003).

28. M. Twisk, F. van de Veen, S. Repping *et al.*, Preferences of subfertile women regarding elective single embryo transfer: additional in vitro fertilization cycles are acceptable, lower pregnancy rates are not. *Fertil. Steril.*, **88** (2007), 1006–1009.

29. J. M. Smeenk, C. M. Verhaak, A. M. Stolwijk, J. A. Kremer and D. D. Braat, Reasons for dropout in an in vitro fertilization/intracytoplasmic sperm injection program. *Fertil. Steril.*, **81** (2004), 262–268.

30. T. J. Child, A. M. Henderson and S. L. Tan, The desire for multiple pregnancy in male and female infertility patients. *Hum. Reprod.*, **19** (2004), 558–561.

31. C. R. Newton, J. McBride, V. Feyles, F. Tekpetey and S. Power, Factors affecting patients' attitudes toward single- and multiple-embryo transfer. *Fertil. Steril.*, **87** (2007), 269–278.

32. A. Pinborg, A. Loft, L. Schmidt and A. N. Andersen, Attitudes of IVF/ICSI-twin mothers towards twins and single embryo transfer. *Hum. Reprod.*, **18** (2003), 621–627.

33. G. L. Ryan, S. H. Zhang, A. Dokras, C. H. Syrop and B. J. Van Voorhis, The desire of infertile patients for multiple births. *Fertil. Steril.*, **81** (2004), 500– 504.

34. M. van Wely, M. Twisk, B. W. Mol and F. van de Veen, Is twin pregnancy necessarily an adverse outcome of assisted reproductive technologies? *Hum. Reprod.*, **21**, (2006), 2736–2738.

35. N. Gleicher, A. Weghofer and D. Barad, Update on the comparison of assisted reproduction outcomes between Europe and the USA: the 2002 data. *Fertil. Steril.*, **87** (2007), 1301–1305.

36. A. Fagerlin, P. A. Ubel, D. M. Smith and B. J. Zikmund-Fisher, Making numbers matter: present and future research in risk communication. *Am. J. Health Behav.*, **31**: Suppl 1 (2007), S47–S56.

37. C. C. Hunault, J. D. Habbema, M. J. Eijkemans *et al.*, Two new prediction rules for spontaneous pregnancy leading to live birth among subfertile couples, based on the synthesis of three previous models. *Hum. Reprod.*, **19** (2004), 2019–2026.

38. A. Templeton, J. K. Morris and W. Parslow, Factors that affect outcome of in-vitro fertilization treatment. *Lancet.*, **348** (1996), 1402–1406.

39. J. W. van der Steeg, P. Steures, M. J. Eijkemans *et al.*, Pregnancy is predictable: a large-scale prospective external validation of the prediction of spontaneous pregnancy in subfertile couples. *Hum. Reprod.*, **22** (2007), 536–542.

40. S. K. Kalra, M. P. Milad, S. C. Klock and W. A. Grobman, Infertility patients and their partners: differences in the desire for twin gestations. *Obstet. Gynecol.*, **102** (2003), 152–155.

41. L. Baor and I. Blickstein, En route to an "instant family": psychosocial considerations. *Obstet. Gynecol. Clin. North Am.*, **32** (2005), 127–139, x.

42. H. L. Bekker, J. Hewison and J. G. Thornton, Understanding why decision aids work: linking process with outcome. *Patient. Educ. Couns.*, **50** (2003), 323–329.

43. M. M. Schapira, A. B. Nattinger and C. A. McHorney, Frequency or probability? A qualitative study of risk communication formats used in health care. *Med. Decis. Making.*, **21** (2001), 459–467.

44. L. J. Trevena, H. M. Davey, A. Barratt, P. Butow and P. Caldwell, A systematic review on communicating with patients about evidence. *J. Eval. Clin. Pract.*, **12** (2006), 13–23.

45. G. Scotland, P. McNamee, V. Peddie and S. Bhattacharya, Safety versus success in elective single embryo transfer: women's preferences for outcomes of in vitro fertilization. *BJOG*, **114** (2007), 977–983.

46. S. Gordts, R. Campo, P. Puttemans *et al.*, Belgian legislation and the effect of elective single embryo transfer on IVF outcome. *Reprod. Biomed. Online*, **10** (2005), 436–441.

47. P. Saldeen and P. Sundstrom. Would legislation imposing single embryo transfer be a feasible way to reduce the rate of multiple pregnancies after IVF treatment?. *Hum. Reprod.*, **20** (2005), 4–8.

48. H. W. Jones, Jr. and J. Cohen, IFFS surveillance 07. *Fertil. Steril.*, **87** (2007), S1–S67.

49. V. C. Wright, J. Chang, G. Jeng, M. Chen and M. Macaluso, Assisted reproductive technology surveillance – United States, 2004. *MMWR Surveill. Summ.*, **56** (2007), 1–22.

50. E. C. Haagen, W. L. Nelen, R. P. Hermens *et al.*, Barriers to physician adherence to a subfertility guideline. *Hum. Reprod.*, **20** (2005), 3301–3306.

51. S. M. Mourad, R. P. Hermens, W. L. Nelen *et al.*, Guideline-based development of quality indicators for subfertility care. *Hum. Reprod.*, **22** (2007), 2665–2672.

52. C. C. Hunault, E. R. te Velde, S. M. Weima *et al.*, A case study of the applicability of a prediction model for the selection of patients undergoing in vitro fertilization for single embryo transfer in another center. *Fertil. Steril.*, **87** (2007), 1314–1321.

53. W. A. Grobman, M. P. Milad, J. Stout and S. C. Klock, Patient perceptions of multiple gestations: an assessment of knowledge and risk aversion. *Am. J. Obstet. Gynecol.*, **185** (2001), 920–924.

14

Single embryo transfer: the Swedish experience

Christina Bergh, Per-Olof Karlström and Ann Thurin-Kjellberg

Background

In vitro fertilization (IVF) is the most successful treatment for infertility, independent of cause. Since the first baby using IVF was born in England in 1978 [1] and in Sweden in 1982, more than three million IVF children have been born worldwide (more than 25 000 in Sweden). In vitro fertilization children represent 3% of all newborns in Sweden.

Although there are high success rates with IVF, there are also certain side effects. During the last decade two of the main focuses in relation to assisted reproductive technology (ART) have been safety and quality, both for mothers and offspring.

Multiple births have been recognized as the main side effect of ART worldwide. Registry data from Europe and the USA indicate multiple births of 25% and 35% respectively, including not only twins but also triplets and higher-order multiple birth babies [2, 3]. Today it is well known from several large registry studies and meta-analyses that IVF children have poorer obstetric and neonatal outcomes than children born after spontaneous conception [4–7], particularly higher rates of prematurity, low/very low birth weight and perinatal death.

Swedish studies have contributed a great deal to this knowledge. There have long been several population registries in Sweden, covering almost 100% of the population: i.e. the Medical Birth Registry, Malformation Registry, Cause of Death Registry, Hos-pital Discharge Registry and an IVF Registry for all children born after IVF. Because Sweden has individual identification numbers for each person, cross-linking between these registries has been possible. To date, three such cross-linkings have been performed between the IVF Registry and the other population registries, revealing important knowledge. A four to six times higher prematurity rate and a six to eight times higher rate of low/very low birth weight was observed for the IVF children, mainly owing to the higher rate of multiple births [4]. It is true, however, that also IVF singletons, after adjustment for maternal age, parity and years of infertility, have an increased risk of adverse outcome compared with spontaneously conceived singletons but this risk is considerably lower as compared with the total IVF cohort [4–6]. Another large Swedish study found that the risk of neurological sequelae was increased among IVF children, particularly among multiple birth babies [8]. Similar risks were identified in the latest cross-linkings [9, 10] including infants born from 1982 to 2001, although the rate of multiple births had decreased.

These large registry studies influenced the attitudes of Swedish IVF doctors, obstetricians, pediatricians, politicians and the general population greatly and demands were made to have these risks reduced. Multiple birth rates are mainly attributable to the number of embryos transferred. A reduction in the number of embryos transferred from three to two did take place in the early 1990s, and this decreased the multiple birth rates from 35% to 25%, but the number of multiple births rose for each year because of the increasing IVF volumes. However, the delivery rate remained stable after this shift in the number of embryos transferred.

The Scandinavian single embryo transfer (SET) study

The pioneering report from Finland in 1999 [11] showed encouraging results after elective transfer of only one embryo. However, most doctors at that time hesitated to reduce the number of embryos transferred to only one owing to the fear of lowering the pregnancy and delivery results considerably. A retrospective study was performed where mother's age and the number of good quality embryos transferred were identified as independent predictors of live births [12]. The challenge was to maintain the overall delivery rates and at the same time dramatically reduce the multiple birth rates. Cut-off limits were calculated for women's age for applying single embryo transfer (SET) with the aim of halving the rate of multiple births in the total IVF population while maintaining overall delivery rates by adding a frozen-thawed SET to patients not achieving a live birth in the fresh cycle. These calculations were then used when designing the Scandinavian SET study [13]. In the later study it was hypothesized that transferring one fresh embryo and if that did not result in a live birth, transferring one frozen-thawed embryo would yield the same live birth rate as transferring two embryos on one occasion and this would simultaneously reduce the multiple birth rates considerably. The study was designed as an equivalence study, where equivalence was defined as the upper limit of the 95% confidence interval for the difference in live births not exceeding 10%. A live birth rate of 30% was assumed in each group. Thus 330 patients per group were needed.

In order to be eligible for randomization in the Scandinavian SET study women were to be less than 36 years of age, performing their first or sec-

ond IVF cycle and have at least two good quality embryos available for transfer or cryopreservation. Good quality embryos were defined as embryos with less than 20% fragmentation and 4–6 cells at day 2, 6–10 cells at day 3, or expanded blastocysts on day 5 or 6. Eleven Scandinavian clinics, both public and private, participated. The patients were randomized to participate between May 2000 and October 2003.

A total of 661 women were randomized, 331 women in the double embryo transfer (DET) group and 330 women in the SET group. An intention-to-treat analysis was performed and in the SET group 128 women had a pregnancy resulting in at least one live birth (38.8%) and in the DET group 142 women (42.9%). The 95% confidence interval for the difference was −3.4% to 11.6%. When only the fresh cycles were compared, the rate of live births was significantly lower in the SET group as compared to the DET group (27.6% vs. 42.9%, $p < 0.001$). The rate of multiple births was 47 of 142 in the DET group compared to 1 of 128 in the SET group (33.1% vs. 0.8%, $p < 0.001$). The study showed that a single fresh embryo transfer, followed (if no live birth) by the transfer of one cryopreserved embryo, markedly reduced the multiple birth rate, while there was no substantial reduction in the pregnancy rate resulting in live births.

In a further analysis of this randomized controlled study, maternal and pediatric outcomes between the SET and the DET group were compared [14]. The rates of prematurely born and low birth weight children were, as expected, significantly lower with the SET strategy, 15/129; 11.6% versus 55/189; 29.1% and 10/129; 7.8% versus 52/189; 27.5% respectively. More maternal complications occurred in the DET group, including severe hemorrhage, preterm labor and preterm rupture of the membranes as well as more Cesarean sections. A higher number of severe neonatal complications, requiring neonatal hospital care was found in the DET group [14, 15].

In a multivariate regression analysis, including cycles with 0% or 100% implantation ($n = 520$) maternal and embryo variables were analyzed. The variables first IVF cycle, conventional IVF as

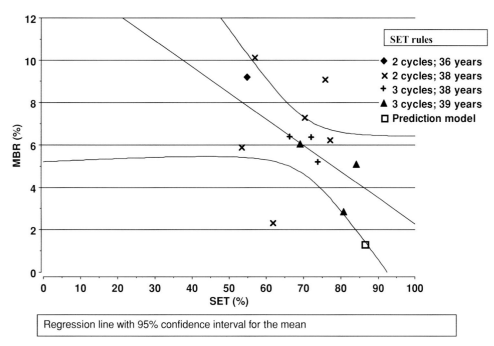

Figure 14.1 Multiple birth rates (MBR) in relation to the percentage of SET for women below 40 years at different IVF units in Sweden 2004 (From [17] with permission from *Hum. Reprod.*)

fertilization method, 4-cell embryos and ovarian sensitivity all correlated independently with ongoing implantation [16].

Observational studies

In parallel with the recruitment to the Scandinavian SET study, and owing to the intensive debate in Sweden concerning the high multiple birth rate after IVF, the law concerning assisted reproduction was changed in the year 2003 and in the guidelines from the Swedish Board of Health and Welfare the number of embryos to be transferred was regulated. This was preceded, however, by a voluntary shift by the IVF doctors themselves using the SET rules according to the Scandinavian SET study. The regulations state that one embryo should be the normal routine and only when the risk of twins is regarded low two embryos may be transferred.

Before the new regulations were issued, in 2002, the multiple birth rates on a national level were only reduced to just below 20% with an elective SET (eSET) rate of 21.2% and a total SET rate of 30.6%. The guidelines of 2003 proposed, by the IVF doctors, that eSET be used for women of less than 38 years if there was one embryo of good quality in the first two cycles. During 2003, with implementation of the new legislation, the multiple birth rates decreased to 11.8% and the eSET and SET rates increased to 41.3% and 54.3% respectively. The 14 Swedish IVF units continued to revise their eSET criteria further, according to the legend in Figure 14.1, during the next year, 2004. National data shown in Figure 14.1 describe the multiple birth rates with regression line at different IVF units and the corresponding SET frequencies for women below the age of 40. To achieve a multiple birth rate of maximum 5%, a SET rate of at least 75% is needed for women below 40 years of age according to the regression equation

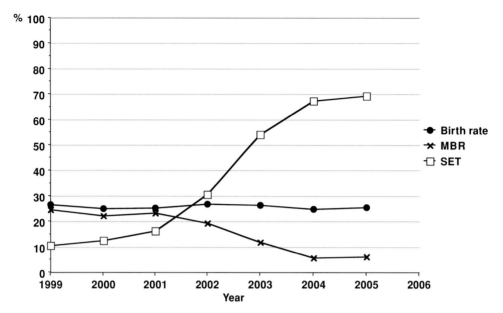

Figure 14.2 Birth per embryo transfer and multiple birth rates (MBR) in relation to the percentage of SET in Sweden 1999–2005.

MBR = 17.4–0.166 x% SET. One clinic developed a prediction model based on patient and cycle characteristics together with embryo scores for predicting the chance of pregnancy and the risk of twin births. The model was used to establish a cut off level of 10% risk for twin pregnancy to decide between SET and DET [18, 19]. The clinic using the predicting model achieved the lowest multiple birth rate. In 2004 the multiple birth rates continued to decrease dramatically in Sweden to 5.7% with a SET level of 67.4%, and similar figures were noted for 2005 (Figure 14.2).

A comparison was made between the year 2000 (when eSET and SET constituted 4.3% and 12.6% of all transfers) with year 2004 (when more than 50% of the transfers were eSET) (Table 14.1). The SET level in different age cohorts is of special interest. A considerable decrease in multiple birth rate was observed for all age groups below 40, while the birth rate remained unchanged.

The multiple birth rate after DET decreased from 27.2% to 20.4% and the birth rate from 29.2% to 22.3% during the six years between 1999 and 2005. A large variation in the multiple birth rates (5–25%) between the different IVF units was, however, still observed [17]. Probably the multiple birth rates in Sweden can be further reduced, without impairment of the overall delivery rate, by less restrictive SET rules. Such a development is supported by findings from a recent observational study in Finland [20].

Before these national data were available similar results were published by Saldeen and Sundström [21] representing one large IVF unit. In this debate article the authors showed results before and after the new regulations and discussed whether legislation or voluntary SET is the most feasible way to proceed.

When SET has been introduced more embryos will be available for cryopreservation and thus SET requires a well-functioning freezing program. In a retrospective analysis it was recently shown that although DET results in a slightly higher live birth rate than SET for fresh cycles, when calculating

Table 14.1 Number of embryo transfers (ET), percentage of SET, delivery and multiple birth rates (MBR) in different age cohorts in Sweden, year 2000 and 2004

Age	Number of ET		SET (%)		Delivery rate (%)		MBR (%)	
	2000	2004	2000	2004	2000	2004	2000	2004
< 30	965	1211		82.7	32.3	31.0	25.3	4.0
30–34	2424	2937		76.5	30.0	29.7	25.0	6.0
35–37	1596	2005		69.8	22.8	24.0	18.5	5.6
38–39	771	1032		49.9	17.3	17.9	15.8	5.4
40–41	469	603		38.3	14.5	12.9	10.3	7.7
> 41	361	348		26.1	5.8	10.3	6.2	13.9
Total	6586	8136	12.6	67.4	25.1	25.0	22.2	5.7

Reproduced from [17] with permission from *Hum. Reprod.*

cumulative results for one fresh and the following frozen-thawed cycles from one oocyte pick-up, the overall live birth rates were very similar, 33.5% and 34.8% for DET and SET, respectively [22].

Attitudes

Another important aspect of IVF when trying to reduce complications for the children, is patients' and doctors' attitudes towards SET and multiple births. Some studies have shown that patients prefer twins compared to singletons [23] while other studies have indicated that increased knowledge and awareness of the complications of multiple births seemed to influence patient's attitudes towards a preference for SET [24]. In addition, in a recent systematic review from the Netherlands concerning women's attitudes, most women seemed to deal effectively with the burden of successive IVF cycles [25].

In a Nordic survey we investigated doctors' attitudes towards SET and multiple births [26]. It was found that the SET and multiple birth rates in the different Nordic countries reflected the attitudes of the Nordic IVF doctors to SET and multiple births well. A twin rate of > 10% was accepted by only 5% of Swedish IVF doctors while in the other Nordic countries between 21% and 35% of the doctors found such a multiple birth rate acceptable.

Quality of life

In the Scandinavian SET study quality of life of mothers was assessed. The patients were asked to answer two well-known and validated questionnaires, SF-36 [27, 28] and SPSQ (Swedish Parenthood Stress Questionnaire) [29, 30] six months after delivery. The questionnaires were answered by 98.1% of the patients. No significant differences were found between the SET and DET groups and the results were also comparable to a normal Swedish population [14] (Figure 14.3a, b).

Costs

The Scandinavian trial showed superiority for SET versus DET concerning costs, when costs were compared per randomized woman or per delivery with live born child/children [14]. The incremental cost-effectiveness ratio (ICER) was also in favor of SET, indicating that SET was cost-effective as compared with DET. A recent systematic review [31] of financial assessments of SET versus DET including four studies [14, 32–34] provides a good illustration of all the problems associated with trying to compare studies of a financial nature from different countries. Despite the fact that three of these four studies were randomized controlled trials, there were large differences between them concerning study

(a)

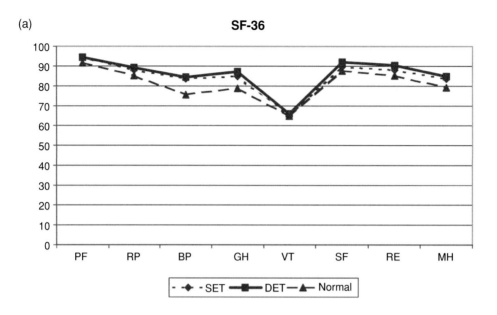

(b)

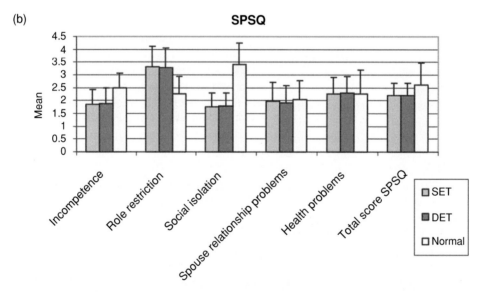

Figure 14.3 (a) SF-36. Comparison of the SF-36 questionnaire between the SET and DET study groups: physical functioning (PF; $p = 0.885$); role physical (RP; $p = 0.708$); bodily pain (BP; $p = 0.835$) general health (GH; $p = 0.197$); vitality (VT; $p = 0.736$); social functioning (SF; $p = 0.304$); role emotional (RE; $p = 0.492$); mental health (MH; $p = 0.594$). Higher values indicate better health. A comparison with a Swedish normal population of women 30–35 years of age is also shown.(b) SPSQ (Swedish Parenthood Stress Questionnaire). Comparison of the SPSQ questionnaire between the SET and DET study groups: Incompetence ($p = 0.707$); Role restriction ($p = 0.968$); Social isolation ($p = 0.655$); Spouse relationship problems ($p = 0.422$); Health problems ($p = 0.841$) and Total score ($p = 0.923$). Higher values indicate higher stress levels. A comparison with a Swedish normal population of mothers with children 21.4 months of age in average is also shown. (From [14] with permission from *Hum. Reprod.*)

population, inclusion/exclusion of frozen cycles, differences in costs in the specific country and methods of cost estimation, etc. All studies included the costs of IVF treatment, pregnancy and delivery and a certain postnatal period, although the length of the latter differed considerably (1–6 months) between studies. Owing to this heterogeneity it was not possible to pool the studies and calculate a common cost estimate for SET and DET. However, eSET in combination with an additional frozen SET appeared to be cost-effective as compared to DET, while when only fresh cycles were compared, the situation was less clear.

REFERENCES

1. P. C. Steptoe and R. G. Edwards, Birth after the reimplantation of a human embryo. *Lancet*, **2**: 8085 (1978), 366.
2. A. N. Andersen, V. Goossens, L. Gianaroli *et al.*, Assisted reproductive technology in Europe, 2003. Results generated from European registries by ESHRE. *Hum. Reprod.*, **22** (2007), 1513–1525.
3. Society for Assisted Reproductive Technology; American Society for Reproductive Medicine, Assisted reproductive technology in the United States: 2000 results generated from the American Society for Reproductive Medicine/Society for Assisted Reproductive *Technology Registry Fertil Steril*, 2004; **81**:1207–1220.
4. T. Bergh, A. Ericson, T. Hillensjö, K.-G. Nygren and U.-B. Wennerholm, Deliveries and children born after in-vitro fertilization in Sweden 1982–95: a retrospective cohort study. *Lancet*, **354** (1999), 1579–1585.
5. F. M. Helmerhorst, D. A. Perquin, D. Donker and M. J. Keirse, Perinatal outcome of singletons and twins after assisted conception: a systematic review of controlled studies. *BMJ*, **328** (2004), 261–265.
6. R. A. Jackson, K. A. Gibson and M. S., Croughan, Perinatal outcomes in singletons following in vitro fertilization: a meta-analysis. *Obstet. Gynecol.*, **103** (2004), 551–563.
7. U. B. Wennerholm and C. Bergh, Outcome of IVF pregnancies. *Fetal Matern. Med. Rev.*, **15** (2004), 27–57.
8. B. Strömberg, G. Dahlquist, A. Ericson, *et al.*, Neurological sequelae in children born after in-vitro fertilisation: a population-based study. *Lancet*, **359**: 9305 (2002), 461–465.
9. B. Källen, O. Finnström, K.-G. Nygren and P. O. Olausson, In vitro fertilization (IVF) in Sweden. Infant outcome after different fertilization methods. *Fertil. Steril.*, **84** (2005a), 611–617.
10. B. Källen, O. Finnström, K.-G. Nygren and P. O. Olausson, In vitro fertilization (IVF) in Sweden. Child morbidity including cancer risk. *Fertil. Steril.*, **84** (2005b), 605–610.
11. S. Vilska, A. Tiitinen, C. Hyden-Granskog and O. Hovatta, Elective transfer of one embryo results in an acceptable pregnancy rate and eliminates the risk of multiple birth. *Hum. Reprod.*, **14**:9 (1999), 2392–2395.
12. A. Strandell, C. Bergh and K. Lundin, Selection of patients suitable for one-embryo transfer reduces the rate of multiple births by half without impairment of overall birth rates. *Hum. Reprod.*, **15** (2000), 2520–2525.
13. A. Thurin, J. Hausken, T. Hillensjö *et al.*, Elective single-embryo transfer versus double-embryo transfer in in-vitro fertilization. *N. Engl. J. Med.*, **351** (2004), 2392–2402.
14. A. T. Kjellberg, P. Carlsson and C. Bergh, Randomized single versus double embryo transfer: obstetric and paediatric outcome and a cost-effectiveness analysis. *Hum. Reprod.*, **21** (2006), 210–216.
15. C. Bergh, How to promote singletons. Contributions from the Bertarelli Foundation Meeting: "Triplets End Point" (online only publication). *Reprod. Biomed. Online*, **15**: Suppl. 3 (2007). www.rbmonline.com/Article/2749.
16. A. Thurin, T. Hardarsson, J. Hausken *et al.*, Predictors of ongoing implantation in IVF in a good prognosis group of patients. *Hum. Reprod.*, **20** (2005), 1876–1880.
17. P. O. Karlström and C. Bergh, Reducing the number of embryos transferred in Sweden-impact on delivery and multiple birth rates. *Hum. Reprod.*, **22**:8 (2007), 2202–2207. Epub 2007 Jun 11.
18. J. Holte, T. Bergh, J. Tilly, H. Petterson and L. Berglund, The construction and application of a prediction model to minimize twin implantation rate at a preserved high pregnancy rate. *Hum. Reprod.*, **19**: Suppl. 1 (2004), Abstract Book. 20th Annual Meeting of the ESHRE, P-394.
19. J. Holte, L. Berglund, K. Milton *et al.*, Construction of an evidence-based integrated morphology cleavage embryo score for implantation potential of embryos scored and transferred on day 2 after oocyte retrieval. *Hum. Reprod.*, **22** (2007), 548–557.

20. Z. Veleva, S. Vilska, C. Hydén-Granskog *et al.*, Elective single embryo transfer in women aged 36–39 years. *Hum. Reprod.*, **21** (2006), 2098–2102.

21. P. Saldeen and P Sundström, Would legislation imposing single embryo transfer be a feasible way to reduce the rate of multiple pregnancies after IVF treatment? *Hum. Reprod.*, **20** (2005), 4–8.

22. K. Lundin and C. Bergh, Cumulative impact of adding frozen-thawed cycles to single versus double fresh embryo transfers. *Reprod. Biomed. Online*, **15** (2007), 742–748.

23. A. Pinborg, A. Loft, L. Schmidt and A. N. Andersen, Attitudes of IVF/ICSI-twin mothers towards twins and single embryo transfer. *Hum. Reprod.*, **18** (2003), 621–627.

24. C. R. Newton, J. McBride, V. Feyles, F. Tekpetey and S. Power, Factors affecting patients' attitudes towards single- and multiple-embryo transfer. *Fertil. Steril.*, **87** (2007), 269–278.

25. C. M. Verhaak, J. M. J. Smeenk, A. W. M. Evers *et al.*, Women's emotional adjustment to IVF: a systematic review of 25 years of research. *Hum. Reprod. Update*, **13** (2007), 27–36.

26. C. Bergh, V. Söderström-Anttila, A. Selbing *et al.*, Attitudes towards and management of single embryo transfer among Nordic IVF doctors. *Acta Obstet. Gynecol. Scand.*, **86** (2007), 1222–1230.

27. J. E. Ware, K. K. Snow, M. Kosinski and B. Gandek, *SF-36 Health Survey Manual and Interpretation Guide.* (Boston, MA: New England Medical Center, The Health Institute, 1993).

28. M. Sullivan and J. Karlsson, SF-36 Hälsoenkät. *Swedish Manual and Interpretation Guide.* (Sektionen för vårdforskning, Medicinska fakulteten, Göteborgs Universitet och Sahlgrenska sjukhuset, 1994).

29. R. R. Abidin, *Parenting Stress Index (PSI) – Manual.* (Odessa, FL: Psychological Assessment Resources, Inc., 1990).

30. M. Östberg, B. Hagekull and S. Wettergren, A measure of parental stress in mothers with small children: dimensionality, stability and validity. *Scand. J. Psychol.*, **38** (1997), 199–208.

31. A. A. A. Fiddelers, J. L. Severens, C. D. Dirksen *et al.*, Economic evaluations of single versus double-embryo transfer in IVF. *Hum. Reprod. Update*, **13** (2007), 5–13.

32. J. Gerris, P. De Sutter, D. De Neubourg *et al.*, A real-life prospective health economic study of elective single embryo transfer versus two-embryo transfer in first IVF/ICSI cycles. *Hum. Reprod.*, **19**:4 (2004), 917–923.

33. H. G. Lukassen, D. D. Braat, A. M. Wetzels *et al.*, Two cycles with single embryo transfer versus one cycle with double embryo transfer: a randomized controlled trial. *Hum. Reprod.*, **20**:3 (2005), 702–708.

34. A. A. A. Fiddelers, A. P. A. van Montfoort, C. D. Dirksen *et al.*, Single versus double embryo transfer: cost-effectiveness analysis alongside a randomized trial. *Hum. Reprod.*, **21** (2006), 2090–2097.

15

Single embryo transfer: the Dutch experience

Aafke P. A. van Montfoort

Epidemiological background

Following Belgium and Finland, also in the Netherlands concern was raised about the safety and risks of in vitro fertilization (IVF), and especially the risks involved in multiple pregnancies. To give an overall picture of IVF in the Netherlands, the Dutch Society of Obstetrics and Gynecology (NVOG) collects IVF outcome data from the 13 licensed IVF centers. The last few years around 15 000 cycles per year were performed of which 60% was conventional IVF and 40% IVF with intracytoplasmic sperm injection (ICSI) (www.nvog.nl). With 16 million inhabitants, this means that per million inhabitants 938 cycles are performed, which lies around the average number in Europe [1]. From 2003 onwards, besides the number of pregnancies, also the number of multiple pregnancies was collected by the NVOG. In that year, out of 15 769 initiated cycles, 3706 led to an ongoing pregnancy, of which 77.8% was a singleton, 21.7% a twin and 0.5% a triplet (www.nvog.nl). Assuming 3600 live births with a similar distribution of multiples and singletons, this would result in 4417 children of which 37% were part of a twin or triplet pregnancy. In 2003, in total 200 297 children were born (statline.cbs.nl), so in the Netherlands 2.2% of the newborn children were the result of IVF and with 3686 multiple pregnancies, 21.7% of the multiple pregnancies were the result of IVF.

Regarding the increasing number of IVF treatments, the high number of multiple pregnancies and the complications associated with these pregnancies (see Chapter 1), also in the Netherlands efforts were made to limit the number of embryos per transfer. There is no legislation on the number to transfer, but since 2003 a recommendation exists not to transfer more than two embryos. In 2004, this still resulted in an overall twin pregnancy rate of 20% (ww.nvog.nl). As there is no national registration of the number of embryos transferred, the rate of single embryo transfer (SET) and the influence of the introduction of SET on the overall outcome of IVF for the Netherlands is hard to analyze. Therefore regarding SET in daily practice only data from individual clinics are available, such as those from our own clinic in Maastricht which are presented below.

However, at the end of the year 2001, three Dutch studies were started within the framework of a research program on health technology assessment of infertility under the authority of the Ministry of Health, Welfare and Sports with the joint theme of safer and simpler IVF. Two studies performed a randomized controlled trial (RCT) on SET versus double embryo transfer (DET) [2, 3] and one was a cohort study on natural cycle IVF [4, 5]. Another RCT comparing SET versus DET was performed outside this program [6]. The three RCTs analyzed different patient groups and different SET and DET strategies, which will be discussed below.

Single Embryo Transfer, ed. J. Gerris, G. D. Adamson, P. De Sutter and C. Racowsky. Published by Cambridge University Press.
© Cambridge University Press 2009.

Table 15.1 Live birth rate and costs/effect for several SET and DET strategies

Study	Groups compared		Live birth rate		Costs/effect(€)	
	1	2	1	2	1	2
Lukassen *et al.* [6][a]	Two cycles SET	One cycle DET	41%	36%	13 438	13 680
{ van Montfoort *et al.* [2][b]	One cycle SET	One cycle DET	21%	40%	35 260	27 586
{ Fiddelers *et al.* [7][c]						
Heijnen *et al.* [3][d]	SET in combination with a mild treatment strategy	DET with a traditional stimulation protocol	43%	45%	19 200	24 038

[a] Only good prognosis patients were included in the study (see text for criteria). Cost-effectiveness analysis was based on the healthcare perspective.

[b] Unselected patient population (i.e., irrespective of female age and the availability of a good quality embryo) was included in the study and

[c] the cost-effectiveness analysis was based on the societal perspective.

[d] Only good prognosis patients were included in the study (see text for criteria). The results are presented over a 12-month period in which on average 1.5 embryo transfers were done in the mild treatment group and 1.4 in the standard stimulation group. Cost-effectiveness analysis was based on the societal perspective.

Alongside these RCTs, cost-effectiveness analyses were performed. In the Netherlands, three IVF cycles per ongoing pregnancy are fully reimbursed (including medication) and when a child is born another three cycles are reimbursed. The medical costs of an IVF treatment including medication are around €2500 [6] and when the laboratory phase and the costs outside health care, such as productivity costs or out-of-pocket costs for the patients, are included these costs are around €4500 per cycle [7].

In this chapter the clinical and cost-effectiveness results of the Dutch studies on SET versus DET and the natural cycle IVF will be presented as well as the Maastricht experience with SET in daily practice.

Dutch experience with SET

Clinical outcome

Two cycles SET versus one cycle DET in a selected patient population

The Nijmegen group were the first to publish a Dutch RCT regarding SET [6]. Their aim was to compare the live birth rate after two consecutive cycles of SET with one cycle of DET, excluding cycles with cryopreserved embryos. Only patients < 35 years of age undergoing their first cycle after primary or secondary subfertility with a basal follicle-stimulating hormone (FSH) level < 10 IU/L and at least two embryos of which one had < 10% fragmentation were included in the study. Of 494 patients younger than 35 years, 387 were excluded. Forty percent did not meet the inclusion criteria, e.g. number and quality of the embryos and 60% refused to participate or had an FSH level ≥ 10 IU/L. Eventually 107 patients were randomized between two cycles SET ($n = 54$) and one cycle DET ($n = 53$). The live birth rate after one cycle of SET was 26% compared to 36% after one cycle of DET (not significant). A second SET cycle in the non-pregnant SET patients led to an increase of the live birth rate to 41%, thereby compensating for the lower live birth rate after the first cycle. By offering two cycles of SET instead of one cycle of DET, the twin pregnancy rate could be reduced from 37% to 0% ($p = 0.002$), but at the expense of an extra IVF cycle for the patients (Table 15.1).

One cycle SET versus one cycle DET in patients irrespective of age and embryo quality

In all published RCTs on SET and DET only patients at high risk for a twin pregnancy were included. The criteria for patients at risk varied between the studies, but were mainly based on female age and the number of good quality embryos available. In this subpopulation of patients, the transfer of one embryo resulted in an equal or lower pregnancy rate as compared to the transfer of two embryos. When in this subpopulation one embryo was transferred and in the remaining older patients or patients with minor quality embryos two embryos were transferred both groups have a similar chance for a pregnancy [2, 8–11]. However, this strategy does not reduce the twin pregnancy rate to the natural level, as in a substantial number of the patients still two embryos are transferred. What would occur when one embryo was transferred in the whole IVF population was however unknown. The aim of our own RCT was therefore to compare the pregnancy rates between one cycle SET and one cycle DET in all IVF patients irrespective of their age and of the availability of a good quality embryo [2]. The only inclusion criteria were that it should be the patient's first IVF cycle and that for a proper randomization at least two embryos had to be available. Patients with a medical reason for SET or patients with a language barrier were excluded. Only transfers with fresh embryos were included in the study. The transfer of cryopreserved embryos was not a part of the randomization.

Of the 621 eligible patients, 56% agreed to participate in the study. Forty patients could not be randomized because only one embryo was available. Eventually 154 patients were randomized to SET and another 154 patients were randomized to DET. As the rate of positive human chorionic gonadotropin (hCG) tests differed significantly already (33.1% after SET vs. 47.4% after DET) and the abortion rate per positive hCG test was significantly higher after SET (35.3% vs. 15.1%), the ongoing pregnancy rate was halved after one cycle SET as compared to one cycle DET (21.4% and 40.3%, respectively) (Table 15.1). However, the twin pregnancy rate was reduced from 21.0% after DET to 0% after SET.

SET in combination with a mild stimulation protocol versus DET with a traditional stimulation protocol analyzed per year in a selected patient population

Another group tested the hypothesis that with a mild ovarian stimulation protocol using a gonadotropin-releasing hormone (GnRH) antagonist, patients were willing to undergo more cycles within a certain time period than patients receiving a traditional GnRH agonist long stimulation protocol [3]. By transferring one embryo in patients treated with the mild stimulation protocol and two embryos in patients treated with the traditional stimulation protocol, in the SET group more cycles per patient per year will be performed, which can compensate for the reduction in live births per cycle as compared to DET in combination with the traditional stimulation protocol. The inclusion criteria for the patients were first cycle, age < 38 years, menstrual cycle length of 25–35 days and a body mass index (BMI) of 18–28 kg/m^2. In total 404 patients were included in this non-inferiority trial and were randomized between a maximum of three IVF cycles with standard ovarian stimulation in combination with DET ($n = 199$) or a maximum of four IVF cycles with mild ovarian stimulation in combination with SET ($n = 205$). In this study the transfer of cryopreserved embryo was included and in both groups the number of transferred cryopreserved embryos was based on patients' preferences.

Although it makes it hard to compare with other studies, in this study the outcome parameter was live birth rate per year of treatment instead of per cycle. Within one year, in the mild treatment group, on average 2.3 cycles per patient were started resulting in 1.5 embryo transfers and a live birth rate of 43.3%. In the traditional treatment group these data were 1.7, 1.4 and 44.7% respectively (Table 15.1). The multiple pregnancy rate after one year was 0.5% per mildly stimulated patient and 13.1% per traditionally stimulated patient. The cumulative live birth rate after three cycles of DET was 50.3% and after four cycles of SET 52.4%, i.e. similar, but with a strong reduction of twins.

Natural cycle IVF

Another way of performing SET is by natural cycle IVF in which the one spontaneously developing oocyte is used for IVF. The Groningen group described their results with natural cycle IVF with minimal stimulation after a maximum of three and nine cycles [4, 5]. The inclusion criteria were 18–36 years of age, first IVF treatment ever or after a pregnancy, a regular menstrual cycle and a BMI between 18 and 28. Only patients requiring IVF and not ICSI were included. The 256 patients that were offered a maximum of nine cycles started a total of 1048 (= 4.1/patient) cycles. Of these, 625 (59.6%) led to a successful oocyte retrieval and 382 (36.5%) to an embryo transfer. In 81 patients a live birth was achieved (31.6% per patient and 7.7% per started cycle). The overall dropout rate of patients was 47.8%. Although natural cycle IVF requires little medication, the oocyte retrieval is easy and only a small risk for ovarian hyperstimulation syndrome (OHSS) exists, the higher number of cycles needed to obtain a pregnancy as compared to IVF with ovarian stimulation and the disappointments when an oocyte retrieval is canceled or unsuccessful, fertilization fails or when there is no embryo transfer led to the decision of patients to quit the study.

Cost-effectiveness

In the three RCTs on SET versus DET the cost-effectiveness of the strategies was analyzed as well (Table 15.1). The costs of the IVF treatment itself, including the medication, was similar between both study groups, whatever the conditions for SET were [3, 6, 7]. What makes the difference are the costs of the pregnancies and deliveries and especially of the twin pregnancies. From the healthcare perspective,

these costs are estimated to be €13 469, whereas for a singleton these are €2 550 [12].

When we compared SET with DET in an unselected patient population (i.e., irrespective of female age and the availability of a good quality embryo) the relative reduction in live birth rate after SET compared to DET is higher than the reduced costs, resulting in higher costs per live birth after SET as compared to DET (€35 260 and €27 586, respectively) as analyzed from the societal perspective [7]. The costs of each additional live birth after DET as compared to SET are therefore relatively low, €19 096 (i.e., incremental cost-effectiveness ratio, ICER). In other words, the costs of the extra SET cycles needed to obtain a similar live birth rate do not weight against the extra costs of twin pregnancies after DET.

However, in a selected patient population, the extra cycles needed to obtain a live birth after SET do weight against the extra costs of twin pregnancies after DET [6] resulting in similar costs per live birth (€13 438 and €13 680, respectively) analyzed from the healthcare perspective.

When analyzing SET in combination with a mild ovarian stimulation protocol and DET with standard treatment for a period of 12 months the costs per live birth are even disadvantageous for DET (€19 200 vs. €24 038) with an ICER of standard compared to mild ovarian stimulation of €185 000 [3].

Counseling the patients

For patients, a twin pregnancy is not always an adverse outcome and the increased pregnancy rate after DET is one of the most important variables positively influencing the patients' choice for DET [13]. In the above-mentioned RCT studies all patients were offered an extra cycle when they would be allocated to the SET group, whether it was a second SET cycle [6], an extra cycle which was not a part of the randomization [2] or a fourth cycle as part of the strategy investigated [3]. Under this condition patients were willing to receive one embryo. Our personal experience in Maastricht is that when the patients are counseled about the risks and

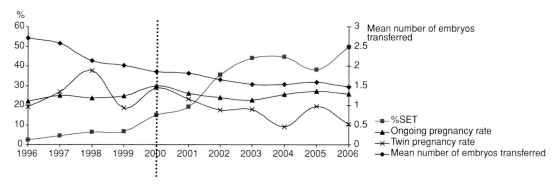

Figure 15.1 Proportion of single embryo transfers (SET), ongoing and twin pregnancies and the mean number of embryos transferred in Maastricht, the Netherlands, 1996–2006. Before 2000 the attention was focused on the reduction of the number of transferred embryos from three to two. From 2000 onwards, SET was gradually introduced.

complications involved in twin pregnancies they are willing to receive one embryo and sometimes even request the transfer of one embryo. Our standard transfer policy at the moment is to transfer one embryo in patients younger than 38 years with at least one good quality embryo (see below). Almost all patients accept this policy. Only 0.26% requests the transfer of two embryos and 3.6% requests the transfer of one embryo irrespective of the availability of a good quality embryo.

Maastricht experience with SET in daily practice

Besides the RCT on SET versus DET [2], SET was introduced gradually in daily practice in Maastricht over the past years. In Figure 15.1 the proportion of SET, which consist of compulsory SET (cSET, i.e. SET when only one embryo is available) and elective SET (eSET, i.e. the transfer of one embryo when more than one embryo is available for transfer), is shown in relation to the ongoing and multiple pregnancy rate. The patients participating in the RCT are not included. Before the year 2000, the number of transferred embryos was gradually reduced from three to two. First only in patients younger than 35 years, but soon the age limit was set to younger than 38 years. The proportion of triple pregnancies was indeed

reduced to zero (except for the exceptional DET, where one of the two implanted embryos divides into a monozygotic twin). The high twin pregnancy rate however remained and also the ongoing pregnancy rate did not suffer from the reduction in embryos transferred. This and the encouraging results from Belgium and Finland with SET made us confident to introduce SET in our clinic. From the year 2000 onwards only one embryo was transferred in the case where the female patient was younger than 37 years of age and at least one embryo of excellent quality was available. Even when applied in the first three cycles of an IVF patient, there was no reduction in pregnancy rate after SET as compared to DET, although the pregnancy rate in both groups was lower in the third cycle when compared to the first two [11]. The overall twin pregnancy rate in 2001 was however still 23.1%, probably due to the fact that the proportion of cycles with SET was relatively small, only 19%. Over the past years, the criteria for a good quality embryo were gradually liberated, and some new parameters for embryo quality, such as the absence of multinucleated blastomeres and early first cleavage, were introduced. Embryos of suboptimal morphology, but positive for these new characteristics were now considered to be a good quality embryo. Also under these conditions the pregnancy rate after SET and DET was similar [14]. Regarding the first cycle only, in 56% of the

SET cycles and in 26% of the DET cycles, embryos could be cryopreserved. After the transfer of these embryos, mostly per two, the ongoing pregnancy rates increased to 42.0% after SET in the fresh cycle and 32.8% after DET [2].

In our six years of experience with SET we increased the proportion of cycles with SET from 15% to 50%, while our overall ongoing pregnancy rate remained around 26%. In 2005 there was an unexplained reduction of the SET rate which immediately resulted in an increase in twin pregnancies. In 2006 the criteria for a good quality embryo were therefore again slightly changed, which increased the SET rate and resulted in only 10% of the ongoing pregnancies to be a twin pregnancy.

Conclusions

As shown by all studies discussed above, the transfer of one embryo will always lead to a lower pregnancy rate per cycle as compared to the transfer of two embryos. This was also shown in a meta-analysis of RCTs on SET versus DET in a selected group of patients [15]. When female age and availability of a good quality embryo are not taken into account, the difference between SET and DET is even higher; the pregnancy rate after SET was halved as compared to the pregnancy rate after DET but the twin pregnancy rate was reduced to 0% [2]. In observational studies, when SET was applied in the good prognosis patients (young with good quality embryos) and DET in the remaining patients (referred to as SET/DET policy), the pregnancy rates between both groups are comparable, even in the second and third IVF cycle [2, 11], with a pregnancy rate around 30%. These data are comparable to other observational studies [8–10].

Hypothetically, the similar pregnancy rates between SET and DET could be expected because the increase in the proportion of SET will not only lead to a decrease in pregnancy rate after SET, as can be concluded from the RCTs, but will also lead to a decrease in pregnancy rate after DET as the pregnancy prognosis of the patients remaining

for DET decreases with less strict criteria for SET. The reason why in studies showing an increase in the SET rate the pregnancy rate over the years still remains stable at around 30% or increases only slightly is probably the improvement of the IVF technique and skills. When still two fresh embryos would have been transferred in all patients, the pregnancy rate would have increased to around 40% as can be concluded from the RCT where DET was applied irrespective of age and the availability of a good quality embryo [2].

A strategy to make up the arrears of SET would be the transfer of cryopreserved embryos [16]. Although the effect of cryopreservation on success rates has not been thoroughly investigated, all Dutch studies showed that after SET more embryos could be cryopreserved. In a retrospective analysis of the SET/DET policy in the non-participants of the RCT in our own clinic, the transfer of cryopreserved embryos increased the ongoing pregnancy rate in the SET group from 33% to 42% and in the DET group from 30% to 33%. The overall twin pregnancy rate after fresh and frozen embryo transfers was 15% [2].

To compensate for the difference in pregnancy rate per cycle between SET and DET, other strategies involving extra treatment cycles were investigated. The RCTs by Lukassen *et al.* [6] and by Heijnen *et al.* [3] both showed that at least one extra cycle with SET could overcome the difference in pregnancy rate, but only in a subpopulation of IVF patients. A Markov model based on the results of the RCT performed in our center with patients irrespective of age and the availability of a good quality embryo showed however that in this patient group six cycles SET could not reach the pregnancy rate obtained after three cycles DET (data not published).

Regarding the cost-effectiveness, it is hard to compare the different studies as the costs were determined differently among the studies and one study was performed from the healthcare perspective and the others from the societal perspective. Nevertheless, it can be concluded that when SET is applied in a selected population only, the costs per live birth are similar or even favor those associated with DET. When applied in the whole IVF population, the costs per live birth after DET are more favorable.

The Dutch experience with SET shows that SET is not a suitable transfer strategy for all IVF patients, unless a substantial decrease of the pregnancy rate is accepted to completely prevent twin pregnancies. It is more preferable to apply SET in a selected patient population, both from a clinical and a cost-effectiveness point of view, although with such a policy the twin pregnancy rate cannot be reduced to the natural level. A balance has to be found between the decrease in pregnancy rate with SET and the decrease in twin pregnancy rate. The question on what are the best selection criteria for SET, leading to the highest overall pregnancy rate with the lowest overall twin pregnancy rate, remains to be solved. Nevertheless, with the current selection criteria, the transfer of cryopreserved embryos or an additional fresh cycle can compensate for the reduced pregnancy rate after SET. As the pregnancy rate remains similar these patients will accept the transfer of one embryo.

What do we know?
Regarding the risks and severe complications associated with twin pregnancies, these should be prevented. To maximally reduce the number of twin pregnancies, in all patients one embryo should be transferred. According to a RCT, this however leads to a halving of the pregnancy rate as compared to DET. When SET is performed in a selected group of good prognosis patients, based on female age and embryo quality, the reduction is less severe, while still a considerable number of twin pregnancies can be prevented. If in daily practice in this selected patient population one embryo is transferred and in the remaining older patients or patients with minor quality embryos two embryos are transferred the pregnancy rate is similar in both groups.

What do we need to know?
The similar pregnancy rates between SET in good prognosis patients and DET in the remaining patients could perhaps be expected, irrespective of the criteria for SET. An increase in the proportion of SET will not only lead to a decrease in pregnancy rate in that subpopulation. It will also lead to a decrease in pregnancy rate in the DET population as the pregnancy prognosis of the patients remaining for DET decreases. On the other hand, strict criteria for SET will increase the overall pregnancy rate but also the twin pregnancy rate. Therefore, a balance has to be found between a decrease in pregnancy rate and a decrease in twin pregnancy rate when applying SET.

What should we do?
To find this balance, the selection criteria for the subpopulation of IVF patients suitable for SET, in which a maximal reduction in twin pregnancies can be obtained with a minimal or acceptable reduction in pregnancy rate, should be determined. A small decrease in pregnancy rate as compared to DET should be associated with a large decrease in twin pregnancy rate. It should be carefully considered whether measures decreasing the twin pregnancy rate only marginally balance the reduction in pregnancy rate as only a percentage of the twins has complications that should be prevented.

REFERENCES

1. A. N. Andersen, V. Goossens, L. Gianaroli *et al.*, Assisted reproductive technology in Europe, 2003. Results generated from European registers by ESHRE. *Hum. Reprod.*, **22** (2007),1513–1525.
2. A. P. van Montfoort, A. A. Fiddelers, J. M. Janssen *et al.*, In unselected patients, elective single embryo transfer prevents all multiples, but results in significantly lower pregnancy rates compared with double embryo transfer: a randomized controlled trial. *Hum. Reprod.*, **21** (2006), 338–343.
3. E. M. Heijnen, M. J. Eijkemans, C. De Klerk *et al.*, A mild treatment strategy for in-vitro fertilisation: a randomised non-inferiority trial. *Lancet*, **369** (2007), 743–749.
4. M. J. Pelinck, N. E. Vogel, A. Hoek *et al.*, Cumulative pregnancy rates after three cycles of minimal stimulation IVF and results according to subfertility diagnosis: a multicentre cohort study. *Hum. Reprod.*, **21** (2006), 2375–2383.

5. M. J. Pelinck, N. E. Vogel, E. G. Arts *et al.*, Cumulative pregnancy rates after a maximum of nine cycles of modified natural cycle IVF and analysis of patient drop-out: a cohort study. *Hum. Reprod.*, **22** (2007), 2463–2470.

6. H. G. Lukassen, D. D. Braat, A. M. Wetzels *et al.*, Two cycles with single embryo transfer versus one cycle with double embryo transfer: a randomized controlled trial. *Hum. Reprod.*, **20** (2005), 702–708.

7. A. A. Fiddelers, A. P. van Montfoort, C. D. Dirksen *et al.*, Single versus double embryo transfer: cost-effectiveness analysis alongside a randomized clinical trial. *Hum. Reprod.*, **21** (2006), 2090–2097.

8. J. Gerris, P. De Sutter, D. De Neubourg *et al.*, A real-life prospective health economic study of elective single embryo transfer versus two-embryo transfer in first IVF/ICSI cycles. *Hum. Reprod.*, **19** (2004), 917–923.

9. H. Martikainen, M. Orava, J. Lakkakorpi and L. Tuomivaara, Day 2 elective single embryo transfer in clinical practice: better outcome in ICSI cycles. *Hum. Reprod.*, **19** (2004), 1364–1366.

10. A. Tiitinen, L. Unkila-Kallio, M. Halttunen and C. Hyden-Granskog, Impact of elective single embryo transfer on the twin pregnancy rate. *Hum. Reprod.*, **18** (2003), 1449–1453.

11. A. P. van Montfoort, J. C. Dumoulin, J. A. Land *et al.*, Elective single embryo transfer (eSET) policy in the first three IVF/ICSI treatment cycles. *Hum. Reprod.*, **20** (2005), 433–436.

12. H. G. Lukassen, Y. Schonbeck, E. M. Adang *et al.*, Cost analysis of singleton versus twin pregnancies after in vitro fertilization. *Fertil. Steril.*, **81** (2004), 1240–1246.

13. S. Murray, A. Shetty, A. Rattray, V. Taylor and S. Bhattacharya, A randomized comparison of alternative methods of information provision on the acceptability of elective single embryo transfer. *Hum. Reprod.*, **19** (2004), 911–916.

14. A. P. van Montfoort, A. A. Fiddelers, J. A. Land *et al.*, eSET irrespective of the availability of a good-quality embryo in the first cycle only is not effective in reducing overall twin pregnancy rates. *Hum. Reprod.*, **22** (2007), 1669–1674.

15. Z. Pandian, A. Templeton, G. Serour and S. Bhattacharya, Number of embryos for transfer after IVF and ICSI: a Cochrane review. *Hum. Reprod.*, **20** (2005), 2681–2687.

16. A. Tiitinen, M. Halttunen, P. Harkki, P. Vuoristo and C. Hyden-Granskog, Elective single embryo transfer: the value of cryopreservation. *Hum. Reprod.*, **16** (2001), 1140–1144.

16

Philosophical and ethical considerations on single embryo transfer

Guido Pennings

Introduction

From the very start of in vitro fertilization (IVF), the increase of effectiveness was a major objective of infertility specialists. Although the success rate has increased considerably, policymakers and healthcare insurers are still not satisfied with the present results. In several countries, this is a major reason for refusing reimbursement of IVF [1]. The focus on effectiveness was reinforced by other factors such as the fact that a high success rate also attracts more patients and allows the physicians to make more money. As a consequence, the goal of maximizing the success rate has dominated the field for many years.

A first crack in this one-track focus was the introduction of single embryo transfer (SET) [2]. Since both practitioners and patients believed that the replacement of several embryos increased the success rate, multiple embryo replacement was the rule. Very slowly one realized that this practice had devastating consequences. The price to be paid for the multiple births is enormous, in terms of financial costs, health complications and psychological suffering [3, 4].

We argued recently that the process that started with SET should eventually result in a global "patient-friendly" approach [5]. Patient-friendly assisted reproductive technology (ART) includes four aspects or criteria: cost-effectiveness, equity of access, risk minimization and minimal burden for the patients. All four criteria have a strong normative ethical basis: cost-effectiveness relies on the optimal use of community resources to maximise well-being; equity of access is based on justice; minimal risk is founded on the non-maleficence principle and minimal burden is largely based on the autonomy principle. Like SET, this proposal is founded on an altered ranking of these criteria compared with effectiveness. It is not enough to give the patient the highest chance to take home a healthy child; one should offer the patient a fair chance to obtain a treatment that combines the highest chance of returning home with a healthy baby taking into account the cost of treatment for patient and society, the risks and the burden for the patient.

I will show that three out of four criteria strongly favor SET. However, burden minimization with its strong link with patient autonomy might point in a different direction. It has become standard practice in the last two decades to stress patients' rights and to allow patients to participate in treatment decisions. This emphasis partially explains the attention and importance attributed to informed consent. However, in the field of reproductive medicine, patient preferences are scarcely studied [6]. Patients are rarely given the choice to opt for a less effective but considerable less burdensome treatment. This choice could prove important in the discussion

Single Embryo Transfer, ed. J. Gerris, G. D. Adamson, P. De Sutter and C. Racowsky. Published by Cambridge University Press.
© Cambridge University Press 2009.

on low or minimal stimulation IVF [7]. An exception to the general lack of studies regarding patient preferences is precisely the desire for multiple pregnancies. Most studies indicate an overwhelming preference of patients for twin pregnancies [8–12]. The question then becomes: how does the patients' preference for twins fit into the patient-friendly model?

Risk minimization

This point needs little elaboration as the effects of multiple pregnancies are extensively discussed in the literature of the last decade. Multiple pregnancies are the cause of a strong increase in obstetric complications, perinatal morbidity, congenital malformations, maternal and fetal morbidity and long-term social, psychological and economic difficulties [13]. In short, multiple pregnancy causes harm to the mother, the future children and society. On the basis of the principle of non-maleficence ("do not harm"), the physician should not transfer several embryos. However, the general justification for causing harm or taking risks is the good that results from the same act. The good in this case is the (slightly) higher chance of pregnancy. Although balancing benefits and disadvantages in the case of embryo transfer is more complicated than it looks at first sight, the general agreement among experts in the case of multiple pregnancies is that the risks outweigh the benefits. Moreover, there are acceptable and even preferable ways of treating the patients which diminish or completely avoid the harm. The existence of alternatives makes it even more difficult to justify the risks.

Cost-effectiveness

It has been shown that the high rate of multiple pregnancies generates an enormous additional financial cost for society which indirectly makes the present practice cost-ineffective. Multiple pregnancies produce a dramatic increase in total med-

ical costs compared with singletons [14]. To calculate the total cost, one should not only take the cost of treatment but also the neonatal costs and the cost of long-term care for severely handicapped children [15]. All these costs weigh heavily on the global healthcare budget. In addition, the costs in social, emotional and psychological terms resulting from life-long complications associated with mental retardation and congenital malformation in the children are tremendous.

The importance of cost-effectiveness is based on the principle of utility. There is strong pressure on the healthcare budget which has a tendency to grow faster than other sectors. No society will be able to cover all healthcare costs for all its citizens. A situation of scarcity forces us to think hard about how the money should be allocated in health care. The available funds should be directed to those sectors where they can create the greatest amount of good. Money spent in one sector (e.g., neonatal intensive care) cannot be spent elsewhere. The scarcity, combined with the principles of beneficence and solidarity, forces the physician as well as the patient to take into account the cost implications of their decisions. Individual patients are not free to choose a therapy that would usurp a disproportional amount of money since this would disadvantage others with equally valid claims on treatment. The physician remains the advocate of his or her patient but not without regard for costs and social obligations. The interests of society and the individual patient have to be balanced in order to be able to maintain a healthcare system that provides a decent level of healthcare services to all.

Equity and access

In most European countries, medically assisted reproduction is at least partially reimbursed. In countries like the United States, infertility is primarily private treatment without public or private insurance coverage. The cost of IVF/ICSI (intracytoplasmic sperm injection) to individual couples can go up to 25% of annual household expenditures in

Canada and the United States [16]. Given the high cost, patients know in advance that they can afford only a very limited number of cycles. The fewer cycles they can handle financially, the more important the success rate becomes. Patients with limited resources will opt for a treatment that gives the highest success rate even if this may result in multiple births and complications such as ovarian hyperstimulation syndrome. The Expert Group on Multiple Births after IVF pointed at the lack of publicly funded IVF as the single greatest obstacle to the introduction of elective SET (eSET) policy in the United Kingdom [17]. Many patients resist the introduction of this policy because they fear that their chances of getting pregnant will be reduced. This is also demonstrated in the trade-offs made by patients. For instance, in Murray *et al.*'s study, a fixed charge for the fresh and frozen embryo transfer cycles after one oocyte retrieval would lead to an increased acceptance of SET by patients [18]. Still, "insurance is not a magic bullet for the multiple birth problem associated with assisted reproductive technology" [19]. Up till now, there is little evidence to support the premise that insurance coverage in itself will result in a lower rate of multiple births. There is a modest effect but the situation is more complex than that [20]. Insurance coverage may decrease the pressure from patients to transfer more embryos because there is a lower financial burden but other factors (like the emotional burden of a failed cycle) remain the same. Moreover, the success rate remains important for the doctors. A combination of factors, among which possibly a legal restriction on the number of embryos that can be transferred, is needed.

Access to infertility treatment on the basis of need and not on the basis of financial capacity is supported by the principle of justice. When patients have to pay all costs or the largest part of the treatment cycle out of their own pockets, poor people will take risks that rich people do not have to take. Ironically, this increases the chance of the poorest people to run into debts if it turns out to be a multiple pregnancy. People without health insurance will have to shoulder the extra costs generated by a multiple birth and the possible expenses caused by complications.

The problem

The available evidence on multiple pregnancies has convinced most practitioners that this is a result that should be avoided. Following this conviction, the professional societies have issued guidelines for good clinical practice that should lead to a significant reduction of multiple pregnancies. However, all surveys show that the patients' wishes deviate from the guidelines. Most authors believe that this discrepancy can be explained by a lack of information. They propose to remedy the problem by improving education of the patients. Interestingly, Gleicher and colleagues make the reverse kind of reasoning: they also notice that patient attitudes are not in agreement with the existing practices but they conclude that re-evaluation of the practices may therefore be indicated [8]. This conclusion is based on the importance attributed to patient autonomy. They believe that decisions about risk acceptance fall within a patient's autonomy. Patients make similar risk/benefit decisions in every area of medicine. Although this may be true in general, it is questionable whether decisions in medically assisted reproduction are similar. Patients in assisted reproduction not only decide for themselves but also for the future offspring. This makes a major difference for the argumentation since a refusal by the physician to respect the patient's wish does not need to be justified by paternalism. To decide whether we should change the patients' desires or not, we have to evaluate the desire.

Rationality and autonomy

The issue of rationality can be separated in two steps: (1) is the wish or desire rational? and (2) is the action that should realize the desire rational? Let us start with the first question: is it rational to want twins? Desires are evaluated on a list of mostly negative criteria. Rational desires should not be grounded in false beliefs or ignorance of fact; they should not be the product of psychological compulsions, emotional disturbances or physical addictions [21]. The desire for twins for instance is irrational when the couple believes that twins always have a special bond or that raising twins is similar to raising singletons. The second question is whether the decision of the couple to have several embryos transferred is rational. In a desire-satisfaction theory of rationality, actions are judged on the basis of their contribution to the realization of the desire. If the couple wants a normal healthy family, it would be irrational to ask for the replacement of a number of embryos that is likely to result in a multiple birth. If the couple, however, explicitly wants twins, it is rational to replace two embryos. In some cases, the desire for twins is not a desire for twins as such but a desire for two children. Most people have an ideal family size in mind when they start their parental project. The surveys indicate that the idea of an "ideal family' plays a role in people's acceptance or preference for twins. Mrs Z, a 47-year-old woman with fertility problems who desires a multiple pregnancy, explains her wish to have two embryos replaced as follows: "I'm an only child and I never liked it, and I really want 2 children and I don't know how many chances I'll have' [22]. When people know that, because of age or financial limitations, they can only have one or a few IVF cycles, it may be rational for them to go for twins. However, it is highly unlikely that their ideal family includes a child with a serious handicap. The decision to have several embryos transferred would also be irrational when the woman without valid reason believes that she will not become pregnant with multiples. Self-exempting beliefs are fairly widespread and predict people's decisions to continue risky behavior such as smoking.

A final and very important element to evaluate the desire is the full information criterion. This criterion states that people need full information on all relevant aspects and that they are competent to understand this information. This criterion itself has different facets that will be discussed in the following pages.

Knowledge about risks and complications

Most researchers believe that the patient's preference is mainly caused by a lack of information about complications, morbidity and mortality rates, psychological and social problems, etc. Several studies have focused on risk perception and knowledge of risks. However, when we look at the results of the different studies, the conclusion that the patients' decisions are caused by a lack of knowledge or ignorance about risks is unwarranted. The acceptance of multiples decreased when the number of children increased, thus showing that risk did affect desire [8]. The desire for twin pregnancies also goes down as risk magnitudes go up [23]. The better educated the women were about increased risks associated with multiple gestation, the less they saw twins as a desirable outcome. Other studies, on the contrary, do not prove a link between risk and preference. Blennborn et al. [24] found that the perceived awareness of risk of multiple pregnancies was equal in patients who chose one or two embryos. In the study by Kalra et al. [10], the patients' estimates of the risks of pregnancy complications associated with twin gestations were higher than the estimates in the medical literature and still 68% felt that a twin pregnancy was desirable or highly desirable. However, it is not always clear in these studies what exactly patients knew about the risks. If one asks whether they are aware of an increased risk for twins, this may be nothing more than an empty statement without real meaning for patients. Still, the study by Murray et al. [18], in which patients were provided with an extra leaflet on risks associated with twin pregnancy and with a face-to-face discussion with a nurse, showed that additional information did not increase patients' acceptance of eSET if it meant a fall in pregnancy rates. The analysis of the responses of the Human Fertilization and Embryology Authority's (HFEA's) Patient Panel corroborated this finding: 72% had received information about the risks to mothers and children resulting from multiple embryo transfer but only 9% changed their attitude [17].

Cognitive dissonance may play an important role in the reception of the information and may be a barrier to informed consent. Patients may try to cope with the evidence by devaluating, minimizing and not noticing the information. This psychological mechanism should be considered when communicating risks [25]. The data provided by the doctor do not fit the existing view most patients have about twins (as attractive, preferable, acceptable) and consequently are largely ignored. The news media may contribute to the coming into being of the original view [17, 26]. Television programs seldom show twins when things turn out badly. There is a strong tendency for (self-)selection. Not surprisingly, neither parents nor clinics and physicians are eager to participate in a message that might raise questions about their responsibility.

The main problem might be that people find it extremely difficult to work with statistical data. It is a well-established fact that patients have great problems understanding and interpreting statistical information. In the case of multiple pregnancies, the information is mostly presented as relative to other statistical data (five times more mortality than in singletons), considers different aspects of the treatment (success rate and complications) and different parties (complications for the mother, health risks for the offspring), and applies to different periods and goals (immediate success, long-term effects). In other words, these are sophisticated statistical data. It is possible that only extensive counseling about the possible adverse outcomes and the real-life implications of raising multiples will have an impact on patients' decision-making [27]. Nevertheless, counseling does not always affect knowledge of the risks. This failure to accurately quantify the risks may be due to patients' lack of familiarity with medical terminology, lack of facility with numeric information and difficulty internalizing the personal relevance of generalized medical situations [23].

Knowledge about the real-life implications

A second problem for the rationality of the desire for twins is the inadequate appreciation of what possible future states will be like. People clearly underestimate the effects of twins on their lives [28]. If people with twins live reasonably happy lives, the patients may rationally desire twins. However, if the contrary is true, there is no reason why doctors should believe that the couple's evaluation of twins is correct. The main difficulty for infertile patients might be to bring the situation clearly before their minds. One could, as has been done in the context of genetic counseling, ask patients to imagine scenarios. Imagine yourself with twins of which one has a mental disability. Would you be able to cope? The impact of twins on a couple's everyday life should be highlighted, not by providing statistics but by including the personal account narratives from families who have twins (Sherry Dale in [29]).

One way to test whether parents know what it is like to raise twins is to question them before and after the birth of twins [4]. If the perception of the parents differs significantly before and after, this would prove that the original preference and consent for transfer of several embryos was ill-informed. However, I believe now that this conclusion does not necessarily follow. Mothers of IVF/ICSI twins are significantly more positive about having twins than non-IVF/ICSI twin mothers [11]. These mothers had 3- to 4-year-old children and hence had firsthand experience of raising twins. The most remarkable thing about this finding is the almost complete contradiction with all studies done on twin mothers and their families. Having twins has been associated with depression, child abuse, anxiety, fatigue, etc. [30]. A number of elements may explain the contradiction. When parents of twins born after assisted reproduction are questioned about their family, it is difficult for them to tell about the problems because they are happy with these children and because in a way they have asked for a multiple pregnancy. They may have insisted on replacing more embryos and they have been doing everything possible for years to have children (Mortimer in [29]). So, information on how parents with twins evaluate their family life is useful but inconclusive. Moreover, in the Pinborg study [11] a relatively large percentage (18%) of patients did not respond; this may have been those couples with (very) bad experiences due to (extreme) prematurity and high morbidity and even mortality of children.

Overwhelming emotions

Another explanation for the patients' acceptance of multiple pregnancies is that they will do anything to become pregnant. If infertile patients are prepared to take huge risks to have a child, the conclusion would be that they are in some way "blinded' by this desire. This blindness prevents them from thinking rationally. Physicians are then the only persons in a position to carefully consider all the complex risks and benefits without the bias of overwhelming emotion [31]. There are indications that infertile people's decision-making is mainly guided by their desire to become parents. Their wish for a child makes them underestimate the difficulties of raising more than one child, among which possibly a child with special needs [32]. The finding that an overwhelming majority of infertile women undergoing IVF would elect to have quadruplets rather than forfeit the opportunity to have children can also be considered as a good indication [9, 32].

Still, there is also evidence that people do balance success rate against other aspects of the procedure. In a Dutch study, a questionnaire was sent to patients and their physicians asking them to choose between one stimulated cycle and three natural cycles [7, 33]. About 30% of both patients and physicians were willing to trade off 6% success in live birth of the stimulated cycle for the three natural cycles. A study by Hojgaard *et al.* [34] confirmed these findings: patients preferred the simplicity and short duration of a low stimulation cycle despite the higher risk of cancellation. These findings show that a lower burden (psychological, time investment, financial) may outweigh a lower success rate. It is remarkable that patients change their attitude towards SET for their own burden but not for possible harmful effects to the offspring. One explanation could be that the additional cycles are perceived as a heavy, immediate and certain burden while the higher risk of complications related to multiple pregnancy is perceived as uncertain and further away in time. It is clear from patient accounts that IVF is a stressful, demanding, invasive and frequently frustrating experience. Psycho-logical stress is the main reason why patients drop out [35]. In addition, "standard' IVF is longer, more demanding, causes more side effects and psychological problems than mild or minimal stimulation protocols [36, 37]. It can be predicted on the basis of these characteristics that patients will find it easier or at least less objectionable to go through additional cycles in case of failure. Reduced stress and discomfort during mild IVF treatment had a positive impact on the psychological status afterwards, even if pregnancy was not achieved [38]. Success rate is not the sole criterion for patients.

Goal replacement

The final point about the rationality of the actions is that it looks as if the patients, without being aware of this themselves, have substituted their original goal (a family) by a new goal (pregnancy and birth). This confusion between the primary or real wish and the pursued wish would make the latter irrational [39]. Some studies indicate that infertile couples may underestimate the long-term consequences and focus too much on their immediate goal, i.e., the pregnancy. Although there have been several surveys on how patients look at multiple pregnancies, this work was not based on the psychological theories on risk attitude. We need that kind of theoretical approach if we really want to understand what patients think. Just one example: prospect theory explains how risk behavior varies depending on whether the outcomes are perceived as gains or losses relative to a reference point. A relative gain combined with a risk calls for risk-aversive behavior while a relative loss combined by a risk evokes risk-seeking behavior [40]. This theory is used to explain patients' choices in other health domains. It would help to know what infertility patients take as a reference point and whether multiples are perceived as a gain or a loss. The only study which used the standard gamble method on possible outcomes of embryo transfer revealed that women waiting for IVF treatment would prefer to give birth to a child with a chronic disability rather than never give birth at all [41]. Some women view severe child disability outcomes associated with double embryo transfer (DET) as being more desirable than having no child. Treatment success (in the sense of a live birth) is more important than future risks to their offspring. This explains why additional information on adverse outcomes will only have a limited effect on patients' preferences for DET. Interestingly, these findings are broadly consistent with other studies conducted to assess the preferences of women for different birth outcomes. There too, infertile women place different values on treatment outcomes than clinicians and the general population. This is an important finding for the discussion: it suggests that it is not the lack of information or the quality of the information (although this information is obviously necessary for autonomous decisions) but the different value placed by physicians and patients on the risks and complications which leads to different conclusions [42].

The focus of patients on pregnancy may be explained by the logic of the infertility treatment: it prevents patients from thinking beyond the first step. In a phenomenological study of women who had to consider multifetal pregnancy reduction, Collopy found that these women very well recalled that they were given precise statistics associated with each treatment option. Yet they were adamant that this information had virtually no meaning to them. They were exclusively focused on overcoming infertility, not on avoiding a multiple birth. They were single-minded in their pursuit of pregnancy. As one of them said: "I couldn't think that far" [43]. Moreover, they estimated their chances of becoming pregnant with multiples as highly unlikely. They were so used to the idea of being infertile that the possible hyperfertility did not even register in their minds.

Shared decision-making

Shared decision-making refers to a process in which both physician and patient participate in the decision-making process [44]. It involves several steps among which are information exchange and negotiation. The concept sounds very nice and positive but what should be done when no agreement can be reached on the treatment to implement? Who has the final word? Although several measures can be taken to reduce these conflicts to a minimum, there will always remain a hard core of situations in which either the patient or the physician will prevail. Many doctors believe that the ultimate decision lies with the patients and that they cannot refuse to replace the embryos because the property rights of the embryos belong to the patients [45]. However, the question is not to whom the embryos belong but what should or can be done with them. The right of the intentional parents to indicate the disposition of their embryos is not unlimited. This right is always embedded in a social and legal context which determines which options are acceptable. This equally applies to decisions about the transfer of embryos. In several countries, legislation determines how many embryos can be transferred. Although many practitioners regret the existence of such laws as limiting their therapeutic freedom, these laws were seen as necessary because the practice hardly changed. Although there are guidelines from professional societies, the multiple pregnancy rate remains unacceptably high. In countries with a law, there is very little room for negotiation between patient and physician. In countries where the decision is still up to them, conflicts may arise. In order to address these conflicts, one needs a general structure of the patient–physician relationship to determine the rights and duties of both parties. The basic structure, according to me, is one of principle and accomplice. The physician participates in the parental project initiated by the intentional parents. Due to his or her contribution, the physician has moral responsibility for the welfare of the patient and the future child. He or she is more than a technical agent executing another person's plan. The doctor cannot argue that he or she carries no responsibility because the parents have the greatest responsibility and because the embryos belong to them. If the physician accepts the infertile couple's wish to transfer two or three (or even more embryos), he or she is also partially responsible for the possible complications and health consequences of this decision. This can be shown by an example: suppose a 33-year-old woman argues that she can only afford one cycle and that she wants four embryos back. Is it all right for the doctor to replace four? Is it enough to verify that the patient knows what she is doing? Attributing absolute priority to the autonomy of the patient comes down to denying autonomy to the physician and vice versa. We should avoid as much as possible the extreme poles of the continuum. A possible way out of the conflict is conditional treatment. Conditional treatment is a way to balance the views of the physician and the patient [46]. These conditions may reduce the risks, improve the success rate, etc. When the physician says that he or she accepts to treat the patient but will only replace two embryos to minimise the complications associated with multiples, he or she is taking his or her own responsibility. This should not be presented as a violation of the patient's autonomy. Still, the physician should not end up in a logic of prevention, where the goal of avoiding risks for both mother and child outweighs all other values. Enforced SET would tip the balance too much in one direction. It would replace the original focus on effectiveness by a similar one-sided emphasis on minimizing medical risks and healthcare costs. Although these are very important criteria for the evaluation of the practice, the risks of twins may in some cases, depending on the characteristics of the woman, be outweighed by the higher chance of pregnancy. Moreover, causal contribution leads to moral responsibility but that does not imply that the physician is to be blamed when a multiple pregnancy results from his or her decision. When the physician has strong indications that a specific woman has a significantly lower chance of pregnancy when only one embryo is replaced (due to maternal age, embryo quality or treatment history), he or she may have acted correctly and cannot be accused of negligence or recklessness. When walking the thin line between low pregnancy rates and multiple pregnancies, however, he or she should err on the safe side. Ultimately, given the doctor's moral

obligation not to cause harm to the offspring and to the patient, he or she should decide how many embryos to transfer. However, this only applies to the maximum. If the patient wishes fewer embryos transferred, this wish should be honored given the impact of a multiple birth on her life.

The future

It is possible that within a time span of 10 years, medically assisted reproduction, and IVF in particular, will have changed completely from the way it is practiced now. The increasing use of "softer" forms of ovarian stimulation may lead to a practice that avoids or greatly reduces some important problems like multiple pregnancies, cryopreservation of embryos and ovarian hyperstimulation syndrome. There are already now ways to bring down the rate of multiple pregnancies considerably but the general framework is not supportive. We need an integrated approach which combines all types of measures: increased patient education and awareness programs; legal measures to restrict multiple pregnancies; inducing responsibility in the fertility specialists, changes in stimulation protocols to diminish the burden on patients and thus their perception of a cycle, alternative ways of reimbursing treatment, etc. A patient-friendly approach will be a large step in the right direction. If there is a real will to do something about this problem, we will get to the minimum level with the consent and support of all people involved.

What do we know?

The costs of multiple pregnancies for patients, future children and society are high and largely preventable. Several fundamental ethical principles, among which non-maleficence, beneficence and justice encourage SET. The main problem lies with the principle of respect for autonomy. All surveys indicate that there is a large discrepancy between the attitude of the patients towards multiple pregnancy and the position adopted in the professional guidelines in recent years. Most authors seem to be convinced that the attitude of patients is irrational because they insufficiently take into account the sharply increased risks associated with multiples.

What do we need to know?

In order to evaluate the wish of patients for multiples, we need to determine whether this desire is rational and, if so, in which circumstances. This requires a further philosophical analysis of the concept. Simultaneously, we need a better understanding of patients' reasoning about multiple births and the associated risks and benefits. In-depth studies (and not mere surveys) among infertile couples should be performed to reveal the principles underlying the patients' decision-making. Without these elements, we do not know whether the physicians should try to convince patients of the necessity to reduce the number of embryos for transfer or whether they should go along with their wishes.

What should we do?

We should balance the ethical principles involved in order to decide when patients' autonomy (presupposing that the wish to have several embryos transferred is rational) overrides other principles like the welfare of the future child and the health of the patient. Within the specific context of medically assisted reproduction, the moral responsibility of the assisting physician should be clarified.

REFERENCES

1. E. G. Hughes and M. Giacomini, Funding in vitro fertilization treatment for persistent subfertility: the pain and the politics. *Fertil. Steril.*, **76** (2001), 431–442.
2. J. M. R. Gerris, Single embryo transfer and IVF/ICSI outcome: a balanced appraisal. *Hum. Reprod. Update*, **11** (2005), 105–121.
3. W. Ombelet, P. De Sutter, J. Van Der Elst and G. Martens, Multiple gestation and infertility treatment: registration, reflection and reaction – the Belgian project. *Hum. Reprod. Update*, **11** (2005), 3–14.
4. G. Pennings, Multiple pregnancies: a test case for the moral quality of medically assisted reproduction. *Hum. Reprod.*, **15** (2000), 2466–2469.
5. G. Pennings and W. Ombelet, Coming soon to your clinic: patient-friendly ART. *Hum. Reprod.*, **22** (2007), 2075–2079.
6. N. Bayram, M. Van Wely, F. Van Der Veen and P. M. M. Bossuyt, Treatment preferences and trade-offs for ovulation induction in clomiphene citrate-resistant patients with polycystic ovary syndrome. *Fertil. Steril.*, **84** (2005), 420–425.
7. E. N. D. Pistorius, E. M. M. Adang, P. F. M. Stalmeier, D. D. M. Braat and J. A. M. Kremer, Prospective patient and physician preferences for stimulation or no stimulation in IVF. *Hum. Fertil.*, **9** (2006), 209–216.
8. N. Gleicher, D. P. Campbell, G. C. L. Chan *et al.*, The desire for multiple births in couples with infertility problems contradicts present practice patterns. *Hum. Reprod.*, **10** (1995), 1079–1084.
9. J. Goldfarb, D. J. Kinzer, M. Boyle and D. Kurit, Attitudes of in vitro fertilization and intrauterine insemination couples toward multiple gestation pregnancy and multifetal pregnancy reduction. *Fertil. Steril.*, **65** (1996), 815–820.
10. S. K. Kalra, M. P. Milad, S. C. Klock and W. A. Grobman, Infertility patients and their partners: differences in the desire for twin gestations. *Obstet. Gynecol.*, **102** (2003), 152–155.
11. A. Pinborg, A. Loft, L. Schmidt and A. N. Andersen, Attitudes of IVF/ICSI-twin mothers towards twins and single embryo transfer. *Hum. Reprod.*, **18** (2003), 621–627.
12. G. L. Ryan, S. H. Zhang, A. Dokras, C. H. Syrop and B. J. Van Voorhis, The desire of infertile patients for multiple births. *Fertil. Steril.*, **81** (2004), 500–504.
13. J. Hazekamp, C. Bergh, U.-B. Wennerholm *et al.*, Avoiding multiple pregnancies in ART: consideration of new strategies. *Hum. Reprod.*, **16** (2000), 1217–1219.
14. T. L. Callahan, J. E. Hall, S. L. Ettner *et al.*, The economic impact of multiple gestation pregnancies and the contribution of assisted-reproduction techniques to their incidence. *N. Engl. J. Med.*, **331** (1994), 244–249.
15. H. G. M. Lukassen, Y. Schonbeck, E. M. M. Adang *et al.*, Cost analysis of singleton versus twin pregnancies after in vitro fertilization. *Fertil. Steril.*, **81** (2004), 1240–1246.
16. J. Collins, An international survey of the health economics of IVF and ICSI. *Hum. Reprod. Update*, **8** (2002), 265–277.
17. Expert Group on Multiple Births after IVF, One child at a time. Reducing multiple births after IVF (2006).

www.hfea.gov.uk/docs/MBSET_report_Final_Dec_06. pdf.

18. S. Murray, A. Shetty, A. Rattray, V. Taylor and S. Bhat- tacharya, A randomised comparison of alternative methods of information provision on the acceptabil- ity of elective single embryo transfer. *Hum. Reprod.*, **19** (2004), 911–916.

19. M. A. Reynolds, L. A. Schieve, G. Jeng and H. B. Peter- son, Insurance is not a magic bullet for the mul- tiple birth problem associated with assisted repro- ductive technology. *Fertil. Steril.*, **80** (2003b), 32– 33.

20. M. A. Reynolds, L. A. Schieve, G. Jeng and H. B. Peter- son, Does insurance coverage decrease the risk for multiple births associated with assisted reproductive technology? *Fertil. Steril.*, **80** (2003a), 16–23.

21. A. Superson, Deformed desires and informed desire tests. *Hypatia*, **20** (2005), 109–126.

22. R. J. Stillman, A 47-year-old woman with fertility prob- lems who desires a multiple pregnancy. *JAMA,* **297** (2007), 858–867.

23. W. A. Grobman, M. P. Milad, J. Stout and S. C. Klock, Patient perceptions of multiple gestations: an assess- ment of knowledge and risk aversion. *Am. J. Obstet. Gynecol.*, **185** (2001), 920–924.

24. M. Blennborn, S. Nilsson, C. Hillervik and D. Hell- berg, The couple's decision-making in IVF: one or two embryos at transfer? *Hum. Reprod.*, **20** (2005), 1292– 1297.

25. A. Steckelberg, J. Kasper, M. Redegeld and I. Mülhlhauser, Risk information – barrier to informed consent? A focus group study. *Soz Praventivmed.*, **49** (2004), 375–380.

26. G. S. Letterie, Multiple births: does the news media influence public perceptions? *Hum. Reprod.*, **19** (2004), 2680–2681.

27. J. Wang, M. Lane and R. J. Norman, Reducing multi- ple pregnancy from assisted reproduction treatment: educating patients and medical staff. *Med. J. Aust.*, **184** (2006), 180–181.

28. D. A. Hay, C. Gleeson, C. Davies *et al.*, What informa- tion should the multiple birth family receive before, during and after the birth? *Acta Genet. Med. Gemellol.* (Roma), **39** (1990), 259–269.

29. Canadian Fertility and Andrology Society. Incidence and complications of multiple gestation in Canada: proceedings of an expert meeting. *Reprod. Biomed. Online*, **14** (2007), 773–780.

30. M. Garel, B. Blondel and M. Kaminski, Multiple births in couples with infertility problems. *Hum. Reprod.*, **10** (1995), 2748–2753.

31. G. L. Ryan and B. J. Van Voorhis, The desire of infertil- ity patients for multiple gestations – do they know the risks? *Fertil. Steril.*, **81** (2004), 526.

32. S. R. Leiblum, E. Kemmann and L. Taska, Atti- tudes toward multiple births and pregnancy concern in infertile and non-infertile women. *J. Psychosom. Obstet. Gynaecol.*, **11** (1990), 197–210.

33. D. Braat and J. Kremer, National experience with elec- tive single-embryo transfer. D. The Netherlands. In J. Gerris, F. Olivennes and P. De Sutter, eds., *Assisted Reproductive Technologies: Quality and Safety* (Boca Raton: Parthenon Publishing Group, 2004), pp. 123– 125.

34. A. Hojgaard, H. J. Ingerslev and J. Dinesen, Friendly IVF: patient opinions. *Hum. Reprod.*, **16** (2001), 1391– 1396.

35. C. Olivius, B. Friden, G. Borg and C. Bergh, Why do couples discontinue in vitro fertilization treatment? A cohort study. *Fertil. Steril.*, **81** (2004), 258–261.

36. M. J. Pelinck, N. E. A. Vogel, A. Hoek *et al.*, Cumulative pregnancy rates after three cycles of minimal stimula- tion IVF and results according to subfertility diagnosis: a multicentre cohort study. *Hum. Reprod.*, **21** (2006), 2375–2383.

37. B. C. J. M. Fauser, P. Devroey, S. S. C. Yen *et al.*, Min- imal ovarian stimulation for IVF: appraisal of poten- tial benefits and drawbacks. *Hum. Reprod.*, **14** (1999), 2681–2686.

38. C. De Klerk, N. S. Macklon, E. M. E. W. Heijnen *et al.*, The psychological impact of IVF failure after two or more cycles of IVF with a mild versus standard treat- ment strategy. *Hum. Reprod.*, **22** (2007), 2554–2558.

39. M. D. Bayles, *Reproductive Ethics.* (Englewood Cliffs, New Jersey: Prentice-Hall, 1984).

40. S. M. C. Van Osch, W. B. Van Den Hout and A. M. Stiggelbout, Exploring the reference point in prospect theory: gambles for length of life. *Med. Decis. Making*, **26** (2006), 338–346.

41. G. S. Scotland, P. McNamee, V. L. Peddie and S. Bhattacharya, Safety versus success in elective single embryo transfer: women's preferences for outcomes of in vitro fertilisation. *BJOG*, **114** (2007), 977–983.

42. G. M. Hartshorne and R. J. Lilford, Different perspec- tives of patients and healthcare professionals on the potential benefits and risks of blastocyst culture and

multiple embryo transfer. *Hum. Reprod.*, **17** (2002), 1023–1030.

43. K. S. Collopy, "I didn't think that far": infertile women's decision making about multiple reduction. *Res. Nurs. Health*, **27** (2004), 75–86.

44. C. A. Charles, T. Whelan, A. Gafni, A. Willan and S. Farrell, Shared treatment decision making: what does it mean to physicians? *J. Clin. Oncol.*, **21** (2003), 932–936.

45. R. G. Edwards, Ethics of preimplantation genetic diagnosis: recordings from the Fourth International Symposium on Preimplantation Genetics. *Reprod. Biomed. Online*, **6** (2002), 170–180.

46. G. Pennings, M. Bonduelle and I. Liebaers, Decisional authority and moral responsibility of patients and clinicians in the context of preimplantation genetic diagnosis. *Reprod. Biomed. Online*, **7** (2003), 509–513.

SECTION 3

Controversies

17

What is the optimum day of transfer for single embryo transfer? Success rates, monozygotic twinning and epigenetic issues

Christine C. Skiadas and Catherine Racowsky

Introduction

Over the past 30 years, in vitro fertilization (IVF) has made remarkable strides in terms of improving success rates. The clinical mainstay of IVF is controlled ovarian hyperstimulation, the goal of which is to retrieve a higher number of oocytes than would be obtained in a natural cycle. The higher number of oocytes retrieved has been associated with an improved pregnancy rate, as there is normally a natural attrition at each stage in the process of IVF. Indeed, not all retrieved oocytes will be mature, not all mature oocytes will fertilize normally, and not all zygotes will become developmentally competent embryos. Moreover, extending the day of culture to the blastocyst stage likely results in loss of viability of some embryos, although this must be counterbalanced against the possibility that the more robust embryos proceed to blastulation in vitro.

In the initial years of IVF, multiple embryos were transferred back to patients and only modest pregnancy rates resulted. With the improvements in stimulation protocols, medications and laboratory techniques, patients and physicians are now able to focus on achieving a successful singleton pregnancy, as opposed to any pregnancy, without regard to the number of developing fetuses.

The overall success of single embryo transfer (SET) depends on several factors, including patient selection (see Chapter 4) and embryo selection

(see Chapter 8), as well as cryo-augmentation (see Chapter 9A) to achieve cumulative pregnancy rates. Although initial fresh cycle pregnancy rates may be decreased following SET, several studies have shown equivalent pregnancy rates on a cumulative basis (including fresh and frozen embryo transfers) with an expected significant reduction in twins. These studies have shown equivalence following day 2 [1, 2], day 3 [3] or day 5 transfer [4, 5].

Single embryo transfer is evolving as the new gold standard in IVF with several European countries having governmental mandates on how many embryos to transfer. In the United States, the Society of Assisted Reproductive Technology Practice Committee has recently published a revised set of guidelines which recommend SET for specific patient populations. However, several questions remain [6]. In this chapter, our goal is to review the literature on the optimal day of transfer for SET as well as the potential complications or unforeseen outcomes associated with SET (such as monozygotic twinning and epigenetic effects).

The optimal day of embryo transfer

The optimal day of embryo transfer has been controversial in IVF over the past few years even without the additional complicating factor of only transferring one embryo. Pregnancies have been reported

Single Embryo Transfer, ed. J. Gerris, G. D. Adamson, P. De Sutter and C. Racowsky. Published by Cambridge University Press.
© Cambridge University Press 2009.

from transfers of embryos on day 1 through day 6 of development. In the initial reports of IVF, due to recognized inadequacies of the culture medium, the aim was to replace the embryos into the maternal environment as quickly as possible. Accordingly, most embryo transfers occurred on day 2. Subsequently, with recognition that benefit to embryo selection might be achieved by extending the duration of culture, transfer on day 3 became commonplace. In the past few years, improvements in laboratory techniques and culture media have also allowed for improved in vitro survival. These improvements have opened the possibility of day 5 transfer which, in and of itself, may have the additional benefit of improved synchrony between the embryo and uterus (by approximating when the embryo would naturally enter the uterus from the Fallopian tube).

The most common days to perform embryo transfer currently are on day 3 and day 5, although there is continued debate in the literature regarding the optimal day of transfer. Several retrospective analyses have demonstrated that blastocyst transfer leads to a higher implantation rate and pregnancy rate, when compared with day 3 transfers [7–9]. However, the majority of prospective randomized studies have revealed no difference in pregnancy rates [10–14], although at least one such study has shown increased pregnancy rates following blastocyst transfer [15]. A Cochrane review of blastocyst transfers versus day 3 embryo transfers identified 16 trials for meta-analysis and concluded that there was no significant difference in live birth rate, pregnancy rate, incidence of multiple gestations or miscarriage rates. However, they did find that those patients who underwent a day 3 transfer were more likely to have additional embryos available for cryopreservation and patients undergoing a day 5 transfer were more likely not to have any embryos available for transfer [16]. Similarly, investigators who randomized patients to a day 3 or day 5 transfer at the time of counseling prior to the start of the cycle found no difference in pregnancy rates, but again confirmed that fewer embryos were available for cryopreservation following day 5 transfer

[17]. The greatest confounding factor in all of these studies is the transfer of more than one embryo. In this context, the increased implantation rate that some studies have shown after blastocyst transfer [10, 11] has led investigators to look at single cleavage stage versus single blastocyst transfer. Therefore, these same results may not hold true for the patient population who is eligible for SET.

Studies comparing day 3 SET versus blastocyst SET

Only a handful of studies, to date, have prospectively evaluated pregnancy rates following day 3 or day 5 transfer with only one embryo transferred and with pregnancy rates following fresh embryo transfer being the outcome variable of interest. Papanikolaou et al. [18] conducted a randomized controlled trial of infertile women to evaluate outcomes of single cleavage stage embryo transfer versus single blastocyst transfer. Inclusion criteria were: patient age less than 36 years, first or second trial of IVF or intracytoplasmic sperm injection (ICSI) with serum follicle-stimulating hormone (FSH) ≤ 12 mIU/mL. In this cohort, patients who had a single blastocyst transfer were significantly more likely to have an ongoing pregnancy at 12 weeks, compared with those patients undergoing cleavage stage SET (33.1% vs. 21.6%, with $p = 0.02$) [18]. Zech et al. [19] also conducted a randomized trial of SET either on day 3 or day 5, in a similar cohort of women (age ≤ 36 years, first or second IVF or ICSI attempt and ≥ 5 fertilized oocytes). Embryos were randomized after the day 1 fertilization check. In the presence of excellent quality embryos (judged by morphology on day of transfer), day 5 embryo transfer was associated with a significantly higher ongoing pregnancy rate per cycle when compared with day 3 embryo transfer (40.8% vs. 25.6%, $p < 0.05$) [19]. These two randomized controlled trials both suggest that for fresh cycles, a single blastocyst transfer leads to an improved pregnancy rate. However, several controversies remain with regards to performing transfer on day 5.

Controversies of day 3 versus day 5 transfer

Does delaying transfer to day 5 result in fewer embryos available for cryopreservation?

The two randomized trials presented above, comparing the optimal day of SET, indicate that in a favorable prognosis patient population, blastocyst SET is associated with higher pregnancy rates from the fresh cycle. However, one of the potential downsides of maintaining the embryos in culture media until day 5 is the decrease in number of embryos available for freezing. In the Papanikolaou study, patients who underwent cleavage stage transfer had a higher number of cryopreserved embryos (4.2 vs. 2.2, $p = 0.001$) and the live birth rate was higher following transfer of thawed day 3 embryos when compared with blastocysts (15% vs. 11%) [18]. The cumulative pregnancy rate (fresh and frozen transfers) was not calculated in this study. Furthermore, many programs have difficulty with successful blastocyst freezing and therefore have reverted to performing day 3 transfers.

Does prolonged culture decrease the likelihood of any embryo transfer?

The decreased survival rates associated with prolonging culture to the blastocyst stage may compromise a successful outcome that would otherwise be achieved following a day 3 transfer. Racowsky *et al.* reported that in patients with three or more 8-cell embryos on day 3, it may be beneficial to consider day 5 transfer, but with fewer than three 8-cell embryos on day 3, a day 3 transfer improves pregnancy rates [20]. These results are further supported by Zech *et al.*, who demonstrated that when patients had three or fewer than three excellent quality embryos on day 3, fewer patients were eligible for transfer on day 5 and there was a drop in the pregnancy rate [19]. Taken together, these observations suggest that the uterus may provide a superior environment compared to that of the in vitro system, and a day 3 embryo transfer may "rescue" embryos that otherwise may not survive in culture.

Does day 3 embryo transfer lead to increased pregnancy loss?

Papanikolaou *et al.* [18] evaluated day 3 SET and day 5 SET and assessed the rate of pregnancy loss between the two groups. Those patients undergoing day 5 SET had a significantly lower rate of pregnancy loss than those patients who had day 3 SET (17.2% vs. 26.8%, $p = 0.017$). Patients also had a higher likelihood of ongoing pregnancy after day 5 transfer. One concern in this study is whether or not the two groups were truly equivalent. The day 5 SET group had a significantly higher number of oocytes retrieved (12.9 vs. 11.2; $p = 0.001$) and a higher number of mature oocytes (8.1 vs. 7.0; $p = 0.001$). The day 5 SET cohort also was younger than the day 3 SET group (30.9 years vs. 31.3 years; $p = 0.01$) although there was no statistically significant difference in age in the women who conceived (31.2 years vs. 30.8 years; $p > 0.05$). A logistic regression was conducted to adjust for female age and the number of mature oocytes and the only factor that remained significant was day 5 SET [21]. However, in this population the proportion of elective SET was 77% of patients having day 5 SET and only 69% of those having day 3 SET ($p < 0.05$), an observation indicating that more patients on day 3 had a non-elective SET, due to only one embryo being available. Despite these limitations, the potential for increased pregnancy loss after day 3 SET warrants further investigation.

Does day 5 transfer lead to an increase in monozygotic twinning?

As early as the mid 1980s, there were reports of an increased incidence of monozygotic (MZ) twins after IVF [22, 23], which some authors have suggested may be up to ten times higher than the natural incidence of MZ twins [24]. Monozygotic twins have been reported in several trials evaluating the efficacy of SET and in a review article, Gerris calculated the cumulative incidence of MZ twins from four randomized trials on SET as 2.16%

Days

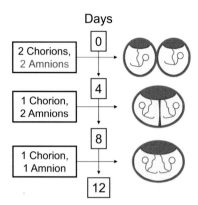

2 Chorions, 2 Amnions — 0

1 Chorion, 2 Amnions — 4

1 Chorion, 1 Amnion — 8

12

Figure 17.1 Time-sensitive placental development in monozygotic twins. Skiadas *et al.* [37]. With permission from Oxford University Press. See color plate section.

[25]. The exact mechanism leading to this increased incidence is unknown, but authors have linked MZ twinning to gonadotropin treatment [26], maternal age (either younger [27] or older [28]) as well as to conditions in the laboratory. Of specific concern are the MZ twins that also share a placenta (monochorionic) or both a placenta and an amniotic sac (monoamniotic). The former are thought to result from an embryo that splits into two after 4 days of development and the latter from an embryo that splits into two after 8 days respectively (Figure 17.1). Monochorionic twins and even more so monoamniotic twins have a higher morbidity than MZ twins that separate early and hence have separate placentas resembling dizygotic twins [29–32].

Given that the vast majority of patients will undergo gonadotropin treatment prior to a fresh embryo transfer, and that maternal age is not modifiable, the only variables that can be altered to affect the rate of MZ twins are in the embryology laboratory. Laboratory techniques, such as micromanipulation of the embryo, including both assisted hatching and ICSI [27, 28, 33–7] have been linked to increased MZ twinning, although this relationship has not been identified in all studies [38, 39]. In addition, culture conditions [40] and prolonged time in embryo culture may artificially induce twins due to abnormal hatching [41] or apoptosis in the embryo [42]. Finally, day 5 embryo transfer [38, 43–

45] has been linked with increased MZ twins [37]. Interestingly, none of the prospective randomized trials comparing day of embryo transfer (day 3 or day 5) have shown this increase, although given the low incidence of MZ twins, these studies may be underpowered to do so.

Should epigenetic and imprinting issues impact the day of SET?

The success of an assisted reproductive technology (ART) procedure is typically measured by the take-home baby rate, whether this is defined as the number of deliveries according to the number of cycles initiated, the number of egg retrievals or the number of embryo transfers. However, mounting evidence indicates that critical attention should be paid not only to this outcome measure, but also to the health of the children born (reviewed by [46]). In particular, concerns regarding ART-associated increased risks of epigenetic alternations and imprinting disorders raise questions as to whether embryo culture duration should be minimized. In other words, given these concerns, should day 3 be considered the preferred day for SET rather than day 5?

While most ART neonates appear normal, several recent studies emphasize an increased risk for adverse pregnancy outcomes compared with those of non-ART conceived pregnancies (reviewed by [47]). Particular attention has focused on the increased rates of perinatal complications of singleton pregnancies, including small-for-gestational-age infants, preterm delivery and perinatal mortality, in addition to maternal complications [48–50]. Evidence is also accumulating that there are increased risks of syndromes involving epigenetic alterations in children born from ART [51, 52]. The etiologies underlying such increased risks are unknown and could relate to underlying reproductive pathologies inherent to the infertile couple, the pharmaceutical agents used for ovarian stimulation and/or to in vitro technologies per se. Of note, however, mouse experiments have definitively shown culture medium-associated epigenetic disturbances during preimplantation development [53, 54], which raise the question whether SET after prolonged culture to the blastocyst stage is desirable.

Epigenetic reprogramming, imprinting disorders and ART

Epigenetic reprogramming involves heritable alterations in the structure of DNA resulting from changes in the chromatin structure that do not involve disruption in the nucleotide sequence per se (reviewed by [52]). The major forms of epigenetic modification are DNA methylation and histone deacetylation, and typically involve condensed chromatin states and gene silencing. Differential DNA methylation leading to expression of only one of two parental alleles is a mechanism of gene regulation known as genomic imprinting. Defects in imprinting may cause either over- or underexpression of certain genes, leading to specific syndromes such as Beckwith–Wiedemann syndrome [55–57] and Angelman syndrome [58, 59] and to cancers such as retinoblastoma [60]. The incidence of each of these imprinting disorders in children born from ART appears to be higher than background (reviewed by [51, 52]) although it is important to stress that the relative risks are inferred from small case studies and extrapolations to estimations of ART usage in the population at large.

Epigenetic disturbances in cultured embryos

Preimplantation embryos, whether from mouse or man, can develop in media that vary widely in their composition, from simple balanced salt solutions and carbohydrates (for e.g. P1 in human IVF) to very complex media such as Ham's F10, Global, or the G-series media. The embryos that result are developmentally competent because live offspring are born following their transfer. However, studies with mouse indicate that gene expression can be per-

turbed by the culture conditions [54, 61], and that genes regulating protein synthesis and cell proliferation are differentially expressed depending upon the medium used for culture. Moreover, the expression and methylation of the imprinted gene *H19* in mouse embryos is likewise dependent on the type of culture medium used [53, 62]. Although not proven, these medium-induced effects may be due to differences in methionine content of the media, which can affect DNA methylation and imprinting [63, 64].

Similar genetic studies have not been performed in human embryos for obvious ethical reasons. Nevertheless, indirect evidence that culture medium type may induce genetic reprogramming in human preimplantation embryos is suggested by the observation that culture medium type was associated with the level of human chorionic gonadotropin secretion early in pregnancy following transfer of day 3 embryos [65].

To date, there is no direct evidence in the human that any laboratory intervention, including the day of embryo transfer, is responsible for the apparent increased incidence of the imprinting disorders associated with ART. Indeed, in a recent review of the national Beckwith–Wiedemann registry, Chang *et al.* concluded that the only common variable among the index cases was the use of ovarian stimulation [57]. In this context, a recent study has revealed methylation changes in the oocytes of some infertility patients after controlled ovarian stimulation, and also changes in methylation in oocytes of superovulated mice [66]. Nevertheless, in light of compelling data with mouse embryos, further research is required to investigate a possible association of culture-induced epigenetic alterations with ART.

Conclusions

Whether SET should be performed on day 5 involves weighing the possible advantages of improved embryo selection and embryo/uterine synchrony against the likelihood of fewer cryopreserved embryos and an increased risk of MZ twins. In addition, the possibility of culture-induced perturbations in epigenetic reprogramming must not be disregarded. Despite the very small absolute number of pregnancies affected by monozygosity and imprinting disorders, we should minimize the occurrence of these severe conditions at all costs. Therefore, it would seem advisable to perform SET routinely on day 3, at least until we have further assurance that the in vitro technologies do not increase the risk of epigenetic disturbances.

What do we know?

- Randomized controlled trials and a large meta-analysis have shown no difference in pregnancy rates when day 3 versus day 5 transfers (including more than one embryo) were evaluated.
- The two randomized controlled trials comparing day 3 to day 5 SET have shown a significantly higher fresh cycle pregnancy rate following day 5 transfers.
- Patients planning on having a day 5 transfer have an increased risk of not having an embryo transfer, and of having fewer embryos available for cryopreservation. Therefore, the decision of which day to perform embryo transfer should not be made until embryo number and quality have been assessed on day 3.
- In the human ART population, available data show an overall increase in the incidence of imprinting disorders involving Beckwith–Wiedemann syndrome, Angelman syndrome and retinoblastoma.
- There are compelling data in animal models that culture conditions induce epigenetic disturbances by modulation of DNA methylation, resulting in imprinting defects.
- Aberrant DNA methylation is present in some human oocytes following controlled ovarian stimulation.

What do we need to know?

- Do cumulative (fresh + frozen) pregnancy rates per cycle vary following day 3 versus day 5 SET?
- What selection criteria should be used to determine who should have a day 3 versus a day 5

embryo transfer – does it depend on the patient and/or on the laboratory?
- Do culture conditions affect gene expression in human preimplantation embryos, including global DNA methylation patterns and the modulation of the regulatory regions of imprinted genes?
- If so, are these effects more pronounced as the duration of culture increases from day 3 to day 5?

What should we do?

- Undertake additional research to compare the incidence of MZ twinning, gestational ages, perinatal risks, maternal complications and birth weights for pregnancies established following day 3 versus day 5 SET.
- Continue research assessing the possible association between ART and epigenetic defects. If such an association is proven, research must focus on distinguishing among the possible explanations, including possible increased risks imposed by epigenetic defects in the gametes of infertility patients, the ovarian stimulation regimens used and culture systems employed, including possible exacerbation with prolonged embryo culture. To this end, ART registries should establish prospective collections of cord blood for epigenetic testing in ART deliveries for linkage back to the type of culture medium used and the day that embryos were transferred.

REFERENCES

1. H. Martikainen, A. Tiitinen, C. Tomás *et al.*, One versus two embryo transfer after IVF and ICSI: a randomized study. *Hum. Reprod.*, **16**:9 (2001), 1900–1903.
2. A. Thurin, J. Hausken, T. Hillensjo *et al.*, Elective single-embryo transfer versus double embryo transfer in in vitro fertilization. *N. Engl. J. Med.*, **351**:23 (2004), 2392–2402.
3. D. Le Lannou, J. Griveau, M. Laurent *et al.*, Contribution of embryo cryopreservation to elective single embryo transfer in IVF-ICSI. *Reprod. Biomed. Online*, **13**:3 (2006), 368–375.

4. J. Catt, T. Wood, M. Henman and R. Jansen, Single embryo transfer in IVF to prevent multiple pregnancies. *Twin Res.*, **6**:6 (2003), 536–539.

5. M. Henman, J. Catt, T. Wood *et al.*, Elective transfer of single fresh blastocysts and later transfer of cryostored blastocysts reduces the twin pregnancy rate and can improve the in vitro fertilization live birth rate in younger women. *Fertil. Steril.*, **84**:6 (2005), 1620–1627.

6. Practice Committee of the Society for Assisted Reproductive Technology; Practice Committee of the American Society for Reproductive Medicine, Guidelines on number of embryos transferred. *Fertil. Steril.*, **86**:Suppl. 4 (2006), S51–S52.

7. D. Gardner, P. Vella, M. Lane *et al.*, Culture and transfer of human blastocyst increases implantation rates and reduces the need for multiple embryo transfers. *Fertil. Steril.*, **69**:1 (1998), 84–88.

8. P. Schwarzler, H. Zech, M. Auer *et al.*, Pregnancy outcome after blastocyst transfer as compared to early cleavage stage embryo transfer. *Hum. Reprod.*, **19**:9 (2004), 2097–2102.

9. M. Wilson, K. Hartke, M. Kiehl *et al.*, Integration of blastocyst transfer for all patients. *Fertil. Steril.*, **77**:4 (2002), 693–696.

10. D. Gardner, W. Schoolcraft, L. Wagley *et al.*, A prospective randomized trial of blastocyst culture and transfer in in vitro fertilization. *Hum. Reprod.*, **13**:12 (1998), 3434–3440.

11. M. Scholtes and G. Zeilmaker, A prospective, randomized study of embryo transfer results after 3 or 5 days of embryo culture in in vitro fertilization. *Fertil. Steril.*, **65**:6 (1996), 1245–1248.

12. M. Bungum, L. Bungum, P. Humaidan and C. Yding Andersen, Day 3 versus day 5 embryo transfer: a prospective randomized study. *Reprod. Biomed. Online*, **7**:1 (2003), 98–104.

13. S. Coskun, J. Hollanders, S. Al-Hassan *et al.*, Day 5 versus day 3 embryo transfer: a controlled randomized trial. *Hum. Reprod.*, **15**:9 (2000), 1947–1952.

14. J. Hreinsson, B. Rosenlund, M. Fridstrom *et al.*, Embryo transfer is equally effective at cleavage stage and blastocyst stage: a randomized prospective study. *Eur. J. Obstet. Gynecol. Reprod. Biol.*, **117** (2004), 194–200.

15. I. Van Der Auwera, S. Debrock, C. Spiessens *et al.*, A prospective randomized study: day 2 versus day 5 embryo transfer. *Hum. Reprod.*, **17**:6 (2002), 1507–1512.

16. D. Blake, M. Proctor, N. Johnson and D. Olive, Cleavage stage versus blastocyst stage embryo transfer in assisted conception. *Cochrane Database Syst. Rev.*, **4** (2005), CD002118.pub2.

17. E. Kolibianakis, K. Zikopoulos, W. Verpoest *et al.*, Should we advise patients undergoing IVF to start a cycle leading to a day 3 or day 5 transfer. *Hum. Reprod.*, **19**:11 (2004), 2550–2554.

18. E. Papanikolaou, M. Camus, E. Kolibianakis *et al.*, In vitro fertilization with single blastocyst-stage versus single cleavage-stage embryos. *N. Engl. J. Med.*, **354**:11 (2006), 1139–1146.

19. N. Zech, B. Lejeune, F. Puissant *et al.*, Prospective evaluation of the optimal time for selecting a single embryo for transfer: day 3 versus day 5. *Fertil. Steril.*, **88**:1 (2007), 244–246.

20. C. Racowsky, K. Jackson, N. Cekleniak *et al.*, The number of eight-cell embryos is a key determinant for selecting day 3 or day 5 transfer. *Fertil. Steril.*, **73**:3 (2000), 558–564.

21. E. Papanikolaou, M. Camus, H. Fatemi *et al.*, Early pregnancy loss is significantly higher after day 3 single embryo transfer than after day 5 single blastocyst transfer in GnRH antagonist stimulated IVF cycles. *Reprod. Biomed. Online*, **12**:1 (2006), 60–65.

22. J. Yovich, J. Stanger, A. Grauaug *et al.*, Monozygotic twins from in vitro fertilisation. *Fertil. Steril.*, **41**:6 (1984), 833–837.

23. R. Edwards, L. Metler and D. Walters, Identical twins and in vitro fertilization. *J. In Vitro Fert. Embryo Transf.*, **3** (1986), 114–117.

24. B. Behr, J. Fisch, C. Racowsky *et al.*, Blastocyst-ET and monozygotic twinning. *J. Assist. Reprod. Genet.*, **17** (2000), 349–351.

25. J. Gerris, Single embryo transfer and IVF/ICSI outcome: a balanced appraisal. *Hum. Reprod. Update*, **11**:2 (2005), 105–121.

26. M. Schachter, A. Raziel, S. Friedler *et al.*, Monozygotic twinning after assisted reproductive techniques: a phenomenon independent of micromanipulation. *Hum. Reprod.*, **16** (2001), 1264–1269.

27. L. Schieve, S. Meikle, H. Peterson *et al.*, Does assisted hatching pose a risk for monozygotic twinning in pregnancies conceived through in vitro fertilization? *Fertil. Steril.*, **74** (2000), 288–294.

28. N. Abusheika, O. Salha, V. Sharma and P. Brinsden, Monozygotic twinning and IVF/ICSI treatment: a report of 11 cases and review of the literature. *Hum. Reprod. Update*, **6** (2000), 393–396.

29. N. Sebire, R. Snijders, K. Hughes, W. Sepulveda and K. Nicolaides, The hidden mortality of monochorionic twin pregnancies. *Br. J. Obstet. Gynecol.*, **104** (1997) 1203–1207.

30. A. Adegbite, S. Castille, S. Ward and R. Bajoria, Neuromorbidity in preterm twins in relation to chorionicity and discordant birth weight. *Am. J. Obstet. Gynecol.*, **190** (2004), 156–163.

31. J. Dube, L. Dodds and B. Armson, Does chorionicity or zygosity predict adverse perinatal outcomes in twins? *Am. J. Obstet. Gynecol.*, **186** (2002), 579–583.

32. K. Hack, J. Derks, V. de Visser, S. Elias and G. Visser, The natural course of monochorionic and dichorionic twin pregnancies: a historical cohort. *Twin Res. Hum. Genet.*, **9**:3 (2006), 450–455.

33. M. Alikani, N. Noyes, J. Cohen and Z. Rosenwaks, Monozygotic twinning in the human is associated with the zona pellucida architecture. *Hum. Reprod.*, **9** (1994), 1318–1321.

34. R. Slotnik and J. Ortega, Monoamniotic twinning and zona manipulation: a survey of U. S. IVF centers correlating zona manipulation procedures and a high-risk twinning frequency. *J. Assist. Reprod. Genet.*, **13** (1996), 381–385.

35. K. Yakin, B. Balaban and B. Urman, Risks of monochorionic pregnancies after assisted hatching. *Fertil. Steril.*, **79**:4 (2003), 1044–1046.

36. A. Hershlag, T. Paine, G. Cooper *et al.*, Monozygotic twinning associated with mechanical assisted hatching. *Fertil. Steril.*, **71**:1 (1999), 144–146.

37. C. C. Skiadas, S. A. Missmer, C. B. Benson *et al.*, Risk factors associated with pregnancies containing a monochorionic pair following ART. *Hum Reprod* (2008), PMID:8378561.

38. V. Wright, L. Schieve, A. Vahratian and M. Reynolds, Monozygotic twinning associated with day 5 embryo transfer in pregnancies conceived after IVF. *Hum. Reprod.*, **19**:8 (2004), 1831–1836.

39. E. Scott Sills, M. Moomjy, N. Zaninovic *et al.*, Human zona pellucida micromanipulation and monozygotic twinning frequency after IVF. *Hum. Reprod.*, **15**:4 (2000), 890–895.

40. G. Cassuto, M. Chavrier and Y. Menezo, Culture conditions and not prolonged culture time are responsible for monozygotic twinning in human in vitro fertilization. *Fertil. Steril.*, **80**:2 (2003), 462–463.

41. H. Malter and J. Cohen, Blastocyst formation and hatching in vitro following zona drilling of mouse and human embryos. *Gamete Res.*, **24** (1989), 67–80.

42. Y. Menezo and D. Sakkas, Monozygotic twinning: is it related to apoptosis in the embryo? *Hum. Reprod.*, **17** (2002), 247–248.

43. J. Jain, R. Boostanfar, C. Slater, M. Francis and R. Paulson, Monozygotic twins and triplets in association with blastocyst transfer. *J. Assist. Reprod. Genet.*, **21**:4 (2004), 103–107.

44. E. Sheiner, I. Har-Vardi and G. Potashnik, The potential association between blastocyst transfer and monozygotic twinning. *Fertil. Steril.*, **75**:1 (2001), 217–218.

45. A. da Costa, S. Abdelmassih, F. de Oliveira *et al.*, Monozygotic twinning and transfer at the blastocyst stage after ICSI. *Hum. Reprod.*, **16**:2 (2001), 333–336.

46. U. Reddy, R. Wapner, R. Rebar and R. Tasca, Infertility, assisted reproductive technology, and adverse pregnancy outcomes: executive summary of a National Institute of Child Health and Human Development workshop. *Obstet. Gynecol.*, **109**:4 (2007), 967–977.

47. V. Wright, J. Chang, G. Jeng, M. Chen and M. Macaluso, Assisted reproductive technology surveillance – United States, 2004. *MMWR Surveill. Summ.*, **56**:SS06 (2007), 1–22.

48. F. Helmerhorst, D. Perquin, D. Donker and M. Keirse, Perinatal outcome of singletons and twins after assisted conception: a systematic review of controlled studies. *BMJ*, **328** (2004), 261–265.

49. R. Jackson, K. Gibson, Y. Wu and M. Croughan, Perinatal outcomes in singletons following in vitro fertilization: a meta-analysis. *Obstet. Gynecol.*, **103** (2004), 552–563.

50. A. Van Montfoort, A. Fiddelers, J. Janssen *et al.*, In unselected patients, elective single embryo transfer prevents all multiples, but results in significantly lower pregnancy rates compared with double embryo transfer: a randomized controlled trial. *Hum. Reprod.*, **21** (2006), 338–343.

51. E. Niemitz and A. Feinberg, Epigenetics and assisted reproductive technologies: a call for investigation. *Am. J. Hum. Genet.*, **74** (2004), 599–609.

52. S. Jacob and K. Moley, Gametes and embryo epigenetic reprogramming affect developmental outcome: implication for assisted reproductive technologies. *Pediatr. Res.*, **58** (2005), 437–446.

53. A. Doherty, M. Mann, K. Tremblay, M. Bartolomei and R. Schultz, Differential effects of culture on imprinted H19 expression in the preimplantation mouse embryo. *Biol. Reprod.*, **62** (2000), 1526–1535.

54. P. Rinaudo and R. Schultz, Effects of embryo culture on global pattern of gene expression in preimplantation

mouse embryos. *Reproduction*, **128** (2004), 301–311.

55. M. DeBaun, E. Niemitz and A. Feinberg, Association of in vitro fertilization with Beckwith-Wiedemann syndrome and epigenetic alterations of LIT1 and H19. *Am. J. Hum. Genet.*, **72** (2003), 156–160.

56. E. Maher, L. Brueton, S. Bowdin *et al.*, Beckwith-Wiedemann syndrome and assisted reproductive technology (ART). *J. Med. Genet.*, **40** (2003), 62–64.

57. A. Chang, K. Moley, M. Wangler, A. Feinberg and M. DeBaun, The association between Beckwith-Wiedemann syndrome and assisted reproductive technology: a case series of 19 patients. *Fertil. Steril.*, **83** (2005), 349–354.

58. J. Clayton-Smith and L. Laan, Angelman syndrome: a review of the clinical and genetic aspects. *J. Med. Genet.*, **40**:2 (2003), 87–95.

59. K. Orstavik, K. Eiklid, C. Van Der Hagen *et al.*, Another case of imprinting defect in a girl with Angelman syndrome who was conceived by intracytoplasmic sperm injection. *Am. J. Hum. Genet.*, **72** (2003), 218–219.

60. A. Moll, S. Imhof, J. Cruysberg *et al.*, Incidence of retinoblastoma in children born after in vitro fertilisation. *Lancet*, **361** (2003), 309–310.

61. Y. Ho, K. Wigglesworth, J. Eppig and R. Schultz, Preimplantation development of mouse embryos in KSOM: augmentation by amino acids and analysis of gene expression. *Mol. Reprod. Dev.*, **41** (1995), 232–238.

62. M. Mann, S. Lee, A. Doherty *et al.*, Selective loss of imprinting in the placenta following preimplantation development in culture. *Development*, **131** (2004), 3727–3735.

63. G. Wolff, R. Kodell, S. Moore and C. Cooney, Maternal epigenetics and methyl supplements affect agouti gene expression in Avy/a mice. *FASEB J.*, **12** (1998), 949–957.

64. R. Waterland and R. Jirtle, Transposable elements: targets for early nutritional effects on epigenetic gene regulation. *Mol. Cell. Biol.*, **23** (2003), 5293–5300.

65. B. Orasanu, K. Jackson, M. Hornstein and C. Racowsky, Effects of culture medium on hCG concentrations and their value in predicting successful IVF outcome. *Reprod. Biomed. Online*, **12**:5 (2006), 590–598.

66. A. Sato, E. Otsu, H. Negishi, T. Utsunomiya and T. Arima, Aberrant DNA methylation of imprinted loci in superovulated oocytes. *Hum. Reprod.*, **22** (2007), 26–35.

18

Cost-effectiveness of single embryo transfer in assisted reproductive technology cycles

John Collins

Summary

Single embryo transfer (SET) is the most direct means of reducing the frequency of multiple pregnancies in assisted reproductive technology (ART) cycles. Multiple pregnancies are associated with increased frequency of preterm birth, and thereby with increased perinatal mortality and morbidity, both immediately and later during childhood. The burden of morbidity is reflected in the cost of health care: newborn hospital costs are four times higher for twin births and more than ten times higher for triplet births than singleton births. Cost-effectiveness analyses based on randomized controlled trials (RCTs) show that in good prognosis cycles, the transfer of a single embryo involves sufficient cost saving to support additional treatment cycles involving SET cycles. Single embryo transfer policies arising from legislation, negotiation or clinic decisions in Sweden, Belgium and the United States have reduced multiple birth rates without impairing overall live birth rates.

Introduction

Concern about costs is integral to modern clinical practice. Along with effectiveness, side effects and patient preferences, cost is a key element in the selection of treatment. The balance between effec-tiveness and harm is quite evident with SET, because transferring two embryos instead of one may be associated with higher overall live birth rates, which are due to higher twin birth rates. Cost-effectiveness studies may be especially relevant in this situation because the excess costs of the more effective intervention could be applied to increase the effectiveness of the less harmful intervention.

This chapter will outline the principles of health-economic analysis, discuss the incremental cost-effectiveness ratio (ICER), summarize cost analyses of multiple births, review the trials that provide evidence for cost-effectiveness of SET, summarize the cost-effectiveness data and provide a clinical practice context for decision-making about SET.

Principles of health-economic analysis

Health-economic analysis describes the costs arising from the prevention, diagnosis and treatment of disease. While costs of care, by themselves, are interesting mainly to economists and healthcare policy analysts, costs also can be interpreted by clinicians to reflect the severity of disease or the extent of treatment. Larger expenditures generally imply a greater allotment of healthcare services, which in turn implies more severe or more widespread disease.

The most common types of economic analysis are cost descriptions and cost–outcome descriptions,

Single Embryo Transfer, ed. J. Gerris, G. D. Adamson, P. De Sutter and C. Racowsky. Published by Cambridge University Press.
© Cambridge University Press 2009.

Table 18.1 Types of full economic evaluation

Cost-effectiveness analysis
Cost-minimization analysis
Cost–utility analysis
Cost–benefit analysis

usually derived from a case series, which enumerate costs without reference to outcomes. Case series also can give rise to cost–outcome descriptions, which do evaluate costs and outcomes. These may be identified as cost-effectiveness studies, but fall short of this definition because case series do not include a comparison with an alternative. The term cost-effectiveness implies a comparison of both costs and effects, preferably within a RCT. Cost-effectiveness also may be estimated from the data of cohort comparative studies (cost comparisons) or from models based on known costs and published treatment effects [1].

Cost-effectiveness analyses are one of four types of full economic assessment (Table 18.1). Cost-effectiveness analyses estimate the costs in each intervention of an outcome benefit measured in natural units. The natural units are usually events, such as fewer deaths or, in the case of infertility treatment, more live births. The other types of full economic assessment are cost-minimization studies, cost–utility studies, and cost–benefit studies. Cost-minimization studies are cost-effectiveness studies where the effects are known to be similar, so the least costly alternative would be preferred. Cost–utility analyses consider the cost per common natural unit of measurement. The measurement may be quality-adjusted life years (QALY), or disability-adjusted life years (DALY), neither of which applies readily to event outcomes such as those associated with infertility treatment. Cost–benefit analyses consider the cost per increment of comprehensive benefit measured in monetary terms such as dollars or yen. Converting treatment benefits to monetary terms is not a simple matter, and the monetary results may not be meaningful to clinicians.

The viewpoint or perspective chosen by the analysts affects the interpretation of the analysis. The perspective may be that of the patient, of healthcare professionals, of the pharmaceutical industry, of insurers (public and private) or of society as a whole. The societal perspective has the advantage that the whole population uses health care. Also, a societal viewpoint allows different economic analyses to be compared in a fair manner [2].

Which direct and indirect costs to include in the analysis is largely determined by the viewpoint. Direct costs are the procedure, physician, drug and hospital costs that arise in the course of the diagnosis, treatment and follow-up of the medical condition under study. Direct costs would be relevant to most economic analyses. Ideally direct costs would include the actual cost of each process in the care of each patient and an appropriate proportion of the overhead or fixed costs in the institution. Often, however, costs have to be inferred from charges to individuals or insurers, and these charges may not be identical to actual costs. Indirect costs typically include time lost from work and travel costs [1]. Indirect costs would be of greater interest from a patient or societal perspective.

The incremental cost-effectiveness ratio

The ICER is the expression used by cost-effectiveness analysis to compare a new approach with a standard approach. The new approach may be better, the same or worse; it may cost more, the same or less. Ideally, the new intervention would be better than the current standard and cost less. In this case the new intervention "dominates" the standard intervention. Such clear superiority is rarely seen – most often, the greater benefit with a new intervention also costs more. In this case a judgment has to be made about whether the extra cost is worth the gains achieved. To assist with this judgment the ICER states how much one has to pay for each additional unit of effectiveness [1].

The ICER is the ratio of the difference in costs to the difference in effects between the new and the standard intervention. If the new drug costs $20 000

Table 18.2 Hospital newborn and maternal costs per family

Authors	Currency	Cost Year	Cost		
			Singletons	Twins	Triplets
Callahan *et al.*, 1994 [3]	USD	1991	9 845	37 974	109 765
Chelmow *et al.*, 1995 [4]	USD	1993	–	–	64 837
Luke *et al.*, 1996 [5]	USD	1991	9 326	88 891	–
Ruiz *et al.*, 2001 [6]	USD	1995	–	46 796	–
Cassell *et al.*, 2003 [7]	CAD	2001	6 750	39 430	222 000
Lukassen *et al.*, 2005 [8]	euro	2002	2 550	13 469	–
Ledger *et al.*, 2006 [9]	GBP	2005	3 313	9 122	32 354

USD, US dollar; CAD, Canadian dollar; GBP, Great Britain pound.

to treat 100 women compared with $18 000 for the standard drug, the difference in costs is $2000. If there are 20 births with the new drug and 15 with the old drug, the difference between treatments is 5 births. The ICER is 2000/5 = $400. In other words, the cost of each additional birth with the new treatment is $400.

Cost of multiple births

Estimates of the cost of singleton, twin and triplet births vary according to time and country. Hospital charges per family in the United States were less than $10 000 for singleton pregnancies, and at least fourfold higher for twins and sixfold higher for triplet births (Table 18.2). The dates for the costs were 1991 to 1995. Costs for 2972 twins in 2002 were $29 797 for the larger twin to $37 443 for the smaller twin [10]. In the Netherlands, singleton and twin birth costs were €2550 and €13 469, respectively. In the United Kingdom costs were £3313, £9122 and £32 354 for singleton, twin and triplet births respectively. Compared with singleton births, the overall average costs are around fourfold higher for twin births, up to 18-fold higher for triplet births and 22-fold higher for quadruplet births.

The relatively higher costs for multiple births continue into mid childhood. From birth to 5 years of age, based on 276 897 children in the United King-

dom, the adjusted mean cost of all hospitalizations was £1532 for singletons, £3826 for twins and £8156 for higher-order multiple births [11]. Up to 7 years of age, based on 303 in vitro fertilization (IVF) births including 153 singletons and 121 twins, the cost per child of post-neonatal hospital care was €206 for an IVF singleton, which was 2.6-fold higher than a control singleton (€80). For a twin the cost was three- to fourfold higher whether the twin was IVF (€224) or control (€302) [12]. Although costs of multiple birth are greatest immediately after birth, continuing costs for care of the additional burden of disease and disability accrue during childhood.

Randomized controlled trials with cost-effectiveness analyses

Four RCTs have compared SET with double embryo transfer (DET), each with a different strategy in the SET arm and differences in eligibility (Table 18.3). The SET strategy in the earliest Dutch trial was to select good prognosis patients and allow an additional SET cycle (54 patients) [8]. The SET strategy in the second Dutch trial encouraged enrolment of all patients with two embryos regardless of age [14]. The third Dutch trial compared two different approaches to cycle management: four cycles of minimal stimulation with a gonadotropin-releasing hormone (GnRH) antagonist and SET versus three

Table 18.3 Randomized controlled trials of single embryo transfer (SET) versus double embryo transfer (DET)

Source	Strategy	Number of patients	Total live births (%)
Lukassen *et al.*, 2005 [8]	SET + SET	54	22 (41)
	DET	53	19 (36)
Thurin *et al.*, 2004 [13]	SET + 1 cryo[a]	330	120 (36)
	DET	331	142 (43)
van Montfoort *et al.*, 2006 [14]	Elective SET	154	32 (21)
	DET	154	73 (47)
Heijnen *et al.*, 2007 [15]	4 cycles minimal stimulation + SET	205	91 (44)
	3 cycles standard stimulation + DET	199	102 (51)

[a] cryo = one cycle of cryopreserved SET if necessary.

Table 18.4 Multiple birth rates in RCTs of SET versus DET

Source	Strategy	Singleton births (%)	Multiple births (%)
Lukassen *et al.*, 2005 [8]	SET + SET	22 (41)	0 (0)
	DET	12 (23)	7 (37)
Thurin *et al.*, 2004 [13]	SET + 1 cryo[a]	119 (36)	1 (0.8)
	DET	95 (29)	47 (33)
van Montfoort *et al.*, 2006 [14]	Elective SET	32 (21)	0 (0)
	DET	58 (37)	15 (21)
Heijnen *et al.*, 2007 [15]	4 cycles minimal stimulation + SET	91 (44)	1 (1.1)
	3 cycles standard stimulation + DET	76 (38)	26 (25)

[a] cryo = one cycle of cryopreserved SET if necessary.

cycles of standard stimulation with GnRH agonist and DET [15]. The SET strategy in the Swedish trial included SET and one cryopreserved embryo transfer cycle [13].

In three of four RCTs the overall birth rate per cycle was lower with SET than with DET (Table 18.3). In the second Dutch trial, the likelihood of a live birth was only 21% with SET and 47% with DET because no judgments were allowed as to which patients were best for SET. For selected good prognosis patients outside the trial in the same center, however, SET and DET results were similar, in part because poor prognosis patients received DET [14].

Singleton and multiple birth rates are shown in Table 18.4 by intention to treat, with all patients included in the group to which they were randomly allocated. In three of the four RCTs, the singleton birth rate was higher with SET. There were virtually no multiple births in the SET groups, but the DET group in all four trials experienced a high rate of multiple births (Table 18.4). Interestingly, the SET group in the Swedish trial included a spontaneous twin birth [16] and the SET group in the third Dutch trial included a triplet pregnancy in a woman whose IVF cycle was canceled for monofollicular development who had intrauterine insemination [15].

Table 18.5 Costs per patient for SET and DET

| Authors | Costs included | Cost per patient (euros) | |
		SET	DET
Lukassen *et al.*, 2005 [8]	6 weeks	5 475	4 904
Kjellberg *et al.*, 2006 [16]	6 months	9 309	12 318
Fiddelers *et al.*, 2007 [18]	4 weeks	7 334	10 924
Heijnen *et al.*, 2007 [15]	6 weeks	8 333	10 745

Table 18.6 Incremental costs for SET versus DET

Authors	Strategy	ICER (euros)[a]
Lukassen *et al.*, 2005 [8]	(SET + SET) or DET	−11 905
Kjellberg *et al.*, 2006 [16]	(SET + 1 cryo[b]) or DET	71 940
Fiddelers *et al.*, 2007 [18]	SET or DET	19 096
Heijnen *et al.*, 2007 [15]	Minimal stimulation + SET or Standard stimulation + DET	42 999

[a] ICER = incremental cost-effectiveness ratio: cost per additional live birth with DET.

[b] cryo = one cycle of cryopreserved SET if necessary.

Cost-effectiveness analyses based on the published trials

Costs and effects were published separately for three of the trials. Costs for the first Dutch trial were derived from an earlier publication [17]. The cost-effectiveness analyses were published after the effects were reported for the second Dutch trial and the Swedish trial [16, 18]. The costs of all four RCTs were published in euros and cost estimates were based on prices in 2002 [8], 2003 [18] and 2004 [15, 16]. The costs included were those for ART in all cases and for subsequent costs of pregnancy up to 4 weeks postpartum [19], 6 weeks postpartum [15, 17] and 6 months postpartum [16].

Three of four RCTs reported costs per patient and in the other study that information could be calculated from costs per birth [8] (Table 18.5). Costs per patient were higher for SET than DET in the first Dutch trial because there were 94 cycles of SET and 54 cycles of DET [8]. In the remaining trials, DET costs were higher because of the multiple births.

Table 18.6 shows the ICERs, either as reported [16, 18] or as calculated from the data supplied by the authors, using the methods discussed above [8, 15]. These ICER estimates indicate that it costs anywhere from minus €12 000 to plus €72 000, depending on the clinical strategy, to get one additional birth with a DET cycle.

Thus, although pregnancy rates with DET are generally higher than with SET, the cost per additional pregnancy in three of four clinical scenarios is high enough to consider avoiding DET in good prognosis patients. Childhood costs may substantially increase the cost of multiple births [11, 12], and if known would further increase the ICER. Depending on the method of funding ART, the cost per additional DET live birth alternatively could be used to fund many SET cycles.

Clinical practice context for decision-making

Economic analysis can inform clinical practice by reflecting the severity of a condition in the greater costs associated with its care. For example, the costs of care for preterm newborns reveal the serious burden of disease linked to preterm births after assisted reproduction. Economic analysis also helps in making choices about where to allocate limited health-care funds to achieve the optimal benefit, that is, the most benefit for the greatest possible number of people. The ICERs indicate that spending on incentives to increase the frequency of SET may be offset by savings on the cost of treatment for preterm multiple births.

A reduction in multiple birth rates was achieved in Sweden, where SET rates increased from 10% to

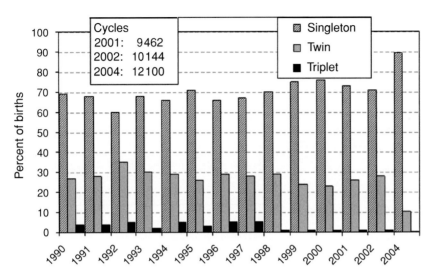

Figure 18.1 Live birth rate and multiple birth rates in Belgium, 1990–2004 (www.Belrap.be).

65% of ART cycles from 1999 to 2004 [20]. Because active peer pressure was reducing the number of embryos transferred, legislation introduced in 2003 accelerated only modestly the rising trend in SET. Despite the reduction in the average number of embryos transferred, overall delivery rates did not fall below 25%, and multiple birth rates decreased dramatically from about 25% in 1999 to 5% in 2004.

On July 1, 2003, the Belgian government began to reimburse ART laboratory costs for couples with female age less than 43 years for a maximum of six treatment cycles. In return, ART programs adopted a liberal SET transfer policy aiming at reduced multiple pregnancy rates and associated costs [21]. Data from the Belgian Register of Assisted Procreation show that the reduction in the cost to couples has increased the utilization of ART, from 10 144 cycles in 2002 to 12 100 cycles in 2004 (9.6% increase per year), as would be expected. The cost of the added cycles is offset by the reduced costs of a falling twin rate, from more than 25% to less than 10% in the same years. Overall live birth rates were not changed (Figure 18.1) (www.Belrap.be).

In the United States peer pressure and guidelines are having an effect, although the response has not been so dramatic as the response after legislation in Sweden and government incentives in Belgium [22]. One clinic introduced an educational program for couples together with a mandatory SET policy for good prognosis patients [23]. Knowledge of twin risks improved among the couples, overall ongoing pregnancy rates were similar before and after the policy change (63% vs. 58%) and the multiple-gestation rates declined from 35% to 19%.

While the cost-effectiveness analyses indicate that SET is usually cheaper than DET, effectiveness is optimal when clinical judgment is applied to select good prognosis patients. Female age less than 38 years, no evidence of a previous poor response and a satisfactory number of embryos available for transfer are commonly held to be good prognosis factors. Rigid legislation or clinical policies requiring SET in all patients are likely to result in much lower ART birth rates, as shown by the second Dutch trial [14].

What do we know now?
Single embryo transfer is the most direct means of reducing the frequency of multiple pregnancies in ART cycles. Cost studies based on RCTs show that one SET cycle is cheaper than one DET cycle

mainly because of the DET cost associated with twin pregnancy.

What do we need to know?

Because the incremental cost of DET over SET varies with study design, clinical setting and healthcare policies, studies are needed in more settings to provide information that can be generalized to most patients.

What should we do?

It will be necessary to convince patients and policy analysts around the world that SET should be adopted wherever possible because the increased burden of morbidity associated with twin births is the reason for the extra cost of DET.

REFERENCES

1. M. F. Drummond, M. J. Sculpher, G. W. Torrance, B. J. O'Brien and G. L. Stoddart, *Methods for the Economic Evaluation of Health Care Programmes*, 3rd edn. (Oxford: Oxford University Publishing, 2005).
2. S. Byford and J. Raftery, Perspectives in economic evaluation. *BMJ*, **316** (1998), 1529–1530.
3. T. L. Callahan, J. E. Hall, S. L. Ettner *et al.*, The economic impact of multiple gestation pregnancies and the contribution of assisted reproduction. *N. Engl. J. Med.*, **331** (1994), 244–249.
4. D. Chelmow, A. Pensias, G. Kaufman and C. Cetrulo, Costs of triplet pregnancy. *Am. J. Obstet. Gynecol.*, **172** (1995), 677–682.
5. B. Luke, H. R. Bigger, S. Leurgans and D. Sietsema, The cost of prematurity: a case-control study of twins vs singletons. *Am. J. Public Health*, **86** (1996), 809–814.
6. R. J. Ruiz, C. E. Brown, M. T. Peters and A. B. Johnston, Specialized care for twin gestations: improving newborn outcomes and reducing costs. *J. Obstet. Gynecol. Neonat. Nurs.*, **30** (2001), 52–60.
7. K. A. Cassell, C. M. O'Connell and T. F. Baskett, The origins and outcomes of triplet and quadruplet pregnancies in Nova Scotia: 1980 to 2001. *Am. J. Perinatol.*, **21** (2003), 439–445.
8. H. G. M. Lukassen, D. Braat, A. M. M. Wetzels *et al.*, Two cycles with single embryo transfer versus one cycle with double embryo transfer: a randomized controlled trial. *Hum. Reprod.*, **20** (2005), 702–708.
9. W. L. Ledger, D. Anumba, N. Marlow, C. M. Thomas and E. C. Wilson, The costs to the NHS of multiple births after IVF treatment in the UK. *BJOG*, **113** (2006), 21–25.
10. B. Luke, M. B. Brown, P. K. Alexandre *et al.*, The cost of twin pregnancy: maternal and neonatal factors. *Am. J. Obstet. Gynecol.*, **192** (2005), 909–915.
11. J. Henderson, C. Hockley, S. Petrou, M. Goldacre and L. Davidson, Economic implications of multiple births: inpatient hospital costs in the first 5 years of life. *Arch Dis Child Fetal Neonatal Ed*, **89** (2004), F542–F545.
12. S. Koivurova, A. L. Hartikainen, M. Gissler, E. Hemminki and M. R. Jarvelin, Post-neonatal hospitalization and health care costs among IVF children: a 7-year follow-up study. *Hum. Reprod.*, **22** (2007), 2136–2141.
13. A. Thurin, J. Hausken, T. Hillensjo *et al.*, Elective single-embryo transfer versus double-embryo transfer in in vitro fertilization. *N. Engl. J. Med.*, **351** (2004), 2392–2402.
14. A. P. van Montfoort, A. A. Fiddelers, J. M. Janssen *et al.*, In unselected patients, elective single embryo transfer prevents all multiples, but results in significantly lower pregnancy rates compared with double embryo transfer: a randomized controlled trial. *Hum. Reprod.*, **21** (2006), 338–343.
15. E. M. Heijnen, M. J. Eijkemans, C. De Klerk *et al.*, A mild treatment strategy for in-vitro fertilisation: a randomised non-inferiority trial. *Lancet*, **369** (2007), 743–749.
16. A. T. Kjellberg, P. Carlsson and C. Bergh, Randomized single versus double embryo transfer: obstetric and paediatric outcome and a cost-effectiveness analysis. *Hum. Reprod.*, **21** (2006), 210–216.
17. M. H. G. Lukassen, Y. Schonbeck, E. M. M. Adang *et al.*, Cost analysis of singleton versus twin pregnancies after in vitro fertilization. *Fertil. Steril.*, **81** (2004), 1240–1246.
18. A. A. Fiddelers, J. L. Severens, C. D. Dirksen *et al.*, Economic evaluations of single- versus double-embryo transfer in IVF. *Hum. Reprod. Update*, **13** (2007), 5–13.
19. A. A. Fiddelers, A. P. van Montfoort, C. D. Dirksen *et al.*, Single versus double embryo transfer: cost-effectiveness analysis alongside a randomized clinical trial. *Hum. Reprod.*, **21** (2006), 2090–2097.

20. P. O. Karlstrom and C. Bergh, Reducing the number of embryos transferred in Sweden-impact on delivery and multiple birth rates. *Hum. Reprod.*, **22** (2007), 2202–2207.

21. W. P. Ombelet, P. De Sutter, J. Van der Elst and G. Martens, Multiple gestation and infertility treatment: registration, reflection and reaction – the Belgian project. *Hum. Reprod. Update*, **11** (2005), 3–14.

22. J. E. Stern, M. I. Cedars, T. Jain *et al.*, Assisted reproductive technology practice patterns and the impact of embryo transfer guidelines in the United States. *Fertil. Steril.*, **88** (2007), 275–282.

23. G. L. Ryan, A. E. Sparks, C. S. Sipe *et al.*, A mandatory single blastocyst transfer policy with educational campaign in a United States IVF program reduces multiple gestation rates without sacrificing pregnancy rates. *Fertil. Steril.*, **88** (2007), 354–360.

19

Defining success in assisted reproduction

Siladitya Bhattacharya

Defining success

Defining success in assisted reproductive technology (ART) has proved to be surprisingly contentious. Traditionally the prerogative of clinics, rather than patients, the choice of criteria for success has been shaped by clinical and laboratory considerations, ease of collecting and reporting data, and the need to appear competitive. Pregnancy rates per fresh cycle of treatment were the original favored indicator of treatment success, but live birth is now perceived to be a more robust end point. In recent years, the thinking surrounding in vitro fertilization (IVF) has matured to an extent where safety is acknowledged as an important end point of treatment and multiple pregnancies perceived as complications of ART. The logical extension of this is the view that the ideal outcome of ART should be a singleton live birth [1], but this concept has generated much debate within the specialty [2]. This chapter will review the case for reporting outcomes in ART, assess the appropriateness of those in current use and consider alternative ways of defining success.

Why report success in ART?

An outcome parameter has been defined as a "measure enabling the clinician to study, understand and eventually control variables that influence the success of a therapy" [3]. Reasons for defining and reporting success in ART are summarized in Table 19.1. Without a clear understanding of the desired end point of an intervention, it is impossible to gauge the effect of treatment, compare alternative modalities, evaluate clinic performance, identify adverse events, perform research or organize service delivery. Yet it is easy to see how individual components of a complex intervention such as ART have their own relevant end points. Accepted outcomes of ART have traditionally included efficacy, safety, patient satisfaction, social acceptability and costs [4]. In recent years many clinicians have begun to feel strongly that complications of treatment, such as multiple pregnancy, undermine any gains in terms of pregnancies/births and this should be reflected in any comment on the outcome of treatment. Others feel that the two are quite independent of each other and should be reported on separately.

Most current outcomes deal with clinical end points rather than the process of treatment. While this is what most health service providers as well as consumers are familiar with, outcome indicators are influenced by extraneous factors such as the clinical case mix [5]. For example, a clinic treating a large number of poor prognosis women who are older and who have multiple failed previous treatments will have lower pregnancy and live birth rates. A culture of evaluation based on outcome alone could

Single Embryo Transfer, ed. J. Gerris, G. D. Adamson, P. De Sutter and C. Racowsky. Published by Cambridge University Press.
© Cambridge University Press 2009.

Table 19.1 Reasons for reporting success in ART

- To provide a measure of the effectiveness of treatment
- To measure quality of care
- To audit clinical practice
- To identify complications
- To facilitate clinical decision-making
- To allow comparison results across clinics, countries
- To allow patients and purchasers to compare clinics
- To facilitate publication and dissemination of research

Table 19.2 What is a good outcome measure?

- Unambiguous
- Easily understood by all
- Valid
- Reproducible
- Easy to calculate
- Clinically relevant

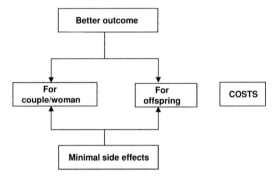

Figure 19.1 Defining success.

lead to a natural reluctance on the part of clinics to treat such women. An outcome-based approach can also be questioned on the grounds that clinical care in infertility encompasses a number of clinical, social and laboratory domains. Evaluation of each of these is important, given that a successful clinical outcome, i.e. pregnancy or live birth, occurs in fewer than 50% patients.

One solution is to use process indicators of quality of care [6] – based on evidence-based guidelines [7], which are, arguably, more sensitive and unlikely to be confounded by factors beyond the clinic's control [5]. These also have the potential to be used constructively to improve delivery of care [8]. However, for meaningful day-to-day reporting, there is no real substitute for clinical outcomes. The main problem with commonly used measures is their multiplicity, suggestive of a lack of a single universally accepted end point. This stems from the different objectives for reporting outcomes, different aspects of treatment reported on and priorities of different stakeholder groups.

Criteria for a good outcome measure

Generic criteria for a good outcome measure are summarized in Table 19.2. In ART an outcome measure needs to be relevant, and incorporate clinical- and cost-effectiveness, efficiency, acceptability and safety (Figure 19.1). In addition, it should be valid, i.e. measure what it is meant to measure, and reliable, i.e. provide consistent measurements at different time periods. Outcomes should ideally reflect

the intrinsic worth of a treatment as well as the ability of a clinical team to provide it. Finally, outcome measures should be user-friendly. Any relevant statistics should be easy for a clinic to calculate and for patients to understand.

Outcome measures deconstructed: numerators and denominators

Most outcome measures involve a numerator and denominator (Figure 19.2). Numerators reflect the parameter which is being evaluated (e.g., pregnancy, live birth), while the denominator defines the context in which the numerator is assessed (e.g., treatment cycles, women, time horizon).

Numerators

A list of commonly used numerators is shown in Table 19.3. It is generally, but not universally, accepted that the measures of treatment effect

Table 19.3 Proposed numerators

Worse

- Follicle number
- Estradiol levels
- Oocyte number
- Fertilization rate
- Embryo number
- Implantation
- Conception
- Ongoing pregnancy
- Live birth
- Live singleton birth
- Term birth
- Term singleton birth

Better

$$\text{Outcome} = \frac{\text{numerator}}{\text{denominator}}$$

Figure 19.2 Outcome measures deconstructed.

occurring at the start of treatment are less useful clinically than those occurring at the end of treatment, i.e. follicle number is less relevant than pregnancy.

Markers of successful ovarian stimulation

Parameters such as numbers of follicles, estradiol levels and oocyte numbers are surrogate markers which reflect ovarian response, but brisk response is not necessarily correlated with the best clinical outcome. Sometimes excessive response may be inversely correlated with a positive outcome, e.g. ovarian hyperstimulation leading to cycle cancellation.

Embryological outcomes

Fertilization rate, embryo number and embryo quality are again predictive of a good outcome but lack sufficient precision in terms of predicting pregnancy and live birth. While important in themselves, they are liable to reflect subjective interobserver variations. As intermediate outcomes they are of limited interest to consumers and purchasers.

Pregnancy

Pregnancy has been used for decades to reflect the success of IVF treatment. Many practitioners feel very strongly that it is the outcome most immediate to ART, as obstetric outcomes may be influenced by non-ART factors. The main criticism of pregnancy as an outcome is twofold: the term "pregnancy" is not without a significant degree of ambiguity due to the problems of disentangling biochemical, clinical and ongoing pregnancy. The first suffers from a need to define the level of beta-human chorionic gonadotropin (βhCG) which is compatible with pregnancy, the second and third rely on ultrasound identification of a fetal heart and agreement on a suitable gestational age at scan. In addition, there is some debate about the value of reporting on subsets such as "term" pregnancy or "successful" pregnancy. The latter should refer to cases which result in live birth but could include extremely preterm infants born as early as 20–24 weeks which show signs of life.

Live birth

The main advantage of live birth as an outcome is its unambiguity. It is generally accepted as the most robust parameter of success [9] and represents the desired end point for infertile couples. Unfortunately, it has been criticized by some ART practitioners as being too remote from the original treatment and susceptible to the confounding effects of obstetric complications and co-interventions. It also groups singletons and multiples together although, in reality, multiples fare significantly worse.

Singleton live birth

This recognizes the complications that are associated with multiple births and is perceived to be a desirable end point by many clinicians [2]. It balances effectiveness and safety in ART, but falls short of capturing the full range of perinatal complications by, for example, not making a distinction between term and preterm births.

Singleton term live birth

Birth emphasising successful singleton at term (BESST) is seen by many as possessing greatest discriminative ability to detect a favorable outcome from the maternal and perinatal point of view [2]. As a whole there is much support for the use of a variable such as this, which defines safety. At the same time, it is acknowledged that singleton, term singleton and healthy term singleton all carry an element of uncertainty [10].

However, despite its undoubted value its role as an ideal outcome has been challenged by other authors [3, 10–14] on a number of different issues. Some authors feel that the sheer scale and complexity of ART means that it is simplistic to expect a single parameter to do justice to it all. Griesinger *et al.* [3] argue that the outcome measure should be context specific and should reflect the specific question being asked at the time. Pinborg *et al.* [15] propose a minimum of three parameters covering stimulation, laboratory and embryo transfer outcome. They suggest that appropriate measures of success are: number of oocytes per aspiration, number of ongoing implantations per embryo transferred and number of deliveries per embryo transferred. If a single parameter had to be chosen, they would opt for singleton live birth per oocyte as their preferred outcome, but accept that this is difficult for non-experts to comprehend and would have very limited practical use.

Other authors feel that selective reporting of term singletons as the only outcome has limitations. The etiology of preterm births in singletons is multifactorial [16, 17]. A measure which incorporates gestational age cannot be presented without the background patient and treatment characteristics associated with preterm delivery [10]. Additionally, if we agree to focus on neonatal well-being as an end point, preterm delivery is only one of a number of

risk factors including low and very low birth weight as well as growth restriction. The literature suggests that even singletons born after ART are at increased risk of low birth weight in comparison with naturally conceived infants [18, 19]. By the same token, many adverse outcomes do not manifest themselves till much later. At the same time it is not feasible to monitor children born through ART for an indefinite period of time.

Some clinicians may feel that it is inappropriate to exclude births between 34 and 37 weeks as the outcome in terms of intact survival in many of these infants is good and the need for neonatal care minimal. There is also a lack of recognition that in many obstetric complications, such as preeclampsia, antepartum hemorrhage and growth restriction, extending pregnancy to term may be detrimental to the fetus. Finally it can be argued that the term "successful" in this definition is unclear although it is assumed to mean healthy. This can be seen to be a misrepresentation of the truth as any potential long-term complications are disregarded.

Dickey *et al.* [12] do not accept that multiples (especially twins) should be excluded from statistics of success of ART. Although this may change in years to come, the net contribution of ART to total multiple births at the present time is very limited. Thus, a few ART-related multiples are unlikely to change the safety profile of the treatment as a whole. Second, it is mainly triplets (not twins) which contribute to high morbidity and mortality, and it is inappropriate to combine the two when compiling morbidity statistics.

While it is true that twins due to ART account for a small proportion (12% in the USA but > 50% in Western Europe) of all preterm births [20], many believe that these are a few too many as they are entirely avoidable. Given the rapid increase in the worldwide uptake of IVF, the first argument may also rapidly become out of date.

Denominators

If agreement on a numerator is difficult, consensus on a denominator is virtually impossible. Whether

Table 19.4 Proposed denominators

- Per cycle
- Per started cycle
- Fresh cycle vs. fresh + frozen cycle
- Per oocyte recovery
- Cumulative (lifetime) outcomes
- Per embryo transfer
- Per woman

this is per cycle, per oocyte retrieval, per transfer, per embryo, or per woman over a specified time horizon is debatable (Table 19.4). Min *et al.* [2] suggest a per cycle approach while Vail and Gardner [21] stated that the only relevant denominator was per woman.

Fresh cycle

The suggested denominator for the BESST outcome is a fresh cycle. This is mainly historical and reflects the ease of analysis based on routinely collected cycle data available in most clinics.

Cumulative outcome fresh + frozen

The number of cryopreservation cycles is rising. In Europe more than 45 000 frozen embryo transfers are performed each year [22]. The contribution of frozen embryo transfers has been significant, resulting in cumulative live birth rates of 52.8% per oocyte retrievals [23] and 41.8% in women 36–39 [24]. As a result, it has been proposed that it is important to take into account the effect of all embryos achieved during a single oocyte retrieval procedure [25, 26]. Cumulative delivery rate should therefore be calculated per stimulated cycle after all embryo transfers, fresh and frozen, have been performed. This strategy also emphasizes the critical role of cryopreservation programs in the context of elective single embryo transfer (eSET) strategies.

Outcome per woman

It has been argued that expressing outcomes per treatment (either fresh or frozen) represents a myopic and misleading view of outcomes. The most clinically meaningful denominator is the woman undergoing IVF treatment [21]. From a purely statistical viewpoint, the hierarchical nature of infertility data (multiple oocytes, embryos per cycle and multiple cycles per woman) dictates that it should be the woman who should be the unit of analysis rather than cycles. Having more than one observation per woman in a dataset encourages error due to the possibility of spurious narrow confidence intervals and low p values.

Complex outcomes

The idea that the goal of ART is to maximize maternal and neonatal health gain has led to more sophisticated (and complex) ways of defining outcomes. One approach is to highlight effectiveness in terms of healthy singleton live births as a positive end point and multiple embryo transfer as a negative outcome. This translates into the somewhat formidable corrected singleton live birth per cycle. This is calculated by subtracting the multiple live birth from the singleton live birth rate per cycle and would challenge the abilities of most clinics and patients. The sum (S) of cumulative singleton delivery rate (CUSIDERA) and cumulative twin delivery rate (CUTWIDERA) has been suggested as a measure of efficacy [27] while the ratio of (S/CUTWIDERA) expressed as a percentage is a measure of safety.

Perception of outcomes

While absolute measures of success may seem self-evident to members of the medical profession, consumers of health services may see things differently. Maternal mortality rates are two to three times higher in multiples [28] the absolute risk is low (10 per 100 000) and neonatal mortality is 31 per 1000 in twins compared to 6 per 1000 in singletons [29]. Many clinicians see this as unambiguous proof of the dangers of multiples and discount these complications from perceived success. Some patients see success as an independent end point and complications a necessary price they are willing to pay for it.

Clinicians may feel that a high twin rate in IVF is unacceptable [30], but couples may have different views [31]. The safe delivery of healthy twins for example, while not ideal, may be seen as a positive indicator of success [11]. Some women, especially mothers of IVF twins, may actually see twins as a desirable outcome [15, 32]. Others who are paying for their treatment, may feel that having twins represents a cost-effective way of completing their family. Many are willing to take risks in order to achieve this goal. This may be due, in part, to insufficient information about the potential risks of a twin pregnancy. Yet, improved methods of communicating risks to couples do not always change couples' opinions. Fewer than a third of UK women in their early thirties, embarking on their first IVF cycle, felt that a hypothetical policy of eSET was acceptable, if it meant slightly reduced pregnancy rates [33]. Just over half were willing to consider eSET, provided they were not charged for cyropreservation and subsequent replacement of spare embryos.

Despite the awareness that multiple pregnancies are associated with maternal and perinatal complications, many infertile couples see a twin delivery as a positive outcome [34]. To many couples undergoing IVF treatment, the immediate threat is failure to get pregnant rather than the more remote risk of feto-maternal complications. Some women waiting for IVF treatment view severe child disability outcomes associated with double embryo transfer as being more desirable than having no child at all. Women embarking on IVF may be influenced more strongly by considerations of "treatment success" rather than future risks to their offspring [35].

Reasons for alternative measures

The evolution of many of the alternative outcomes in common use can be ascribed to the different and sometimes conflicting perspectives of the various members of the ART team. For example, many clinicians and patients find it intuitive to report outcomes as pregnancy or live birth per cycle started. Many embryologists, however, can legitimately claim that the outcome which best reflects their input is pregnancy/live birth per embryo transfer, as they are unable to influence events prior to this stage of the treatment cycle. In actual fact this is not necessarily true. While failure to transfer embryos can be due to poor stimulation and monitoring, poor oocyte recovery or poor gamete quality, it can also reflect suboptimal laboratory practice and conditions which can affect fertilization embryo quality.

Many clinicians and researchers will argue that a single outcome is simply too blunt for the purposes of assessing the diverse steps involved in ART and it is simplistic to push for such an approach [3]. This is a reasonable view, which reflects the reality of ART where the process of treatment involves a number of steps which should ideally be captured in any evaluation of the whole. In practice, this would work if all reported results incorporated all the agreed end points. In fact this does not occur, and the freedom to choose some outcomes and not others has been confusing and unhelpful.

Sometimes it is the ease of collecting and analyzing data (e.g., per cycle) which can influence the choice of outcome. This is particularly true of large national datasets such as the Human Fertilization and Embryology Authority (www.hfea.gov.uk), where the process of data collection is kept simple in order to encourage participation by IVF clinics.

Finally, it is understandable that clinics may choose to present outcomes which are most likely to show them in a positive light. Thus clinics which have a relatively poor cryopreservation program are unlikely to wish to present cumulative data per oocyte recovery.

Yet, while individual measures of success are of interest to different stakeholders and may continue to have a place in our lexicon, there needs to be a single outcome which is relevant to patients and meaningful to clinicians. There are a number of reasons why an agreed end point is necessary.

Clarity and consistency

While each historical indicator of success has a genuine place in the evaluation of the treatment process, the rationale for its use has been less than explicit. As we have seen, variation in each numerator and denominator results in inconsistency and confusion – something that may not always be unwelcome in terms of putting a gloss on any statistics. This creates a climate of uncertainty among clinics and consumers who need to have a common goal and an agreed set of standards.

Evaluating effectiveness of treatments

Unless success can be defined, it will be impossible to decide which treatments or interventions are successful. This has relevance in terms of reporting of research findings, clinical audit and clinic performances. It is also important in terms of evaluating the strength of the evidence base underpinning alternative treatments [36].

Consequences of status quo

One of the consequences of the present situation is our current practice of inconsistent reporting of clinical and research findings [21]. In terms of combating iatrogenic multiples associated with ART, recommendations based on safety [37] come into conflict with conventional indices of success. The present system provides a degree of freedom to clinics and clinicians but the lack of clarity leads to loss of confidence on the part of doctors and patients, and unwillingness on the part of funders to engage with the fraternity. Lack of uniformity in terms of reporting success rates also makes it difficult to evaluate clinics and treatments. It can also impede interpretation of research findings and delay implementation of potentially beneficial treatments. Finally, the present emphasis on immediate outcomes such as pregnancy per fresh cycle as opposed to concern about the societal implications of maternal and perinatal complications could be damaging as ART becomes more common. The suggestion, therefore, that the status quo is satisfactory and that clinicians and researchers should be free to choose appropriate primary outcome measures [3] is untenable.

Towards a consensus

It is true to say that no single criterion will capture all the different quality aspects of ART. We have to agree on a common primary criterion for success that everyone can subscribe to, and satisfy our desire for detail with a number of secondary measures. Ideally, outcomes of relevance should be agreed by all stakeholders including consumers, clinicians, service providers, purchasers, regulating bodies (where relevant) and the general public. Until such time, live birth appears to be an outcome that many can relate to. From a clinical as well as a statistical point of view, there is much support for expressing such an outcome per woman than per cycle [9, 21, 26, 38]. Unqualified, this is difficult to report and it needs a time horizon. An alternative is to report cumulative live birth rates per woman, for each fresh oocyte retrieval. This has the benefit of simplicity and unambiguity but does not address the issue of safety, which should be addressed in the context of secondary outcomes such as rates of multiple and singleton live births.

Assessment of a clinic's performance is best performed by means of a process outcome. For example, it has been suggested that the percentage of eSETs performed by a clinic is a statistic which captures the efficiency and confidence of a clinic. Only clinics with high live birth rates would be confident enough to decrease number of embryos per transfer without compromising live birth rates [9]. This outcome has the benefit of incorporating an element of safety which is missing from the clinical outcome – i.e. live birth per woman. It has been pointed out that such a measure may not be relevant to countries where eSET and cryopreservation of spare embryos is not possible for legal reasons [27].

Choice of outcomes of success in infertility is and will continue to be highly sensitive to individual preferences. Yet, as long as there is no unanimity about primary outcomes in ART, the evidence base on the subject will remain open to interpretation. As a profession, we need to be consistent in our approach to this dilemma and aware of our responsibilities to our patients.

REFERENCES

1. J. A. Land and J. L. H. Evers, Risks and complications in assisted reproduction techniques: report of an ESHRE consensus meeting. *Hum. Reprod.*, **18** (2003), 455–457.
2. J. K. Min, S. A. Breheny, V. MacLachlan and D. L. Healy, What is the most relevant standard of success in assisted reproduction? The singleton, term gestation, live birth rate per cycle initiated: the BESST endpoint for assisted reproduction. *Hum. Reprod.*, **19**:1 (2004), 3–7.
3. G. Griesinger, K. Dafopoulous, A. Schultze-Mosgau, R. Felberbaum and K. Diedrich, Is BESST (birth emphasizing a successful singleton at term) truly the best? *Hum. Reprod.*, **19**:6 (2004), 1239–1241.
4. M. J. Davies, J. X. Wang and R. J. Norman, Assessing the BESST index for reproduction treatment. *Hum. Reprod.*, **19**:5 (2004), 1049–1051.
5. J. Mant, Process versus outcome indicators in the assessment of quality of health care, *Int. J. Qual. Health Care*, **13**:6 (2001), 475–480.
6. W. L. D. M. Nelen, R. P. M. G. Hermens, S. M. Mourad *et al.*, Monitoring reproductive health in Europe: what are the best indicators of reproductive health? A need for evidence-based quality indicators of reproductive health care. *Hum. Reprod.*, **22**:4 (2007), 916–918.
7. National Institute for Health and Clinical Excellence. Fertility: *Assessment and Treatment for People with Fertility Problems*. National Collaborating Centre for Women's and Children's Health. Commissioned by NICE, London (2004). www.nice.gov.uk.
8. H. R. Rubin, P. Pronovost and G. B. Diette, From a process of care to a measure; the development and testing of a quality indicator. *Int. J. Qual. Health Care*, **13** (2001), 489–496.
9. J. A. Land and J. L. H. Evers, Defining outcome in ART: a Gordian knot of safety, efficacy and quality. *Hum. Reprod.*, **19**:5 (2004), 1046–1048.
10. L. A. Schieve and M. A. Reynolds, Challenges in measuring and reporting success rates for assisted reproductive technology treatments: what is optimal? *Hum. Reprod.*, **19**:4 (2004), 778–82.
11. W. Buckett and S. L. Tan, The importance of informed choice. *Hum. Reprod.*, **19**:5 (2004), 1043–1045.
12. R. P. Dickey, B. M. Sartor and R. Pyrzak, No single outcome measure is satisfactory when evaluating success in assisted reproduction; both twin births and singleton births should be counted as successes. *Hum. Reprod.*, **19**:4 (2004), 783–787.
13. I. E. Messinis and E. Domali, Should BESST really be the primary endpoint for assisted reproduction? *Hum. Reprod.*, **19**:9 (2004), 1933–1935.
14. U. B. Wennerholm and C. Bergh, Singleton live births should also include preterm births. *Hum. Reprod.*, **19**:9 (2004), 1943–1945.
15. A. Pinborg, A. Loft, L. Schmidt and A. N. Andersen, Attitudes of IVF/ICSI-twin mothers towards twins and single embryo transfer. *Hum. Reprod.*, **18**:3 (2003), 621–627.
16. J. Lumley, Defining the problem: the epidemiology of preterm birth. *BJOG*, **110**:Suppl. 20 (2003), 3–7.
17. J. Moutquin, Classification and heterogeneity of preterm birth. *BJOG*, **110**:Suppl. 20 (2003), 30–33.
18. L. A. Schieve, S. F. Meikle, C. Ferre *et al.*, Low and very low birth weight in infants conceived with use of assisted reproductive technology. *N. Engl. J. Med.*, **346** (2002), 731–737.
19. J. X. Wang, R. J. Norman and P. K. Kristiansson, The effect of various infertility treatments on the risk of preterm birth. *Hum. Reprod.*, **17** (2002), 945–949.
20. M. O. Gardner, R. L. Goldenberg, S. P. Cliver *et al.*, The origin and outcome of preterm twin pregnancies. *Obstet. Gynecol.*, **85** (1995), 553–557.
21. A. Vail and E. Gardner, Common statistical errors in the design and analysis of subfertility trials. *Hum. Reprod.*, **18** (2003), 1000–1004.
22. A. Nyboe Andersen, L. Gianaroli and K. G. Nygren, European IVF-monitoring programme European Society of *Human Reproduction*, and Embryology. Assisted reproductive technology in Europe, 2000. Results generated from European registers by ESHRE *Hum. Reprod.*, **19**:3 (2004), 490–503.
23. C. Hyden-Granskog and A. Tiitinen, Single embryo transfer in clinical practice. *Hum. Fertil.* (camb), **7**:3 (2004), 175–182.
24. Z. Veleva, S. Vilska, C. Hyden-Granskog *et al.*, Elective single embryo transfer in women aged

36–39 years. *Hum. Reprod.*, **21**:8 (2006), 2098–2102; doi:10.1093/humrep/del137.

25. A. Pinborg, A. Loft, S. Siebe and A. N. Andersen, Is there a single 'parameter of excellence'? *Hum. Reprod.*, **19**:5 (2004), 1052–1054.

26. A. Tiitinen, C. Hyden-Granskog and M. Gissler, The value of cryopresentation on cumulative pregnancy rates per single oocyte retrieval should not be forgotten. *Hum. Reprod.*, **19**:11 (2004), 2439–2441.

27. M. Germond, F. Urner, A. Chanson *et al.*, The cumulated singleton/twin delivery rates per oocyte pick-up: the CUSIDERA and CUTWIDERA. *Hum. Reprod.*, **19**:11 (2004), 2442–2444.

28. M. Senat, P. Ancel, M. H. Bouvier-Colle and G. Breart, How does multiple pregnancy affect maternal morbidity and mortality? *Clin. Obstet. Gynecol.*, **41** (1998), 78–83.

29. R. B. Russell, J. R. Petrinin and K. Damus, The changing epidemiology of multiple births in the United States. *Obstet. Gynecol.*, **101** (2003), 129–135.

30. J. Hazekamp, C. Bergh, U. B. Wennerholm *et al.*, Avoiding multiple pregnancies in ART, consideration of new strategies. *Hum. Reprod.*, **15**:6 (2000), 1217–1219.

31. J. Goldfarb, D. J. Kinzer, M. Boyle and D. Kurit, Attitudes of in vitro fertilisation and intrauterine insemination couples towards multiple gestation pregnancy and multifetal pregnancy reduction. *Fertil. Steril.*, **65** (1996), 815–820.

32. N. Gleicher, D. P. Campbell, C. L. Chan *et al.*, The desire for multiple births in couples with infertility problems contradicts present practice patterns. *Hum. Reprod.*, **10** (1995), 1079–1084.

33. S. Murray, A. Shetty, A. Rattray, V. Taylor and S. Bhattacharya, A randomized comparison of alternative methods of information provision on the acceptability of elective single embryo transfer. *Hum. Reprod.*, **19**:4 (2004), 911–916.

34. T. J. Child, A. M. Henderson and S. L. Tan, The desire for multiple pregnancy in male and female infertility patients. *Hum. Reprod.*, **19** (2004), 558–561.

35. G. S. Scotland, P. McNamee, V. Peddie and S. Bhattacharya, Safety versus success in elective single embryo transfer: women's preferences for outcomes of IVF. *BJOG*, **114**:8 (2007), 977–983.

36. S. Bhattacharya and A. Templeton, Redefining success in the context of elective single embryo transfer: evidence, intuition and financial reality. *Hum. Reprod.*, **19**:9 (2004), 1939–1942.

37. P. Braude, Report of the Expert Group on Multiple Births After IVF. One child at a time – reducing multiple births after IVF (2006). www.hfea.gov.uk/docs/MBSET_report_Final_Dec_06.pdf (accessed August 3, 2007).

38. E. M. E. W. Heijnen, N. S. Macklon and B. C. J. M. Fauser, The next step to improving outcomes of IVF: consider the whole treatment. *Hum. Reprod.*, **19**:9 (2004), 1936–1938.

20

Should sperm parameters be considered in patient selection for single embryo transfer?

Denny Sakkas, Hasan M. El-Fakahany and Emre U. Seli

Introduction

Evidence from human egg share models, whereby eggs from the same donor are shared leading to fertilization arising from two different males, indicates that different individual sperm providers can give rise to variations in embryo quality [1, 2]. In one such study examining egg sharing patients we found that when comparing the embryo quality of 104 pairs of patients having shared oocytes embryo quality differed significantly in approximately 15.4% of the pairs. When examining for differences in only the patients transferred embryos, which would be representative of the best embryos available for the patients, embryo quality differed significantly in 14.4% of the pairs. These observations suggest that a paternal influence may impact the chances of an embryo to implant and lead to a live birth. However, it is noteworthy that simple semen characteristics do not explain the difference in embryo quality in egg sharing models [3]. This chapter will therefore examine the indications where a paternal effect exists, and discuss whether treatment strategy in an assisted reproduction setting should be individualized by either altering the time of embryo transfer or increasing the number of embryos to be transferred, depending on male characteristics.

Evidence of a paternal effect in animals

Numerous animal models exist in which a paternal effect has been linked to alterations in embryo development. In the rodent species, it has been shown extensively that paternal cyclophosphamide treatment impacts reproductive outcomes. In one study, paternal cyclophosphamide treatment had no effect on the mean number of embryos per pregnant female. However, as early as day 3 of gestation, there was a significant decrease in cell number among the embryos sired by cyclophosphamide-treated males, leading to a greater than 50% decrease in cell number by day 4 [4]. The cell doubling time in embryos sired by treated males was 33% longer than that of controls. Both the trophectoderm and the inner cell mass cells were proportionally decreased in day 4–5 blastocyst embryos sired by cyclophosphamide-treated males. Thus, paternal cyclophosphamide exposure affected both cell lineages in the conceptus as early as day 3 of gestation. Similar studies have shown that gamma irradiation of mouse spermatozoa also leads to decreased preimplantation embryo development and live births [5, 6].

Other intrinsic anomalies in spermatozoa can also influence embryo development. In the bovine

Single Embryo Transfer, ed. J. Gerris, G. D. Adamson, P. De Sutter and C. Racowsky. Published by Cambridge University Press.

paternally linked differences in the fertilization process, comparing bulls of high and low fertility have been evidenced during the first cell cycle [7]. These authors demonstrated that a beneficial paternal effect from spermatozoa recovered from bulls of high fertility was manifested during the first G1 phase after fertilization. This beneficial effect was then evidenced by an earlier onset and a longer duration of the first DNA replication in both male and female pronuclei, which, more importantly, translated into higher rates of blastocyst formation seven days later. In bulls with low and high fertility capability the percentage of fertilization and overall timing of pronuclear formation was the same, however, it was found that the absence of a beneficial effect in low fertility spermatozoa was linked to a delay in both pronuclei of the onset of the first DNA synthesis, which was subsequently shorter. The origin of this paternal control was later postulated to be linked to a shift in glucose regulation at the time of fertilization [8].

Evidence of a paternal effect in human

In the human, two areas of paternal influences in relation to assisted reproductive technology (ART) have come under investigation. One is the origin of the spermatozoa and whether sperm retrieved from testicular samples give rise to embryos of poorer quality. The second is whether the sperm DNA quality, regardless of origin, influences embryo development.

Testicular spermatozoa and embryo development

Many studies have assessed the efficiency of intracytoplasmic sperm injection (ICSI) using testicular spermatozoa in cases of azoospermia. It is generally believed that testicular retrieval from obstructive azoospermia cases is more successful than that of non-obstructive azoospermia cases [9]. How this translates to embryo quality is however less clear. In one study, 911 ICSI cycles were examined using

fresh sperm obtained after testicular biopsies: 306 ICSI cycles used testicular sperm from men with non-obstructive azoospermia, and 605 ICSI cycles used testicular sperm from men with obstructive azoospermia [10]. Overall, the two pronuclei fertilization rate was lower in the non-obstructive group: 48.5% versus 59.7%. However it was found that there were no differences in in vitro development or morphological quality of the embryos. In the non-obstructive group the clinical implantation rate and clinical pregnancy rate per cycle were significantly lower. Other studies have contradicted the suggestion that pregnancy rates are decreased in non-obstructive azoospermia. A meta-analysis reported a significantly improved fertilization rate and clinical pregnancy rate in men with obstructive azoospermia as compared with non-obstructive azoospermia with a non-significant increase in ongoing pregnancy rate [11]. There was no difference in either implantation rate or miscarriage rate between the two groups. A more recent meta-analysis also revealed a significantly higher fertilization rate among men with obstructive azoospermia compared with those with non-obstructive azoospermia, but no statistically significant difference in clinical pregnancy rates between the two groups [12]. Neither study embarked on any real examination of embryo quality however.

When embryo quality has been examined in relation to sperm origin it was found that embryos arising from non-obstructive azoospermia patients are less likely to lead to good quality embryos. One study examined embryo morphology and found that the number of grade 1 and grade 2 embryos with four blastomeres on day 2 was negatively affected as semen quality was significantly reduced, with the lowest percentage of 4-cell, grade 1 and 2 embryos on day 2 being present in men being treated for non-obstructive azoospermia. This effect was significant in the obstructive and non-obstructive azoospermia groups (10.3% and 7.1% respectively) compared with ICSI controls without azoospermia (19.5%) [13]. Finally, they reported reduced blastocyst formation rates on day 5 in the obstructive azoospermia group compared with controls (58% vs. 32%). No blastocysts were obtained in the non-obstructive azoospermia group due to small numbers of embryos. In a more comprehensive study examining blastocyst rates in relation to origin of sperm, others found that spermatozoa from non-obstructive azoospermic subjects, when utilized for ICSI, resulted in embryos that progress to the blastocyst stage at a lower and slower rate and implant less efficiently [14]. Overall they found the following blastocyst rates after ICSI in ejaculated spermatozoa patients, epididymal, obstructive and non-obstructive azoospermia cases respectively: 1895/3030 (62.5%), 100/190 (52.6%), 77/157 (49%) and 94/235 (40%). Pregnancy and implantation rates tended to be lower in non-obstructive azoospermia patients also. In respect to retrieval and ICSI of round spermatids, outcome results are very poor and the same group [15, 16] has shown that the blastocyst stage is reached by only very few round spermatid ICSI-derived embryos and these embryos do not implant.

Why do testicular spermatozoa and in particular those from non-obstructive azoospermia patients appear to give rise to poorer quality embryos? The actual pathogenesis of azoospermia provides a strong clue to the reason. In studies examining the quality of spermatogenesis and the spermatozoa obtained from these patients it is evident that the nuclear DNA structure is more likely to be impaired. Studies examining testicular sections from azoospermic men have revealed a higher proportion of spermatogenic cells with DNA strand breaks. A number of studies have shown that the most prominent increase in DNA strand breaks is in the testes of men with azoospermia and is actually higher in non-obstructive azoospermia patients [17–19]. This finding is consistent with reports by others and suggests that the pathologies that lead to non-obstructive azoospermia may result in the observed absence of spermatozoa in the ejaculate by using apoptosis as a common final pathway [20]. Interestingly, in one study sperm samples obtained surgically from the epididymis or testis of men with azoospermia or anejaculation were examined and compared with controls obtained by ejaculation in fertile patients [17]. Deoxyribonucleic acid fragmentation was analyzed in the total sample and in a motile fraction that was isolated as in routine ICSI procedures. Breaks in DNA were measured by using the TdT-mediated dUTP nick-end labeling (TUNEL) assay. They found that a higher percentage of cells with DNA breaks was present in men with obstructive azoospermia or anejaculation compared with controls (mean, 18.9% vs. 6.2%). However, a significantly lower degree of DNA fragmentation was observed in the motile fraction from patients compared with donors (0.4% vs. 0.6%). They concluded that in an ICSI setting, the use of motile sperm retrieved from the epididymis or testis of men with obstructive azoospermia does not seem to pose a higher genetic risk to the progeny than do motile ejaculated sperm.

Sperm DNA anomalies and embryo development

The fertilizing spermatozoon may impact the reproductive process at various levels. Both aberrant membrane and cytoskeletal anomalies would be unlikely to cause harm post the fertilization process. Indeed centriolar abnormalities have largely been shown to impede fertilization [21, 22] and are unlikely to lead to inheritable disorders. The two other components of the spermatozoon include the mitochondrial and nuclear components. The mitochondria are believed to be maternally inherited. However some argue that this inheritance could be skewed by micromanipulation techniques such as those utilized in ART [23, 24]. In relation to the contribution of the fertilizing spermatozoon, the nucleus remains as the greatest contributor to the likelihood of success of a reproductive outcome.

Sperm nuclear integrity and in particular the presence of nuclear DNA strand breaks has been more closely examined in the past decade. Their presence was initially reported in the early 1990s [25–27], while their origin and subsequent impact is still not completely understood [28–30]. Their perceived impact has however become increasingly more important in relevance to the use of ICSI.

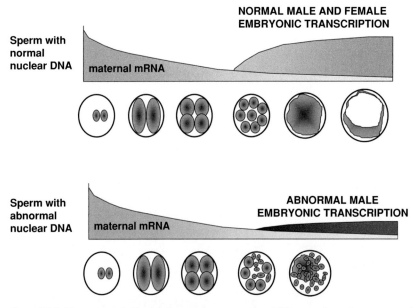

Figure 20.1 The proposed effect of abnormal sperm nuclear DNA on embryonic genome activation. Development until the 4- to 8-cell stage would occur normally under the role of maternal messenger RNA; however once the embryo's own genome is activated abnormalities in paternally inherited DNA may impede development to the blastocyst stage.

Reproductive parameters that could be affected by an increased presence of DNA strand breaks in ejaculated spermatozoa include fertilization, blastocyst development and pregnancy rates. Investigations of the possible association between DNA strand breaks in spermatozoa and fertilization rates in patients undergoing ART have in general found no strong correlation between DNA integrity of ejaculated spermatozoa and in vitro fertilization (IVF) and ICSI fertilization rates. A recent meta-analysis examining eight articles using two different methods which assess sperm DNA damage, the TUNEL assay and sperm chromatin structure assay (SCSA), found that sperm DNA damage did not affect fertilization by IVF or ICSI [31].

For embryo development the results seem to point to differences in growth when sperm DNA damage is increased. In human embryos, activation of embryonic genome expression occurs at the 4- to 8-cell stage [32], suggesting that the paternal genome may not affect embryo development until that stage. Therefore, a lack of correlation between

elevated DNA strand breaks in spermatozoa and fertilization rates is not surprising. A correlation with early embryo development is less clear as a number of studies have failed to find an association between sperm DNA damage and early embryo development [33–34].

In a number of older studies it has been suggested that there was a paternal effect on blastocyst development in relation to sperm quality [35] and when comparing IVF and ICSI [36]. An interesting observation in a number of these papers is that embryo quality was similar until day 2–3 and then the differences in blastocyst development were observed in the day 3 to day 5 stage [36, 37]. This again indicates that a paternal effect may manifest itself post-embryonic genome activation (Figure 20.1).

A number of studies have now examined whether the extent of nuclear DNA damage in ejaculated spermatozoa affects blastocyst development after IVF and ICSI. A negative correlation between blastocyst development and the extent of DNA strand breaks detected using the TUNEL assay to evaluate spermatozoa processed for IVF [38] or SCSA to evaluate unprocessed spermatozoa [39] has been observed. In the former study conducted by ourselves we found that 4 out of 8 patients with sperm DNA damage of $> 50\%$ (as measured by TUNEL) failed to develop blastocysts *in vitro*, compared to only 2 out of the 41 remaining patients, which all had sperm DNA damage of $< 50\%$. In the latter study, males with a $\geq 30\%$ DNA fragmentation index (DFI), as measured by SCSA, were found to be at risk for low blastocyst rates ($< 30\%$) and no ongoing pregnancies. These reports illustrate the importance of DNA integrity and its association with the embryo's ability to develop post-embryonic genome activation, but also indicates that it is not an all-or-none phenomenon as sperm exist in the population which can support embryo development.

Subsequent to embryo development the predictive capacity of sperm DNA integrity tests in relation to pregnancy outcome has shown that pregnancy rates after IVF are reduced in couples who have higher percentages of spermatozoa with DNA strand breaks detected by *in situ* nick translation [40]. Similarly, there is strong evidence for a relationship between sperm nuclear DNA integrity, as assessed with the SCSA, and fertility after both normal intercourse [41, 42] and assisted reproduction techniques [43].

A recent meta-analysis showed that sperm DNA damage, as assessed by the TUNEL assay, significantly decreases only the chance of IVF clinical pregnancy, but not that of ICSI clinical pregnancy [31]. In addition these authors revealed that sperm DNA damage, when assessed by the SCSA, had no significant effect on the chance of clinical pregnancy after IVF or ICSI treatment. All these studies demonstrate that high levels of DNA damage were still compatible with pregnancy and delivery after IVF/ICSI, even if fewer high quality embryos are available.

The increasing number of publications in this field indicates that the relevance of sperm nuclear DNA tests is not completely understood [44]. From the ever-increasing wealth of data collected so far about the SCSA and TUNEL techniques and their

predictive power in ART, we can speculate that an increased fraction of sperm showing DNA damage is certainly a negative trait that reduces the chances of good embryo development and to father a child. However a magic number or percentage of DNA damaged sperm in the population that is not compatible with pregnancy is far from being established.

The contradictory results for ICSI and sperm DNA assessment may be explained on the basis that the DNA integrity of a density gradient-prepared sperm sample and the selection of a single spermatozoon with normal morphology for ICSI by a human operator may lead to the exclusion of many spermatozoa with DNA strand breaks.

In order to increase correlation of these sperm DNA integrity tests with clinical outcome after IVF/ICSI, the sample assessed by the sperm DNA testing techniques should be reflective of how it will be used in the clinical setting. Therefore, whereby assessing DNA damage levels of the semen sample for natural fertility and intrauterine insemination may appear to be predictive, it may be more diagnostically relevant to use the prepared sample for assessment when using IVF or ICSI as a selection method.

Conclusions

The above studies relating a paternal factor to reproductive outcome indicate that the origin of sperm and/or the presence of sperm nuclear DNA strand breaks are not entirely limiting factors to the ability of males to father a child, in particular after ICSI. There are however strong indications that high levels of DNA damage and/or recovery of spermatozoa from non-obstructive azoospermic males may adversely affect blastocyst development. The treatment options available to patients with these indications would therefore be to:
1. culture embryos to the blastocyst stage and/or
2. select in some cases to transfer at least two blastocysts if available and if allowed.

Culture to the blastocyst stage allows the paternal genome to be tested in vitro (Figure 20.1) and will allow a greater sorting of abnormal sperm nuclear DNA as embryos possessing abnormal paternal DNA will more likely fail to form blastocysts. A saving grace for many non-obstructive azoospermic males is that the partner is usually young and the superior egg quality of young females may increase the couple's odds as a whole of achieving pregnancy.

REFERENCES

1. D. Sakkas, Y. D'Arcy, G. Percival *et al.*, Use of the egg-share model to investigate the paternal influence on fertilization and embryo development after in vitro fertilization and intracytoplasmic sperm injection. *Fertil. Steril.*, **82** (2004), 74–79.
2. J. Tesarik, C. Mendoza and E. Greco, Paternal effects acting during the first cell cycle of human preimplantation development after ICSI. *Hum. Reprod.*, **17** (2002), 184–189.
3. D. Bodri, M. Colodron, R. Vidal *et al.*, Prognostic factors in oocyte donation: an analysis through egg-sharing recipient pairs showing a discordant outcome. *Fertil. Steril.*, **88** (2007), 1548–1553.
4. S. M. Austin, B. Robaire, B. F. Hales and S. M. Kelly, **50** (1994) Paternal cyclophosphamide exposure causes decreased cell proliferation in cleavage-stage embryos. *Biol. Reprod.*, **50** (1994), 55–64. [Published erratum appears in *Biol. Reprod.*, **50** (1994), 711.]
5. A. Ahmadi and S. C. Ng, Fertilizing ability of DNA-damaged spermatozoa. *J. Exp. Zool.*, **284** (1999a), 696–704.
6. A. Ahmadi and S. C. Ng, Developmental capacity of damaged spermatozoa. *Hum. Reprod.*, **14** (1999b), 2279–2285.
7. P. Comizzoli, B. Marquant-Le Guienne, Y. Heyman and J. P. Renard, Onset of the first S-phase is determined by a paternal effect during the G1-phase in bovine zygotes. *Biol. Reprod.*, **62** (2000), 1677–1684.
8. P. Comizzoli, F. Urner, D. Sakkas and J. P. Renard, Up-regulation of glucose metabolism during male pronucleus formation determines the early onset of the s phase in bovine zygotes. *Biol. Reprod.*, **68** (2003), 1934–1940.
9. G. D. Palermo, P. N. Schlegel, J. J. Hariprashad *et al.*, Fertilization and pregnancy outcome with intracytoplasmic sperm injection for azoospermic men. *Hum. Reprod.*, **14** (1999), 741–748.
10. V. Vernaeve, H. Tournaye, K. Osmanagaoglu *et al.*, Intracytoplasmic sperm injection with testicular spermatozoa is less successful in men with nonobstructive azoospermia than in men with obstructive azoospermia. *Fertil. Steril.*, **79** (2003), 529–533.
11. J. D. Nicopoullos, C. Gilling-Smith, P. A. Almeida *et al.*, Use of surgical sperm retrieval in azoospermic men: a meta-analysis. *Fertil. Steril.*, **82** (2004), 691–701.
12. M. Ghanem, N. I. Bakr, M. A. Elgayaar *et al.*, Comparison of the outcome of intracytoplasmic sperm injection in obstructive and non-obstructive azoospermia in the first cycle: a report of case series and meta-analysis. *Int. J. Androl.*, **28** (2005), 16–21.
13. K. E. Loutradi, B. C. Tarlatzis, D. G. Goulis *et al.*, The effects of sperm quality on embryo development after intracytoplasmic sperm injection. *J. Assist. Reprod. Genet.*, **23** (2006), 69–74.
14. B. Balaban, B. Urman, A. Isiklar *et al.*, Blastocyst transfer following intracytoplasmic injection of ejaculated, epididymal or testicular spermatozoa. *Hum. Reprod.*, **16** (2001), 125–129.
15. B. Urman, C. Alatas, S. Aksoy *et al.*, Transfer at the blastocyst stage of embryos derived from testicular round spermatid injection. *Hum. Reprod.*, **17** (2002), 741–743.
16. B. Balaban, B. Urman, A. Isiklar *et al.*, Progression to the blastocyst stage of embryos derived from testicular round spermatids. *Hum. Reprod.*, **15** (2000), 1377–1382.
17. L. Ramos, P. Kleingeld, E. Meuleman *et al.*, Assessment of DNA fragmentation of spermatozoa that were surgically retrieved from men with obstructive azoospermia. *Fertil. Steril.*, **77** (2002), 233–237.
18. M. O'Connell, N. McClure and S. E. Lewis, A comparison of mitochondrial and nuclear DNA status in testicular sperm from fertile men and those with obstructive azoospermia. *Hum. Reprod.*, **17** (2002), 1571–1577.
19. E. Seli, O. Moffatt, M. Nijs *et al.*, Apoptosis in testis of normal and azoospermic males: a Fas mediated phenomenon. 49th Annual Meeting of the Society of Gynecologic Investigation, Los Angeles, CA, March 20–23, 2002, Abs No 567.
20. S. Francavilla, M. A. Bianco, G. Cordeschi *et al.*, Ultrastructural analysis of chromatin defects in testicular spermatids in azoospermic men submitted to TESE-ICSI. *Hum. Reprod.*, **16** (2001), 1440–1448.
21. L. Hewitson, C. Simerly and G. Schatten, Cytoskeletal aspects of assisted fertilization. *Semin. Reprod. Med.*, **18** (2000), 151–159.
22. L. Hewitson, T. Dominko, D. Takahashi *et al.*, Unique checkpoints during the first cell cycle of fertilization

after intracytoplasmic sperm injection in rhesus monkeys. *Nat. Med.*, **5** (1999), 431–433.

23. J. St John, D. Sakkas, K. Dimitriadi *et al.*, Failure of elimination of paternal mitochondrial DNA in abnormal embryos [letter]. *Lancet*, **355** (2000), 200.

24. J. C. St John, R. Lloyd and S. El Shourbagy, The potential risks of abnormal transmission of mtDNA through assisted reproductive technologies. *Reprod. Biomed. Online*, **8** (2004), 34–44.

25. P. G. Bianchi, G. C. Manicardi, D. Bizzaro, U. Bianchi and D. Sakkas, Effect of deoxyribonucleic acid protamination on fluorochrome staining and in situ nick-translation of murine and human mature spermatozoa. *Biol. Reprod.*, **49** (1993), 1083–1088.

26. W. Gorczyca, F. Traganos, H. Jesionowska and Z. Darzynkiewicz, Presence of DNA strand breaks and increased sensitivity of DNA in situ to denaturation in abnormal human sperm cells: analogy to apoptosis of somatic cells. *Exp. Cell Res.*, **207** (1993), 202–205.

27. G. C. Manicardi, P. G. Bianchi, S. Pantano *et al.*, Presence of endogenous nicks in DNA of ejaculated human spermatozoa and its relationship to chromomycin A3 accessibility. *Biol. Reprod.*, **52** (1995), 864–867.

28. S. E. Lewis and R. J. Aitken, DNA damage to spermatozoa has impacts on fertilization and pregnancy. *Cell Tissue Res.*, **322** (2005), 33–41.

29. D. Sakkas, E. Seli, G. C. Manicardi *et al.*, The presence of abnormal spermatozoa in the ejaculate: did apoptosis fail? *Hum. Fertil.*, (Camb) **7** (2004), 99–103.

30. D. Sakkas, E. Seli, D. Bizzaro, N. Tarozzi and G. C. Manicardi, Abnormal spermatozoa in the ejaculate: abortive apoptosis and faulty nuclear remodelling during spermatogenesis. *Reprod. Biomed. Online*, **7** (2003), 428–432.

31. Z. Li, L. Wang, J. Cai and H. Huang, Correlation of sperm DNA damage with IVF and ICSI outcomes: A systematic review and meta-analysis. *J. Assist. Reprod. Genet.*, **23** (2006), 367–376.

32. P. Braude, V. Bolton and S. Moore, Human gene expression first occurs between the four- and eight-cell stages of preimplantation development. *Nature* **332** (1988), 459–461.

33. J. G. Sun, A. Jurisicova and R. F. Casper, Detection of deoxyribonucleic acid fragmentation in human sperm: correlation with fertilization in vitro. *Biol. Reprod.*, **56** (1997), 602–607.

34. M. Benchaib, V. Braun, J. Lornage *et al.*, Sperm DNA fragmentation decreases the pregnancy rate in an assisted reproductive technique. *Hum. Reprod.*, **18** (2003), 1023–1028.

35. L. Janny and Y. J. Menezo, Evidence for a strong paternal effect on human preimplantation embryo development and blastocyst formation. *Mol. Reprod. Dev.*, **38** (1994), 36–42.

36. Y. Shoukir, D. Chardonnens, A. Campana and D. Sakkas, Blastocyst development from supernumerary embryos after intracytoplasmic sperm injection: a paternal influence? *Hum. Reprod.*, **13** (1998), 1632–1637.

37. J. C. Dumoulin, E. Coonen, M. Bras *et al.*, Comparison of in-vitro development of embryos originating from either conventional in-vitro fertilization or intracytoplasmic sperm injection. *Hum. Reprod.*, **15** (2000), 402–409.

38. E. Seli, D. K. Gardner, W. B. Schoolcraft, O. Moffatt and D. Sakkas, Extent of nuclear DNA damage in ejaculated spermatozoa impacts on blastocyst development after in vitro fertilization. *Fertil. Steril.*, **82** (2004), 378–383.

39. M. R. Virro, K. L. Larson-Cook and D. P. Evenson, Sperm chromatin structure assay (SCSA) parameters are related to fertilization, blastocyst development, and ongoing pregnancy in in vitro fertilization and intracytoplasmic sperm injection cycles. *Fertil. Steril.*, **81** (2004), 1289–1295.

40. M. J. Tomlinson, O. Moffatt, G. C. Manicardi *et al.*, Interrelationships between seminal parameters and sperm nuclear DNA damage before and after density gradient centrifugation: implications for assisted conception. *Hum. Reprod.*, **16** (2001), 2160–2165.

41. D. P. Evenson, L. K. Jost, D. Marshall *et al.*, Utility of the sperm chromatin structure assay as a diagnostic and prognostic tool in the human fertility clinic. *Hum. Reprod.*, **14** (1999), 1039–1049.

42. M. Spano, J. P. Bonde, H. I. Hjollund *et al.*, Sperm chromatin damage impairs human fertility. The Danish First Pregnancy Planner Study Team. *Fertil. Steril.*, **73** (2000), 43–50.

43. K. L. Larson, C. J. DeJonge, A. M. Barnes, L. K. Jost and D. P. Evenson, Sperm chromatin structure assay parameters as predictors of failed pregnancy following assisted reproductive techniques. *Hum. Reprod.*, **15** (2000), 1717–1722.

44. M. Spano, E. Seli, D. Bizzaro, G. C. Manicardi and D. Sakkas, The significance of sperm nuclear DNA strand breaks on reproductive outcome. *Curr. Opin. Obstet. Gynecol.*, **17** (2005), 255–260.

21

Does self-regulation work for implementation of single embryo transfer?

G. David Adamson

Introduction

Definition of regulation and self-regulation

Regulation is defined as "a rule or order issued by an executive authority or regulatory agency of a government and having the force of law" [1]. Only government or its designated authorities can regulate and impose sanctions. Self-regulation involves guidelines or rules from professional organizations that can recommend certain behaviors, but do not have state authority to force or prevent them. Such organizations may or may not have the ability to impose professional sanctions of variable significance.

Regulation of assisted reproductive technology (ART)

Regulation of ART is complex, because many different aspects of ART can be regulated: (1) production of equipment, instruments and materials, (2) laboratory procedures and inspections, (3) procedure/operating rooms, (4) government/insurance coverage, (5) patients eligible for ART (e.g., based on age, marital status), (6) procedures allowed, (7) number of embryos to transfer, (8) reporting of results, (9) costs of services and payment to donors, (10) research standards, (11) research funding, (12) counseling standards, (13) education standards and (14) other aspects of ART. Most commonly,

regulation is thought to apply to the clinical practice of medicine, although regulation of other aspects of ART can have a profound impact on clinical practice. This chapter will focus on regulation regarding the number of embryos to transfer as well as regulation of other aspects of ART that affect the number of embryos transferred.

To determine whether or not self-regulation works for the implementation of elective single embryo transfer (SET), we need to evaluate the current status of regulation and self-regulation to see if the desired goals were achieved. Whether or not objectives are met depends on our definition of success.

Definition of success

Regulation can be used to attain objectives with respect to any aspect of ART that is regulated (vide supra). Different constituencies, for example, patients, physicians, scientists, counselors, ethicists, the government or the public, often have different measures of success. Examples of regulatory objectives are to meet patient needs, consumer needs, allay public fears, protect embryos/future children, control physicians, or to control research. With many possible objectives there can be multiple definitions of regulatory success, or failure.

The initial success of IVF was defined by the birth of Louise Brown and the babies that followed.

Single Embryo Transfer, ed. J. Gerris, G. D. Adamson, P. De Sutter and C. Racowsky. Published by Cambridge University Press.
© Cambridge University Press 2009.

Subsequently, pregnancy rates per oocyte retrieval or embryo transfer, and also implantation rates per transfer, were considered important. This transitioned somewhat to live birth rates per cycle start, and even long-term follow-up of months or years. Since in many countries these data are not available, the outcome of most interest has remained the number of live births per some denominator of number of ART cycles or patients.

With increasing recognition of complications that can result from multiple birth, a healthy singleton is now considered the ideal outcome [2–5]. Twins are considered a less ideal, but acceptable, outcome by many professionals involved with ART [6]. Additionally, there is increasing recognition that the total reproductive potential from an oocyte retrieval cycle is an important outcome measure of success [7]. This is the number of healthy singleton live births resulting from one oocyte retrieval and fresh transfer as well as any subsequent cryopreserved/thawed embryo transfer cycles using that cycle's embryos. Many consider a secondary measure of success any additional healthy twin live births. Almost everybody considers triplet births to be a serious complication of treatment. In this chapter, a healthy singleton live birth will be considered the desired and ideal outcome, and twin birth an undesired but acceptable outcome. Outcome measurement is actually even more complex, in that it is not only qualitative (healthy singleton), but also quantitative (number of healthy singletons), less the undesired outcomes (unhealthy baby) and the number of undesired outcomes. Since the vast majority of twins are healthy, but the risk of an unwanted outcome is higher, there needs to be some additional accounting for twins as belonging to either the successful or unsuccessful category, or neither (a neutral outcome, in the aggregate). Such measurement involves not only qualitative and quantitative measurements but also value judgments, about which there may be legitimate differences of opinion among patients, physicians, embryologists, scientists, ethicists, politicians and others in society, and especially in the very different societies found around the world.

Regulation and self-regulation: the global situation

Methods for data collection

The most comprehensive review of regulations is compiled by the International Federation of Fertility Societies, which surveys approximately two thirds of the world population [8–11]. The most comprehensive review of ART outcomes is compiled by the International Committee Monitoring ART (ICMART) [12]. These reviews reveal that many different aspects of ART that are regulated can affect the implementation of SET. Additionally, there are great variations and constant change in both regulations and outcomes around the world, reflecting widely divergent and evolving views on ART. It is possible that, with respect to regulation and surveillance, ". . . the details may be unimportant as long as the public believes that some type of surveillance is in place" [11].

Global regulation and self-regulation

In most countries many different interested stakeholders have been involved in the regulation of ART: infertile patients, physicians and other healthcare providers, scientists, reproductive medicine, commercial interests, religious leaders, bioethicists, politicians and the general public. The major, but not only, driving force for much of this activity has been diversity of perspective on the moral status of the embryo, namely, at what point in time and/or development do gametes and the products of conception attain moral status greater than that of human cellular material, and subsequently, the full moral status of a human being.

Legislation and guidelines

Of the 57 countries surveyed by the International Federation of Fertility Societies (IFFS) Surveillance 07, and recognizing the sometimes arbitrary nature of categorization since in some countries there is a spectrum of surveillance for different aspects of ART, 29 had statutes (regulation), 18 had guidelines (self-regulation) and 10 had neither [11]. In many countries with regulations and self-regulation, surveillance consists of periodic reports, and in some on-site inspections. Sanctions in regulated countries include criminal and civil penalties, such as fines and imprisonment, and also loss of medical license and suspension of business [11]. In guideline countries there are no significant penalties for non-compliance, although adverse publicity may result. In the ten countries without regulations or guidelines, "it is notable that practices in these national entities do not differ greatly from those in nations with legislation or voluntary guidelines" [11].

Some countries, for example Italy, have very restrictive legislation and penalties that have caused major changes in clinical practice [13]. It is interesting that legislative penalties apply to practitioners and clinics and not to patients [11]. It is not known the degree to which guidelines are followed in countries that don't have significant penalties. However, "countries with voluntary guidelines appear to enjoy public confidence, and public pressure for a change appears to be very minimal in those countries where guidelines are in vogue" [11].

Insurance coverage

The United States appears to be the only nation in which the only insurance available is through private sources [11]. Approximately 16 states have some type of insurance coverage, ranging from very comprehensive coverage in Massachusetts to simply a mandate to offer infertility insurance to employers in California. Studies have shown that fewer embryos are transferred in states with better insurance coverage but pregnancy rates were also somewhat lower, demonstrating that economic factors can influence the number of embryos transferred and multiple pregnancy rates [14]. Six countries have national health plans that provide complete coverage, including Belgium and Sweden, which have been leaders in SET, again suggesting that financial factors influence strongly multi-

ple pregnancy rates. The Belgian plan is particularly interesting in that coverage for up to six in vitro fertilization (IVF) cycles is dependent on adherence to strict criteria regarding the number of embryos to transfer based on age and cycle number. The number of multiple pregnancies has been reduced from approximately 30% to 10% since 2003 when this plan was initiated, showing that an economic model related to clinical practice, as opposed to strict embryo transfer numbers, can successfully reduce multiple pregnancy rates [11]. Some insurance companies in the United States require practitioners to adhere to the Society for Assisted Reproductive Technology (SART) guidelines in order to be reimbursed. Overall, countries covered by statute have much better insurance coverage than countries covered by guidelines or those without either. Half of all reporting countries have neither private nor public coverage [11]. Financial coverage would, therefore, seem to be a potentially important positive factor affecting the implementation of SET by self-regulation.

Cryopreservation

Cryopreservation of embryos is a critical technology to enhance the overall success rate and to reduce the multiple pregnancy rate by allowing fewer embryos to be replaced at any single transfer. Progress towards SET may influence the rate of cryopreservation [15]. Cryopreservation of blastocysts, to optimize selection of embryos and reduce the number transferred, can also be used to reduce multiple pregnancy rates.

Twenty-five countries have statutes that allow cryopreservation of fertilized eggs. Many countries limit the duration of embryo storage, usually to 5 or 10 years. Italy is the only country to prohibit cryopreservation of embryos. Another 17 countries have guidelines and in 8 cryopreservation is performed without regulation or guidelines [11]. It is known from the experience in Italy that cryopreservation regulations can affect the utilization of SET both in fresh and frozen-thawed cycles, sometimes increasing its utilization and sometimes decreasing it. Time limits on the duration of freezing could potentially affect SET, sometimes causing more embryos to be replaced in order that they be used before the time limit is reached. However, if regulations limit the number of embryos that can be cryopreserved this could reduce the number of embryos available for transfer, but potentially encourage replacement of larger numbers in an effort to achieve pregnancy. Regulations that reduce the number of embryos, either fresh or frozen-thawed, will result in lower pregnancy rates. Efforts to mitigate this by transferring more embryos at each transfer will likely occur.

Gamete and embryo donation

The use of donor sperm has decreased because of ICSI, and also the removal of donor anonymity in some countries, but this should not affect the implementation of SET [16, 17].

Donor eggs for IVF are not allowed by law in 6 countries but are in 21 others. Under guidelines, egg donation is not allowed in 6 countries and is in 11. Of countries without regulations or guidelines, 2 do not practice egg donation and 8 do, sometimes in limited circumstances [11]. Restrictions on anonymity, compensation and other clinical factors have seriously restricted the availability of oocyte donors in some countries. Since oocyte donation from fertile donors has higher success rates than those in the general infertile population, oocyte donation potentially presents an opportunity for increased utilization of SET [12]. For similar reasons, SET should be attractive for embryo donation, although it is uncommonly done.

Blastocyst transfer

Blastocyst transfer has higher implantation rates than day 2 or 3 transfer. When SET is performed, this results in higher live birth rates [18]. However, since only approximately 40% of embryos develop from day 3 to a viable blastocyst, and since many ART clinics experience lower pregnancy rates with cryopreserved/thawed blastocyst transfer than with cryopreserved/thawed day 3 embryo transfer, and because of concerns over increased identical twin-

ning rates with blastocyst transfer and possibly imprinting errors, the desirability of blastocyst stage transfer for SET is still vigorously debated. It is clear that successful SET programs can be developed with day 3 transfer protocols, and it would appear that day 5 or 6 transfer protocols may offer some advantages to some patients. The optimal application of blastocyst to SET merits rigorous scientific study at this time. United States guidelines recommend that fewer blastocysts be replaced than day 3 embryos, and recommends only a single blastocyst be transferred for good prognosis patients less than age 35 years [19].

Welfare of the child

In 2004 the United Kingdom was the only country to take into account the welfare of the child by imposing law, and this law was recently clarified. Greece and New Zealand have recently enacted similar laws, and many countries have required the child have access to sperm, egg and/or embryo donor health information. The American Society for Reproductive Medicine (ASRM) published a guideline from their Ethics Committee in 2004 on "Child Rearing Ability and the Provision of Fertility Services" [11, 20]. There is a significant international trend towards transferring fewer embryos to reduce morbidity and mortality of ART children. This can be seen from the perspective of welfare of the child, family and society. So considerations in addition to the traditional medical outcome for the treated patient are increasingly important and will affect the implementation of SET, whether these are regulations, guidelines or professional/social pressure. Some argue that the best interests of the child must be ART clinicians' priority. While few would disagree on the importance of this outcome, application of this principle can sometimes be complex when attempting to obtain the outcome desired by the patient and protecting her, and his, reproductive rights. There is the potential for laws to be in conflict if the embryo in the laboratory is given a greater moral standing and more rights than the fetus in the womb, and/or those of the intended parents.

Multifetal pregnancy reduction

Multifetal pregnancy reduction (MFPR) is a technique used to reduce the adverse outcome of multiple gestation. Selective termination refers to this technology when fetal reduction is used for a significant developmental abnormality or heterotopic implantation site. Although risks of the procedure are very small and the overall unexpected pregnancy loss rate very low, about 5%, there are clearly difficult ethical, moral and psychological issues for many patients [11, 21–23]. Multifetal pregnancy reduction is not allowed in 1 country with statutes and 7 with guidelines out of 56 surveyed countries, while it was practiced in 20 countries [11]. The widespread utilization of MFPR would tend to work against SET, since multiple pregnancies that resulted from ART transfers could be managed by MFPR, and, conversely, regulations and/or guidelines restricting MFPR would encourage SET. However, such regulations and/or guidelines raise significant issues with respect to reproductive rights and choice, and are therefore very controversial.

Preimplantation genetic diagnosis/screening (PGD/S)

Preimplantation genetic diagnosis (PGD) is allowed by statute in 20 of 29 countries surveyed, not allowed in 3 and not mentioned in 6. It is being performed in 18 countries, with some restrictions in some. Twelve countries with guidelines permit PGD, none prohibit it and 5 don't mention it. It is being performed in 9 countries, in most on a limited basis [11]. It is practiced in 7 additional countries without statutes or guidelines, for a total of 34 countries. Preimplantation genetic screening (PGS) for aneuploidy is being used in 23 of 54 countries surveyed: 13 of 29 with statutes allow it, 6 don't and 10 don't mention it, while only 12 use it; in 5 of 16 with guidelines it is actually used, it is not allowed in 3 and not mentioned in 7; it is used in 6 of 11 countries with neither statutes or guidelines [11]. While many of its benefits are generally accepted and it is widely available, PGD/S is used on a limited basis and has many restrictions. Scientific, technological, clinical, moral, religious and ethical issues have reduced its utilization. If the ability of PGD/S to identify a single healthy embryo, or embryo with very low implantation potential, is improved, it would almost certainly increase live birth rates, healthy baby rates and probably increase the utilization of SET.

Experimentation on the pre-embryo

It would appear that experimentation on the pre-embryo would be very useful to help identify embryos with high versus low implantation potential, and therefore to promote SET. In the IFFS survey, about half the countries found pre-embryo research unacceptable, half based on law and half on societal grounds, and half found it acceptable, often with time-limit restrictions based on embryonic development. The definition of "research" remains unclear. There is no international consensus on this issue [11].

Gamete intrafallopian transfer (GIFT)

Gamete intrafallopian transfer has largely been abandoned as an ART because in almost all clinical situations it has no advantages over IVF and disadvantages of increased invasiveness and cost. In most countries it is not differentiated from IVF by regulations, guidelines or common practice, and in at least seven it is not covered under regulations affecting IVF. In eight countries, it is not used. Some countries limit the number of oocytes that can be replaced. In Italy now it would be legal to transfer two oocytes by GIFT, and then up to three others by IVF embryo transfer, but frozen embryos are not allowed to be used. Therefore, GIFT could potentially be used to circumvent strict SET regulations, although this appears to be uncommonly done, if at all [11, 12].

Status of the conceptus

The moral and legal status of the early developing human conceptus is usually the most important factor determining the regulatory, guideline and practice status of ART procedures in any given country [11]. There is great divergence of opinion on this point, even within countries. This lack of consensus has created legal and other difficulties. Is the pre-embryo a person or a thing, or neither and both at the same time? Different people believe personhood begins anywhere from the time of fertilization to the time of delivery, with many believing that 14 days is when it occurs. But that duration conflicts with commonly accepted reproductive rights in many countries. Many would agree that the embryo has enhanced moral status even if it might not be equal to that of a born person. Many countries with the strictest determination of the personhood of the conceptus have no statutes, while others with statutes have later onset of personhood. There is no international consensus on this issue.

Reproductive travel

Reproductive tourism, or fertility tourism, is a term used to describe travel by a patient outside their own country to receive fertility treatments, almost always because of the lack of availability and/or restrictions on that service in their home country. Some have criticized the term "tourism" because of its definition: "the practice of traveling for recreation" [1]. So perhaps a better term would be "reproductive travel." In any event, it is clear that restrictive legislation in one jurisdiction will result in at least some individuals attempting to circumvent the law. This creates emotional, time, health, financial and perhaps legal hardships for patients. It would be expected that restrictive regulations regarding SET would result in reproductive travel and is, therefore, an argument against regulatory implementation of SET.

Number of embryos for transfer in ART

Twenty-six countries have regulations or guidelines regarding the number of embryos to transfer. Single embryo transfer is proposed in Nordic countries and imposed in Belgium, but only for the first two cycles on women less than 36 years of age. If these two

cycles fail then up to two embryos can be transferred on cycles 3 to 6. For women 36–39 years the first two cycles can involve up to two embryos being transferred or up to three embryos for women > 39 years of age [11]. Insurance coverage is predicated on following these guidelines. Studies from Belgium, Sweden and Finland have shown increases in the proportion of SET [24–26]. These increases in SET have occurred in countries with regulations (e.g., Belgium, Sweden), those with professional guidelines (e.g., Australia) and those with neither (e.g., Finland) [27]. While the proportion of cycles that are SET is still very low in the United States, it is increasing, and the average number of embryos transferred has dropped dramatically in the past decade as the professional guideline recommendations on the number of embryos to transfer have been revised downwards based on analysis of the SART/CDC (Centers for Disease Control and Prevention) registry [28] (Tables 21.1 and 21.2). Furthermore, it has been stated that the observed decreases in numbers of embryos replaced is almost identical in Europe and the United States, despite a more aggressive push toward single embryo transfer in Europe [29–31]. Some American insurance companies are showing interest in providing payment only when physicians follow ASRM/SART guidelines on the number of embryos to transfer.

There appears to be no international consensus on regulations regarding the number of embryos to transfer. The IFFS surveillance concludes that, "On a national basis, self-regulation has not worked so far" [11]. However, it is clear that regulations have not always produced the desired result either, and that implementation of SET can result in lower pregnancy rates than double embryo transfer (DET) [32]. Furthermore, they recognize that, "the worldwide trend appears to be the elective transfer of one embryo for at least the first cycle." They have suggested, "the use of guidelines with sanctions imposed by the medical profession, or the development of specific laws." They have also recognized the need to educate both healthcare professionals and the lay population that multiple gestation is not a desirable outcome of IVF [11]. Therefore, multiple

Table 21.1 Average number of embryos transferred

Age	1996	1997	1998	1999	2000	2001	2002	... 2005
≤ 34	3.9	3.7	3.4	3.0	2.9	2.8	2.7	2.4
35–37	(3.9)	3.8	3.6	3.3	3.2	3.1	3.0	2.6
38–40	(4.0)	3.9	3.7	3.5	3.5	3.4	3.3	3.0
≥ 41	(4.0)	4.0	3.9	3.7	3.7	3.7	3.5	3.3
All	4.0	3.8	3.6	3.2	3.2	3.1	3.0	2.6

$p > 0.001$.
Adapted from Jain *et al.* [28].

Table 21.2 IVF in the United States: 1995–2005

Year	Ret	Deliv/ Ret	Mult/ Deliv	Trips/ Deliv	Triplet Fetuses
1995	35 269	22.5%	37%	5.8%	–
1996	38 432	26.0%	39%	6.9%	–
1997	44 170	27.9%	39%	6.5%	11.4%
1998	53 154	28.9%	38%	6.0%	10.6%
1999	56 835	29.2%	37%	4.9%	8.4%
2000	64 280	29.6%	35%	4.3%	7.7%
2001	66 786	32.3%	36%	4.2%	7.6%
2002	71 402	33.8%	36%	3.9%	7.0%
2003	79 717	33.7%	34%	3.2%	5.9%
2004	82 612	32.6%	33%	2.6%	4.9%
2005	83 935	32.7%	33%	2.3%	4.4%

Adapted from SART data.

approaches other than just regulation of embryo transfer number have been recommended in an effort to reduce the incidence of multiple births.

Summary of international regulations and guidelines surveillance

The IFFS Surveillance 07 documents that approximately half the countries surveyed regulated and controlled ART in some way, but there was great divergence in laws and guidelines because of diversity of religion, tradition, political situation and medical practice. Only three countries felt the situation to be satisfactory (Belgium, Latvia and the United Kingdom). Three countries consider the situation to be disastrous for patients, doctors and

biologists (Germany, Italy and Switzerland) and three felt that they needed laws or guidelines (Bulgaria, Brazil and Chile). In other countries there was a desire to modify the regulations for specific items [11]. The authors, referring to their overall document, stated, "An international 'consensus' appears to be a utopia, and we can imagine that if it existed, it would reflect the lowest common denominator. The actual situation is illogical, unfair to couples, and difficult for doctors and scientists. However, the situation still allows some couples to find solutions that they would never have found with an international consensus. We can hope that in the future, little by little, harmonization of national legislation will benefit from each country's experience and thus avoid outsourcing of this helpful medical procedure" [11].

Regulations and guidelines regarding many aspects of ART can potentially affect the implementation of SET. There are also wide regulatory and guideline variations among and within countries that affect the implementation of SET. Furthermore, some countries with the most regulation have the highest number of embryos transferred, and some with no regulations (e.g., Finland) have the highest implementation of SET and lowest multiple pregnancy rates [12, 27]. Therefore, strict regulation is clearly not the only strategy that can be successful, and sometimes can have unintended consequences. In Italy strict regulation has resulted in higher multiple pregnancy rates and lower overall pregnancy rates. Regulating just the number of embryos transferred may reduce the multiple pregnancy rate, but may reduce the overall pregnancy rate. Furthermore, other ART technologies and issues that are not regulated by number of embryos transferred will potentially influence the pregnancy and multiple pregnancy rate. It can be concluded from this international review that strict regulation of the number of embryos transferred can promote the utilization of SET, but has other, often unintended, consequences and that regulation is not essential to have a high acceptance and implementation of SET.

Current status of regulation in the United States

There is a perception that ART is unregulated in the United States. In fact, ART is very highly regulated in the United States [33, 34]. The Fertility Clinics Success Rate and Certification Act of 1992 was passed with the assistance and support of SART and ASRM, and requires annual reporting of success rates with listing of clinics that don't report [35]. Over 90% of clinics report over 95% of all cycles to SART. Clinic-specific data are published and are subject to validation by professional on-site inspection teams with oversight by the CDC [36, 37]. The Clinical Laboratory Improvement Amendments of 1988 (CLIA88) is mandatory federal regulation of andrology and endocrinology laboratories, requiring on-site inspections with serious sanctions for non-compliance [38]. The Food and Drug Administration (FDA) regulates gamete and embryo donation with rigorous regulations requiring laboratory registration with the FDA, listing of products used in the laboratory, compliance with laboratory and clinical gamete and embryo donor suitability screening, adherence to good tissue practices (currently deferred), unannounced on-site inspections by FDA inspectors and sanctions, including potential criminal charges with imprisonment and heavy fines [39]. The Federal Trade Commission (FTC) oversees advertising by ART programs and has leveled sanctions in the past for inappropriate use of IVF pregnancy rates in advertising by ART programs [34]. Additionally,

federal government regulations from the National Institutes of Health (NIH) cover all human research, the FDA regulates somatic cell nuclear transfer (cloning), the Centers for Medicare and Medicaid Services (CMS) determines some financial components of ART and the Department of Health and Human Services (DHHS) regulates genetic testing and policy, use of gene test data, and embryo research. In short, many aspects of ART are regulated. What is not regulated, and why the perception of lack of regulation persists, is individual reproductive choice regarding clinical care in ART and, in particular, the number of embryos that can be transferred.

However, the professional societies, namely ASRM and its affiliated society, SART, have been very active in establishing practice guidelines and setting practice standards in ART, including those regarding number of embryos to transfer [34]. Minimum standards for IVF were first developed in 1984 and have been regularly updated [40]. These guidelines are extensive and cover all aspects of ART, including laboratory technologies, clinical services, advertising, informed consent, gamete and embryo donation, multiple pregnancy, oocyte donor compensation, ICSI, blastocyst transfer, PGD/S, ovarian tissue and oocyte cryopreservation, and others. The ASRM Ethics Committee has also developed guidelines on many of the important ethical issues involved with the practice of ART, the first being published in 1986. These include disposition of abandoned oocytes, oocyte donation to postmenopausal women, embryo splitting, use of fetal oocytes, posthumous reproduction, financial incentives for oocyte donors, somatic cell nuclear transfer, preconception gender selection, informing offspring of their conception by gamete donation, child-rearing ability and the provision of fertility services, and fertility treatment when the prognosis is very poor or futile [40].

Over the years, SART guidelines have increasingly been followed by SART programs, which constitute over 90% of all IVF clinics. In order to become and retain SART membership, SART now mandates that all SART programs follow strict personnel requirements for program, medical and laboratory directors; have on-site accreditation of the laboratory by the College of American Pathologists (CAP) ASRM, Joint Commission on Accreditation of Hospitals Organization (JCAHO) or New York State; report their pregnancy outcome results to SART; have on-site validation of the results reported to SART; have on-site review of their adherence to SART/ASRM practice, laboratory, advertising and ethical guidelines; and agree to mandatory participation in the SART quality assurance program for IVF clinics with low pregnancy rates or high multiple pregnancy rates. These guidelines have also been introduced into a clinical and scientific environment of constant progress, with increasing pregnancy rates that are among the highest in the world, and a rapidly decreasing multiple pregnancy rate [41].

The most visible practice guideline developed by ASRM and SART has been the guideline on the number of embryos to transfer. This was first published in 1998, and updated in 1999, 2004 and 2006. It is significant that these guidelines have been based on careful and detailed analysis of large volumes of data from the SART database. As laboratory technology and clinical practice improved, so did pregnancy rates, but unfortunately also multiple pregnancy rates. As new SART guidelines have been published there has been a consistent reduction in the number of embryos transferred and a continuous fall in multiple pregnancy rates, while overall pregnancy rates have been increased and then maintained (Table 21.1 and 21.2) [28, 36, 37, 41, 42].

Current guidelines differentiate the number of embryos to transfer based on patient age and "favorable" quality embryos, these being defined as good quality embryos obtained from a woman under age 35 years on a first IVF cycle in sufficient number that excess embryos are available for cryopreservation, or a patient with a previous successful IVF cycle [19] (Table 21.3). These data show that guidelines on number of embryos to transfer can successfully reduce multiple pregnancy rates while maintaining overall pregnancy rates. Programs are subject to review of their embryo transfer number practices when they have on-site validation visits by

Table 21.3 Multiple Birth: ASRM/SART guidelines number of embryos to transfer (2006)

Day 3	< 35	35–37	38–40	> 40
Favorable*	1–2	2	3	5
All Others	2	3	4	5
Day 5	< 35	35–37	38–40	> 40
Favorable*	1	2	2	3
All Others	2	2	3	3

*1st cycle of IVF, good embryo quality, excess embryos available for cryopreservation, or previous successful IVF cycle.
Produced from [19] with permission.

SART, and also annually when their data are analyzed by SART for low pregnancy rates, high number of embryos transferred and/or high multiple pregnancy rates. Clinics with outlying results have to explain the reasons to SART, develop a plan for corrective action and demonstrate improved results in the future, or else lose their SART membership. Participation in this quality assurance program is mandatory for all SART programs. Furthermore, the United States pregnancy rates remain significantly higher than pregnancy rates in most other parts of the world [12, 30, 43]. The goal of SART is to continue to reduce the multiple pregnancy rate, especially the triplet rate, but also the twin rate, while maintaining the overall live birth rate. The last guidelines, published in 2006, were the first to require SET in any of the recommended categories, this being for women less than age 35 years on their first cycle with favorable embryos and a day 5 or 6 blastocyst transfer. The guidelines also recommend that SET be considered and discussed for day 3 transfer in this group of patients.

Regulation vs. self-regulation

Advantages of regulation

Regulation has its advantages. It establishes national standards, recognizes the uniqueness of ART, promotes high quality patient care, ensures minimum standards of care, improves research, protects patients' interests, provides a forum for national debate and participation, allows ethics statements to be mandated by law, enables utilization of precedents in other fields, increases society's confidence in and acceptance of ART, can increase public safety and may increase insurance funding for ART [34]. Regulation may also protect physicians against legal liability for refusing unreasonable treatment requests from patients regarding the number of embryos to transfer or other treatment choices. Regulation is argued to have a role despite the fact it is recognized to be contentious, challenges traditional understandings of family and the status of the embryo, and that professional guidelines are also needed [44]. Regulation is sometimes supported by organized medicine [45].

Furthermore, with respect to multiple pregnancy, it is clear that regulation of SET would dramatically reduce the number of higher-order multiple pregnancies (triplets or higher) to essentially zero, and reduce the twin rate to approximately 5%, if aggressively implemented. Since the adverse outcomes associated with multiple pregnancy have been well established, this would result in benefits to society [2, 46].

Disadvantages of regulation

However, regulation also has its disadvantages. It requires funding, mechanisms of enforcement, support of overseers, clinics and patients, may fail to solve problems, does not prevent psychopathic, sociopathic or illegal behavior, complicates legal issues of intent and due process vis-à-vis criminal versus inadvertent error in the practice of medicine, interferes in the practice of medicine with both intended and unintended consequences, interferes in patients' rights, leads to reproductive travel, discriminates against patients, increases cost to patients and politicizes medical and personal reproductive issues [34, 47].

For example, there is no question that patients who choose to replace more than one embryo do expose themselves to an increased risk of multiple pregnancy, which has potential costs to the

patient, babies and society. But many people in society exhibit risky behavior that has limited benefit to themselves and potentially high costs to family members and society, for example alcoholism, smoking and risky athletic endeavors. Yet consequences of these activities are almost always covered by insurance. Legislators usually do not have expertise and are susceptible to "wheeling and dealing," irrespective of scientific facts, clinical realities, moral uncertainties, or social needs. The West Australia law limiting storage time of human embryos resulted in embryo destruction because extension could not be granted and some couples who were lost to follow-up could not be located in time [48]. While the Human Fertilisation and Embryology Act in the United Kingdom has often been considered a model act, it has also received significant criticism [49]. Regulations can limit the availability of clinical services even when the scientific evidence for such limitation is exceedingly weak [50]. It has been argued that legislative intervention, especially with respect to embryo transfer numbers, might be one cause of the lower pregnancy rates in Europe compared to the United States [30, 31, 43, 51].

Current regulatory structures that have been suggested by some as models have been strongly criticized by others [52, 53]. It has been found that restrictive laws governing "social" issues have a significant impact on the availability of ART services, that reproductive travel is prevalent and that restrictions were circumvented by patients with the assistance of clinics [54]. Reproductive travel can act as a safety valve for patient demand but may affect the quality of services [55]. The challenge for regulations is to balance protection for patients and society with access and freedom for patients to receive the best possible care and professional autonomy for physicians and scientists to provide clinical treatment and perform research. It is not realistic to expect a purely market approach determined by patient choice nor a purely peer self-regulated professional approach to work politically, or be desirable socially, ethically or legally [56]. While there are public interest concerns that would seem to justify some sort of regulatory structure, it has been argued that current regulations that constrain reproductive autonomy of patients and the professional autonomy of physicians and scientists in some jurisdictions are not justified, and that current regulation of ART in some jurisdictions is more burdensome than in other areas of medicine, and cannot be justified based on objective analysis of medical, social, legal, financial and ethical aspects of ART. One is left with the conclusion that religious, moral and political factors, sometimes factional, have been the determining forces in shaping ART regulation in many jurisdictions.

Of course, self-regulation with guidelines also has disadvantages, especially that not all patients or physicians will follow guidelines. But it has important advantages of being less susceptible to outright political pressure, more individualized to patient needs, more quickly changed as technology and scientific understanding progress, and less expensive. Furthermore, social changes and perceptions frequently outdate legislation.

Sixty-nine percent of patients, having been informed of the risks of multiple pregnancy, felt that a multiple pregnancy would be the ideal outcome of IVF [57]. The desire for multiple pregnancy in male and female infertility patients is reduced by patient recognition of the risks of multiple birth, but increased by increasing duration of infertility or previous assisted reproductive treatment [58]. Therefore, SET could potentially increase the desire for multiple pregnancy if early cycles of SET were unsuccessful. This results in psychological, economic and perhaps rarely legal pressure on physicians to replace more embryos than they would recommend. These factors make the argument for some regulation of SET.

Regulation versus self-regulation of SET: general considerations

With respect to regulation versus self-regulation of SET, there are some unique aspects to consider. Primarily, it is very clear from current experience that SET is not the appropriate treatment for all patients at all times. Patients of older age are not appropriate candidates, and will be severely compromised if SET were implemented for all patients. Furthermore, even younger patients may have special medical situations in which it is simply not the best treatment for them because their pregnancy rate will be too low. It is difficult to predict in advance, which strict regulations must do, the myriad of clinical situations faced by the practicing physician. Mandatory SET is potentially unfair to the majority of infertile couples and severely limits the physician's capacity to resolve unfavorable IVF cases. Current IVF technology is imperfect and the impact of SET needs further evaluation, especially in older patients, poor responders, blastocyst transfer and PGD/S. Mandatory SET could solve one problem while creating many new ones [59].

The objective of ART treatment is not to provide services, but to have treatment result in the birth of a healthy singleton baby, while avoiding multiple pregnancy. Many factors besides the number of embryos transferred affect the probability of achieving these outcomes. It is almost impossible for restrictive legislation to take all of these factors into account, especially egg and embryo quality. Furthermore, important prognostic clinical and laboratory information which is obtained during treatment cannot be utilized to benefit the patient.

Other factors affecting implementation of SET include financial coverage which has been associated with decreased number of embryos transferred and pregnancies with three or more fetuses, but also lower pregnancy rates [14]. Financial coverage will almost certainly encourage SET.

Dropout rates also affect the chances of ultimate success [60–64]. One of the issues that must be accounted for is the emotional stress caused by failed cycles, and the impact this has on the probability patients will continue treatment. If patients drop out of treatment, then success rates will be lower. This is a major concern if SET is inappropriately mandated for some patients.

Regulations affecting SET

As noted above, legislation regarding many aspects of ART can affect pregnancy success rates, and/or conflict with other ART regulations. In Germany, The Embryo Protection Act of 1990 states that no more than three eggs can be collected from a patient for fertilization in vitro [65]. After that, all embryos created must be transferred to the patient in order to avoid any embryo cryopreservation or destruction. Only pronuclear stage cryopreservation is allowed. The result of this legislation is lower pregnancy rates because poorer quality embryos are created on average, yet higher multiple pregnancy rates occur because too many good quality embryos must be replaced in some women [66].

Italy passed regulations in 2003 that restrict fertility treatments to heterosexual couples of childbearing age who are living together, prohibits egg or sperm donation or surrogacy, forbids cryopreservation of embryos and mandates that all, but not more than three, embryos must be replaced at embryo transfer. It also prohibits embryo research [67–69].

Spain has regulations that allow cryopreservation but prohibit destroying cryopreserved embryos or donating them to research. As a result, many embryos remain in cryostorage beyond the 5-year storage limit [70].

Canada passed comprehensive regulations in 2004, the Assisted Human Reproduction Agency of Canada [71]. Among its many provisions, the law allows some embryo research, but prohibits payment to gamete or embryo donors or surrogates and has significant fines and imprisonment sanctions. However, despite the fact this is recent regulation and built on other regulatory systems around the world, criticism of the restrictive nature of this regulation has been leveled [72].

Legislation that enabled research on embryos would encourage a better understanding of the implantation potential of any given embryo, which would likely increase the utilization of SET. Preimplantation genetic diagnosis/screening currently has many uses, but its application for aneuploidy screening can potentially enable selection for replacement or cryopreservation of the embryo(s) with the highest implantation rates, thereby encouraging SET. Its efficacy in this regard is yet to be proven, but hopefully technological improvements and a better understanding of embryo physiology and development will enable this to occur in the near future [73]. The moral status of the embryo will affect the application of all ART technologies and legislation in any given country, and will influence the delivery of reproductive services, patients' access to care and quality of the care they receive.

In summary, the purpose of ART is to obtain a healthy singleton live birth with minimal number of adverse outcomes, with multiple pregnancy being the single most important one. While achieving the lowest possible multiple birth rate is very important, ART cannot be considered successful if this objective is achieved through medical practices that cause a significant reduction in cycle pregnancy rates and overall cumulative live birth rate. Legislation is ill-suited to manage patient care because of the multiple factors involved in patient management and the rapid development of new technologies that outdate legislation. Self-regulation by professional guidelines potentially allows the optimal care to be provided to each patient and optimal outcomes to be obtained [74].

How to make self-regulation work

Characteristics of self-regulation

Studies of regulatory systems have suggested that four factors must be addressed for a regulatory system to work: (1) the development of a shared social ethic that helps the needs of the community to be balanced against those of its individual members; (2) the negative impact of intrusive external regulation on scientists and doctors; (3) the requirement for doctors and scientists to review their professional structures reflectively and critically if they are to be entrusted with peer-regulation; and (4) the desirability of constructive dialogue between regulators and regulated rather than the use of coercion and criminal sanctions [56].

Self-regulation with guidelines does not imply absence of oversight. Indeed, it implies sophisticated medical attention to all the issues and development of guidelines by professional organizations that address laboratory, clinical and ethical/social issues. It also does not suggest that each individual physician has the right to make any decision they wish with each patient, but rather gives physicians the flexibility to choose an approach other than that recommended by the guidelines only if they justify such a treatment decision on medical and ethical grounds. Oversight is necessary to ensure that the guidelines are effective in practice, to make improvements to them, and to provide sanctions if physicians do not follow them without sufficient justification for individual patient deviations. Optimally, some type of oversight authority needs to be developed in countries that rely on self-regulation.

An ideal oversight authority has a number of characteristics. It should be a partnership of professionals, patients and the public, and should be independent of any one interested party. It should have few specific regulations, but rather a flexible mandate. It should set standards for care, avoid moral and political agendas and be financed by all the stakeholders. Mandates that an oversight authority should have include mandatory compliance, meaningful sanctions, uniformity in reporting, on-site inspection and validation, practice standards, research standards, education standards, counseling standards, insurance coverage, research funding and limitation of specific regulation [34].

Perspectives on self-regulation

Within the United States, there are many who feel that specific regulation of the number of embryos to transfer is not the best approach: "It seems extremely difficult to control these and unanticipated variables in a legislative manner, and rigidity with regard to the number to be transferred would probably not be in the best interest of the patient." [9]. The CDC recommends guidelines developed by professional organizations: "...efforts are needed...to limit the number of embryos transferred for patients receiving ART. These approaches...should follow guidelines issued by organizations such as the American Society for Reproductive Medicine..." and "A shift to single embryo transfer...may have trade-offs that are unacceptable to many couples and assisted reproduction treatment providers. Given the high costs of assisted reproduction treatment, limited insurance coverage in the USA, and the general perception that the chance for a live birth in a single treatment cycle with single embryo transfer is lower than for treatment cycles with double or more embryo transfer, single embryo transfer is not currently a popular option among couples seeking assisted reproduction treatment" [75, 76]. A multifaceted approach to the multiple pregnancy problem, involving enhanced patient selection, better culturing and selection of top quality embryos, better insurance coverage for IVF, increased physician understanding and appreciation of the risks of multiple birth, better reporting of singleton pregnancy as the ideal outcome and better education of patients about the benefits of limiting the number of embryos transferred, has been recommended [77]. Therefore, there is general consensus that in the United States it is not appropriate to legislate absolute limits to the number of embryos that can be transferred, including SET [74].

Stakeholders in establishing self-regulation for SET

Many parties or stakeholders are interested in regulation and self-regulation of ART. It is difficult to give all stakeholders appropriate representation in one body, and there is overlap of interests in an ever-widening circle of involvement in clinical, laboratory, research, legal, ethical, consumer, financial and public interests (Figure 21.1) [34]. One model for dealing with such a complex situation is to recognize a "hierarchy of interest" (Figure 21.2) [34]. This model suggests that patients, their gametic material and future children have the most standing or interest in ART and its regulation, and their interests should be paramount

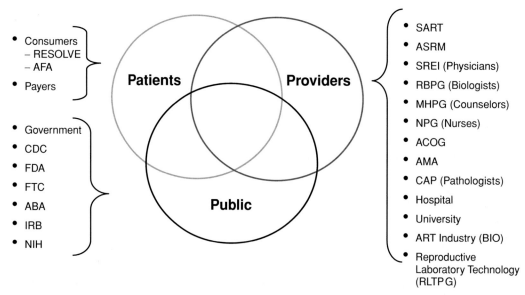

Figure 21.1 Different parties interested in oversight of ART. AFA, American Fertility Association; CDC, Centers for Disease Control and Prevention; FDA, Food and Drug Administration; FTC, Federal Trade Commission; ABA, American Bar Association; IRB, Institutional Review Board; NIH, National Institutes of Health; SART, Society for Assisted Reproductive Technology; ASRM, American Society for Reproductive Medicine; SREI, Society for Reproductive Endocrinology and Infertility; RBPG, Reproductive Biology Professional Group; MHPG, Mental Health Professional Group; ACOG, American College of Obstetricians and Gynecologists; AMA, American Medical Association; CAP, College of American Pathologists; NPG, Nurses Professional Group.

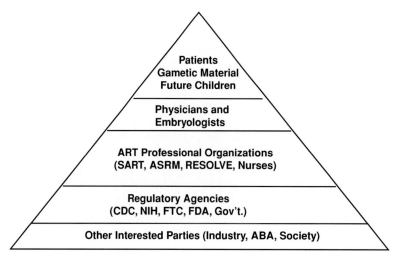

Figure 21.2 The hierarchy of interest. For abbreviations see legend to Figure 21.1.

when developing regulation and oversight. Access to care, reproductive choice, high standards of care, accurate information and informed consent are important to patients. This includes regulations regarding numbers of embryos that can be created, cryopreserved and/or transferred. Physicians, embryologists and scientists who provide ART services have the next highest standing in this hierarchy, which would involve guidelines protecting the patient–physician relationship, confidentiality, medico-legal protection, adequate compensation, minimal restrictions on research, research funding and other professional interests that enhance high quality ART services and their continued improvement. The next level is that of professional organizations that develop practice, laboratory and ethical standards, and should be recognized as having standing except in unusual individual clinical situations. The next level is the regulatory authorities. They develop broad regulatory frameworks but should be responsive to patients, professionals and professional organizations, utilizing their recommendations unless there are compelling alternative social or public interests. The base of this hierarchy is other interested stakeholders and society. They should facilitate the assisted reproductive technologies to the extent they bring good to individual patients, physicians, embryologists and scientists, and to the clinical and scientific benefit of this field of medicine. However, society does have the right and the responsibility to set general limits on the utilization of this technology if it believes its application will be harmful to society as a whole. It should also provide organizational and financial support of the technology, access to it and research if it finds that society will benefit.

With this type of structure, everyone is included in the appropriate way and has a position in developing all aspects of ART. Society sets broad limits through regulations developed with the expertise of professional organizations. Professional organizations set broad guidelines for patient care and laboratory standards, as well as ethics standards, but leaves most of the decisions regarding benefits and harms of individual treatment to those

most affected, the patients and professionals. In this regard, the evidence shows that the United States is moving towards a situation that comprises many of these principles. It is far from perfect, but is flexible and has produced real progress. Therefore, a combination of both regulation and self-regulation is the best approach. This especially applies to regulations regarding the number of embryos to transfer.

Conclusions

Assisted reproductive technology is a complex technological, clinical, scientific and social endeavor. Simple approaches to its problems, for example the multiple birth rate, will not result in the optimal utilization of ART for the overall benefit of all those who need it. In a pluralistic society, it is appropriate to consider a "hierarchy of interest" in balancing patient reproductive choice, the practice of medicine, research and the values, needs and desires of society. Each society will have to develop its own institutions, organizations, structures, processes, legislation, guidelines and practices in order to optimize this for themselves. Hopefully, we can all continue to learn from each other, to evaluate the consequences of successful and unsuccessful strategies and interventions, so that we can constantly increase the benefits of ART to our individual patients, to society, and to the babies we help create. This should be our approach to the problem of multiple pregnancy and the implementation of SET.

What do we know?
1. The desired outcome from ART is a healthy singleton baby. Most patients and many physicians and embryologists consider twins to be an acceptable outcome, but some consider them to be a complication. Triplets are a serious complication.
2. Single embryo transfer is a very effective strategy to reduce multiple births, and is applicable to many, but not all, ART patients.

3. The successful implementation of SET depends on multiple patient, physician, clinical, embryology, cultural, religious, social, economic, legal and ethical factors, and will occur differently in different regions of the world and even within countries. Neither regulation alone nor self-regulation by the profession without the involvement of all the stakeholders will provide optimal care to patients.

What do we need to know?

1. We need better clinical parameters to select patients for SET.
2. We need better embryology parameters to select the best embryos for SET.
3. We need a better understanding of factors that motivate patients in different socioeconomic and cultural environments to undergo ART treatment, to make the choices they do during treatment, and to drop out of treatment.

What do we need to do?

1. We need to perform and evaluate more good studies on countries and practices that have implemented SET, with objective analysis of what worked and what didn't in different clinical, scientific, socioeconomic, cultural and regulatory/self-regulatory environments. We need more support of basic research that will improve our ability to choose an embryo with high versus low implantation potential, and technologies/treatments that will increase implantation and cryopreservation rates.
2. We need to educate patients, physicians and the public on the risks of multiple births, and the benefits of SET.
3. We need to develop systems combining regulation and self-regulation that promote the implementation of SET as broadly as possible for the appropriate patients so that we can minimize multiple births while maintaining optimal live birth rates. This needs to be done while respecting the cultural norms of different societies, protecting the babies born from ART, but not discriminating against infertile patients, multiple birth babies or their parents.

REFERENCES

1. Merriam-Webster Dictionary 2004 version 3.1. Accessed January 2, 2008 at www.m-w.com.
2. J. A. Land and J. L. H. Evers, Risks and complications in assisted reproduction techniques: Report of an ESHRE Consensus Meeting. *Hum. Reprod.*, **18**:2 (2003), 455–457.
3. M. J. Davies, J. X. Wang and R. J. Norman, What is the most relevant standard of success in assisted reproduction? Assessing the BESST index for reproduction treatment. *Hum. Reprod.*, **19** (2004), 1049–1051.
4. R. P. Dickey, B. M. Sartor and R. Pyrzak, What is the most relevant standard of success in assisted reproduction? *Hum. Reprod.*, **19**:4 (2004), 783–787.
5. E. Vayena, P. J. Rowe and P. D. Griffin (eds.), *Recommendations. Medical, Ethical and Social Aspects of Assisted Reproduction: Current Practices and Controversies in Assisted Reproduction.* Report of a WHO meeting. (Geneva, Switzerland: WHO publications, 2001), pp. 381–396.
6. M. Germond, F. Urner, A. Chanson *et al.*, What is the most relevant standard of success in assisted reproduction? The cumulated singleton/twin delivery rates per oocyte pick-up: the CUSIDERA and CUTWIDERA. *Hum. Reprod.*, **19**:11 (2004), 2442–2444.
7. H. W. Jones, Multiple births: how are we doing? *Fertil. Steril.*, **79**:1 (2003), 17–21.
8. IFFS surveillance 98. *Fertil. Steril.*, **71**:5 Suppl. 2 (1999), 1S–34S.
9. H. W. Jones Jr. and J. Cohen, IFFS surveillance 01. *Fertil. Steril.*, **76**: 5 Suppl. 2 (2001), S5–S36.
10. IFFS surveillance 03. *Fertil. Steril.*, **81**: Suppl. 4 (2004), S9–S54.
11. H. Jones, Jr. and J. Cohen, IFFS surveillance 2007. *Fertil. Steril.*, **87**:4 Suppl. 1 (2007), S1–S67.
12. G. D. Adamson, J. de Mouzon, P. Lancaster *et al.*, World collaborative report on in vitro fertilization for year 2000. *Fertil. Steril.*, **85**:6 (2006), 1586–1622.
13. A. P. Feraretti, L. Gianaroli, M. C. Magli *et al.*, Medically assisted conception: an established clinical procedure? In Italy not anymore. *Hum. Reprod.*, **20**: Suppl. (2005), i21–i22.
14. T. Jain, B. L. Harlow and M. D. Hornstein, Insurance coverage and outcomes of in vitro fertilization. *N. Engl. J. Med.*, **347** (2002), 661–666.
15. C. Hydén-Granskog, L. Unkila-Kallio, M. Halttunen and A. Tiitinen, Single embryo transfer is an option in

frozen embryo transfer. *Hum. Reprod.*, **20** (2005), 2935–2938.

16. A. Brewaeys, J. K. de Bruyn, L. A. Louwe and F. M. Helmerhorst, Anonymous or identity-registered sperm donors? A study of Dutch recipients' choices. *Hum. Reprod.*, **20** (2005), 820–824.

17. I. Craft and A. Thornhill, Would all-inclusive compensation attract more gamete donors to balance their loss of anonymity? *Reprod. Biomed. Online*, **10** (2005), 301–306.

18. E. G. Papanikolaou, M. Camus, E. M. Kolibianakis *et al.*, In vitro fertilization with single blastocyst-stage versus single cleavage-stage embryos. *N. Engl. J. Med.*, **354**:11 (2006), 1139–1146. Comment in: *N. Engl. J. Med.*, **354**:11 (2006), 1190–1193.

19. Practice Committee of the Society for Assisted Reproductive Technology; Practice Committee of the American Society for Reproductive Medicine. Guidelines on number of embryos transferred. *Fertil. Steril.*, **86**: 5 Suppl. (2006), S51–S52.

20. Ethics Committee of the American Society for Reproductive Medicine, Child-rearing and the provision of fertility services. *Fertil. Steril.*, **82**: 3 (2004), 564–567.

21. J. Stone, K. Eddleman, L. Lynch and R. L. Berkowitz, A single center experience with 1000 consecutive cases of multifetal pregnancy reduction. *Am. J. Obstet. Gynecol.*, **187** (2002), 1163–1167.

22. M. I. Evans, D. Ciorica, D. W. Britt and J. C. Fletcher, Update on selective reduction. *Prenat. Diagn.*, **25** (2005), 807–813.

23. D. W. Britt, W. J. G. Evans, S. S. Mahta and M. I. Evans, Framing the decision: determinants of how women considering multifetal pregnancy reduction as a pregnancy-management strategy frame their moral dilemma. *Fetal Diagn Ther.*, **19** (2004), 232–240.

24. J. Gerris, Single embryo transfer and IVF/ICSI outcome: a balanced appraisal. *Hum. Reprod. Update*, **11** (2005), 105–121.

25. C. Bergh, Single embryo transfer: a mini-review. *Hum. Reprod.*, **20** (2005), 323–327.

26. A. Tiitinen and M. Gissler, Effect of in vitro fertilization practices on multiple pregnancy rates in Finland. *Fertil. Steril.*, **82** (2004), 1689–1690.

27. C. Hydén-Granskog and A. Tiitinen, Single embryo transfer in clinical practice. *Hum. Fertil.* (Camb.), **7** (2004), 175–182.

28. T. Jain, S. A. Missmer and M. D. Hornstein, Trends in embryo-transfer practice and in outcomes of the use of assisted reproductive technology in the United States. *N. Engl. J. Med.*, **350** (2004), 1639–1645.

29. N. Gleicher and D. Barad, The relative myth of single embryo transfer. *Hum. Reprod.*, **21** (2006), 1337–1344.

30. N. Gleicher, A. Weghofer and D. Barad, Update on comparison of assisted reproduction outcomes between Europe and the USA: the 2002 data. *Fertil. Steril.*, **87**:6 (2007), 1301–1305. Epub 2007 Apr 6.

31. N. Gleicher, A. Weghofer and D. Barad, On the benefit of assisted reproduction techniques, a comparison of the USA and Europe. *Hum. Reprod.*, **22**:2 (2007), 624–626; doi:10.1093/humrep/del405.

32. A. P. A. van Montfoort, A. A. A. Fiddelers, J. M. Janssen *et al.*, In unselected patients, elective single embryo transfer prevents all multiples, but results in significantly lower pregnancy rates compared with double embryo transfer: a randomized controlled trial. *Hum. Reprod.*, **21** (2006), 338–343.

33. G. D. Adamson, Regulation of assisted reproductive technologies in the United States. American Bar Association Family Law Quarterly. **39**:3 (2005), 727–744.

34. G. D. Adamson, Regulation of the assisted reproductive technologies in the United States. *Fertil. Steril.*, **78** (2002), 932–942.

35. The Fertility Clinics Success Rate and Certification Act of 1992; Public Law 102–493.

36. Society for Assisted Reproductive Technology; American Society for Reproductive Medicine, Assisted reproductive technology in the United States: 2001 results generated from the American Society for Reproductive Medicine/Society for Assisted Reproductive Technology registry. *Fertil. Steril.*, **87**:6 (2007), 1253–1266.

37. Centers for Disease Control and Prevention Assisted Reproductive Technology Reports. Accessed January 2, 2008 at www.cdc.gov/reproductivehealth/ART/index.htm.

38. Clinical Laboratory Improvement Amendments of 1988 (CLIA), Pub. L. 100–578.

39. V. L. Baker, M. O. Gvakharia, H. M. Rone, J. R. Manalad and G. D. Adamson, Economic cost for implementation of the U. S. Food and Drug Administration's Code of Federal Regulations Title 21, Part 1271 in an egg donor program. *Fertil. Steril.*, (2007), Oct 20 (Epub ahead of print).

40. www.asrm.org. Accessed January 2, 2008.

41. J. P. Toner, Progress we can be proud of: U. S. trends in assisted reproduction over the first 20 years. *Fertil. Steril.*, **78**:5 (2002), 943–950.

42. J. E. Stern, M. I. Cedars, T. Jain *et al.*, Society for Assisted Reproductive Technology Writing Group. Assisted reproductive technology practice patterns and the impact of embryo transfer guidelines in the United States. *Fertil. Steril.*, **88**:2 (2007), 275–282. Epub 2007 Apr 18.

43. N. Gleicher, A. Weghofer and D. Barad, A formal comparison of the practice of assisted reproductive technologies between Europe and the USA. *Hum. Reprod.*, **21** (2006), 1945–1950; doi:10.1093/humrep/del138.

44. H. Szoke, The nanny state or responsible government? *J. Law Med.*, **9**:4 (2002), 470–482.

45. D. D. M. Braat, J. A. Kremer and W. L. D. M. Nelen, Barriers and facilitators for implementation of single embryo transfer (eSET) in in vitro fertilization (IVF). *Hum. Reprod.*, **20**: Suppl. 1 (2005), i30.

46. U. M. Reddy, R. J. Wapner, R. W. Rebar and R. J. Tasca, Infertility, assisted reproductive technology, and adverse pregnancy outcomes: executive summary of a National Institute of Child Health and Human Development workshop. *Obstet. Gynecol.*, **109**:4 (2007), 967–977.

47. J. Arons, Center for American Progress. Future Choices. Assisted Reproductive Technologies and the Law. December 2007. Accessed January 8, 2008 at www.americanprogress.org.

48. N. Darlington and P. Matson, The fate of cryopreserved human embryos approaching their legal limit of storage within a West Australian in-vitro fertilization clinic. *Hum. Reprod.*, **14**:9 (1999), 2343–2344.

49. Human Fertilization and Embryology Act,1990 (Chapter 37). Accessed January 8, 2008 at www.opsi.gov.uk/acts/acts1990/Ukpga_19900037_en_ 1.htm.

50. D. Mortimer and C. L. Barratt, Is there a real risk of transmitting variant Creutzfeldt-Jakob disease by donor sperm insemination? *Reprod. Biomed. Online*, **13**:6 (2006), 778–790.

51. K. Nygren, A. N. Andersen, R. Felberbaum, L. Gianaroli, J. de Mouzon and Members of ESHRE's European IVF Monitoring (EIM). On the benefit of assisted reproduction techniques, a comparison of USA and Europe. *Hum. Reprod.*, **21**:8 (2006), 2194; doi:10.1093/humrep/del238.

52. K. Petersen and M. H. Johnson, SmARTest regulations? Comparing the regulatory structures for ART in the UK and Australia. *Reprod. Biomed. Online*, **15**:2 (2007), 236–244.

53. K. Petersen, The regulation of assisted reproductive technology: a comparative study of permissive and prescriptive laws and policies. *J. Law Med.*, **9**:4 (2002), 483–497.

54. K. Petersen, H. W. Baker, M. Pitts and R. Thorpe, Assisted reproductive technologies: professional and legal restrictions in Australian clinics. *J. Law Med.*, **12**:3 (2002), 373–385.

55. R. Storrow, Extraterritorial effects of fertility tourism arising from restrictive reproductive laws: what should national parliaments consider? *Hum. Reprod.*, **20**:Suppl. 1 (2005), i48–i49.

56. M. H. Johnson, The art of regulation and the regulation of ART: the impact of regulation on research and clinical practice. *J. Law Med.*, **9**:4 (2002), 399–413.

57. A. Murdoch, Triplets and embryo transfer policy. *Hum. Reprod.*, **12**:Suppl. 11 (1997), 88–92.

58. T. J. Child, A. M. Henderson and S. L. Tan, The desire for multiple pregnancy in male and female infertility patients. *Hum. Reprod.*, **19**:3 (2004), 558–561.

59. E. R. Hernandez, Avoiding multiple pregnancies: sailing uncharted seas. *Hum. Reprod.*, **16**:4 (2001), 615–616.

60. C. Olivius, B. Friden, G. Borg and C. Bergh, Why do couples discontinue in vitro fertilization treatment? A cohort study. *Fertil. Steril.*, **81**:2 (2004), 258–261.

61. J. M. J. Smeernk, C. M. Verhaak, A. M. Stolwijk, J. A. M. Kremer and D. D. M. Braat, Reasons for dropout in an in vitro fertilization/intracytoplasmic sperm injection program. *Fertil. Steril.*, **81**:2 (2004), 262–268.

62. A. S. Penzias, When and why does the dream die? Or does it? *Fertil. Steril.*, **81**:2 (2004), 274–275.

63. A. D. Domar, Impact of psychological factors on dropout rates in insured infertility patients. *Fertil. Steril.*, **81**:2 (2004), 271–273.

64. C. E. Malcolm and D. C. Cumming, Follow-up of infertile couples who dropped out of a specialist fertility clinic. *Fertil. Steril.*, **81**:2 (2004), 269–270.

65. German Act for the Protection of Embryos (1990). *Official Gazette*, 1(1990), 2746.

66. R. Felderbaum, ART laws put patients at risk and should be changed, warns head of Germany's IVF registry. From European Society for Human Reproduction and Embryology 2003. Accessed January 2, 2008 at www.scienceblog.com/community/older/2003/E/20032592.html.

67. European Society for Human Reproduction and Embryology, Italian law on ART brings problems

for doctors and patients. June 22, 2005. Accessed January 2, 2008 at www.medicalnewstoday.com/medicalnews.php?newsid=26443.

68. V. Fineschi, M. Neri and E. Turillazzi, The new Italian law on assisted reproduction technology (Law 40/2004). *J. Med. Ethics*, **31** (2005), 536–539.

69. G. Ragni, A. Allegra, P. Anserini *et al.*, The 2004 Italian legislation regulating assisted reproductive technology: a multicenter survey on the results of IVF cycles. *Hum. Reprod.*, **20** (2005), 2224–2228.

70. J. Tizzard, Restrictive laws in Europe are harming patients. *BioNews*, July 5, 2003. Accessed January 2, 2008 at www.nytimes.com/2004/02/15/international/europe/15SPAI.html?ex=1077823559&ei=1&en=c0095959d6296136.

71. House of Commons of Canada. Bill C-6: An Act respecting assisted human reproduction and related research. Accessed January 2, 2008 at www.parl.gc.ca/common/Bills_ls.asp?Parl=37&Ses=3&ls=C6.

72. C. Rasmussen, Canada's Assisted Human Reproductive Act: is it scientific censorship, or a reasoned approach to the regulation of rapidly emerging reproductive technologies? *Sask Law Rev.*, **67**:1 (2004), 97–135.

73. K. A. de Boer, J. W. Catt, R. P. S. Jansen, D. Leigh and S. McArthur, Moving to blastocyst biopsy for preimplantation genetic diagnosis and single embryo transfer at Sydney IVF. *Fertil. Steril.*, **82**:2 (2004), 295–298.

74. G. D. Adamson and V. L. Baker, Multiple births from assisted reproductive technologies: a challenge that must be met. *Fertil. Steril.*, **81** (2004), 517–522.

75. Centers for Disease Control and Prevention (CDC), Contribution of assisted reproductive technology and ovulation-inducing drugs to triplet and higher-order multiple births – United States, 1980–1997. *MMWR Morb. Mortal Wkly Rep.*, **49** (2000), 535–538.

76. M. A. Reynolds and L. A. Schieve, Trends in embryo transfer practices and multiple gestation for IVF procedures in the USA, 1996–2002. *Hum. Reprod.*, **21**:3 (2006), 694–700.

77. R. J. Stillman, A 47-year-old woman with fertility problems who desires a multiple pregnancy. *JAMA*, **297** (2007), 858–867.

22

An American perspective on single embryo transfer

John M. Norian, Eric D. Levens, Alan H. DeCherney and G. David Adamson

Introduction

Assisted reproductive technology (ART) including in vitro fertilization (IVF) has become increasingly successful in the last 30 years and now is responsible for more than 3 000 000 births worldwide [1, 2]. Despite its global application, ART practice has tremendous regional differences, among them disparate multiple gestation rates [3, 4]. Advances in ART have increased pregnancy rates in addition to reducing multiple birth rates [5]. Nevertheless, the multiple gestation rates following ART remain high. Recognition of the morbidity and mortality associated with multiple births has led to the identification of risk factors for multiple gestations following ART, to providing public education regarding the complications associated with multiples, and to increasing the regulatory involvement in ART practice [3, 6, 7].

Factors associated with multiple births following ART include nulliparity, younger patient age, longer duration of infertility, lower family income

and a lack of knowledge regarding the risks of multiple gestations [8]. In an effort to lower multiple pregnancy rates, many centers now select suitable patients for single embryo transfer (SET) [9, 10]. Today the utilization of SET varies dramatically throughout the world as the result of many factors, such as legislative mandates, insurance coverage and market pressures. Moreover, differing valuations regarding the risks of multiple gestations and lack of knowledge about the risks of multiple gestations complicate the SET issue, in part explaining why global disparities exist [11]. In this chapter, we examine the practice of SET for the reduction of multiple gestations, with an emphasis on the US experience.

Reasons for single embryo transfer

Regardless of the infertility cause, IVF results in the highest pregnancy rate per cycle. However, this advantage is tempered by associated hazards: multiple gestations and its high rate of complications, higher pregnancy-related maternal health risks, family discord and greater health care costs.

Poorer neonatal outcomes

Neonatal complications resulting from multiple pregnancies include prematurity, low birth weight,

This work was supported, in part, by the Reproductive Biology and Medicine Branch, NICHD, NIH, Bethesda, MD.

The opinions or assertions contained herein are the private views of the authors and are not to be construed as official or as reflecting the views of the Department of Health and Human Services, the Department of the Army or the Department of Defense.

and increased perinatal mortality [12]. Approximately 1% of American-born infants are conceived through ART and those infants account for 18% of multiple births nationwide, including 40% of all triplet births [3, 4]. Multiple gestations are responsible for 23% of births prior to 32 weeks' gestation and 26% of infants weighing < 1500 grams [4, 13, 14]. Despite improvements, the infant mortality rate continues to be 4-fold higher for twins (20/1000 live births), 11-fold higher for triplets (47/1000 live births), and 21-fold higher for higher-order multiples (HOM) (94/1000 live births) compared with singletons [15, 16]. Nevertheless, the majority of ART patients report favoring multiple gestations, preferably twins, as a desire to have more than one child and to minimize the physical and psychological stresses associated with ART [17].

Birth outcomes following ART have been the source of significant discussion in the literature. Malformation rates, such as anencephaly, hydrocephalus, esophageal atresia and anal atresia, have been found to be higher among those with multiple gestations than among those with singletons [18–22]. Furthermore, the European Society for Human Reproduction and Embryology (ESHRE) suggested that ART was associated with a 4–8% risk of congenital malformations, leading to greater infant morbidity when compared to natural conceptions [23, 24]. However, the morbidity associated with ART may be more related to the health implications of the underlying subfertile state and less so to ART treatment [25, 26]. Most importantly, much of the morbidity excess associated with ART relates to the prevalence of twins and HOM, often resulting in prematurity [24].

Higher maternal risks and family impact

It is clear that multiple gestations result in greater maternal risks. Of these, pre-eclampsia and eclampsia are especially profound, having upwards of three- to fourfold increased risk among those carrying twin gestations compared with singletons [4, 13, 14]. Furthermore, the relative risk of placental abruption, postpartum hemorrhage, anemia and Cesarean delivery are significantly greater among those with multiple gestations [27, 28].

In addition to the medical complications, there remain family obstacles with rearing twins and triplets including the impairment of the maternal bond, maternal exhaustion and marital disharmony [29–31]. To date, a paucity of expert advice exists as to how to best cope with the stress associated with multiples. Resultantly, major depressive illness and psychological problems are common, persisting for many years. A recent study found that 22% of mothers of multiples following IVF demonstrated severe parenting stress, compared with 5% of mothers with IVF singletons (odds ratio [OR]: 5.1; 95% confidence interval [CI]: 1.6–17.0) and 9% of mothers of naturally conceived singletons (OR: 2.8; 95% CI: 1.0–7.4) [32]. Furthermore, mothers delivering multiples following IVF had a threefold higher risk of depression and were more likely to express negative themes, such as tiredness and questioning parenthood, when compared with those having IVF singletons. On the contrary, those with IVF singletons demonstrated delight toward parenthood [33].

Economic implications

The proportion of IVF cycles resulting in live births have been reportedly higher in states not requiring insurance coverage compared with those states that do require partial or complete coverage. An untoward result, however, was that these states had higher multiple birth rates [34]. Multiple births increase medical care costs [35]. For a single birth, maternal costs are approximately $5000 per pregnancy and neonatal costs are roughly $5000 yielding a total family cost in the order of $10 000, using 2004 inflation-adjusted dollars [35, 36]. For twins, the cost was approximately threefold higher than singleton gestations; while triplets and HOM increased the cost by 11-fold [35]. The ESHRE Working Group has estimated per family costs for IVF twins and IVF quadruplets to be nearly $60 000 and $280 000, respectively [27]. Nevertheless, the economic considerations are apparently unimportant to prospective parents and patients seemingly ignore the aforementioned risks, making statements such as "twins are a nice chance to have two babies at once" and "twins make up for lost time" [9, 17, 37].

Single embryo transfer in practice

Distinguishing between compulsory, medical and elective SET

Prior to discussing the optimal population to offer SET, a distinction must be made between compulsory, medical and elective SET. Compulsory SET (cSET) occurs when only one embryo is available for transfer. In this setting, the resultant outcomes are poor. A study of 1454 cSET cycles found that the mean implantation rate was a dismal 13%, and the ensuing live birth rate was a mere 10% [9, 38]. Medical SET (mSET) is performed when there is an increased a-priori maternal and perinatal risk associated with multiple gestations compared with a singleton gestation. Medical indications for SET include congenital uterine anomalies, poor obstetric history (e.g., incompetent cervix), previous severe premature delivery and severe maternal systemic disease (e.g., insulin-dependent diabetes, cardiac disease, systemic lupus erythematosus) [9, 39].

In contrast, elective single embryo transfer (eSET) has been defined as the transfer of one good quality embryo in cases where ≥ 2 good quality embryos are available. Elective SET implies that a couple has willfully decided upon the transfer of a single embryo after a fresh or frozen IVF cycle [40–43]. The ultimate objective of eSET is to obtain a similar or improved pregnancy rate as compared to multiple embryo transfer, while simultaneously decreasing the risk of multiple gestations.

The declining number of embryos transferred in the United States

In the USA, the number of embryos transferred has been dramatically reduced since the publication of Society for Assisted Reproductive Technol-ogy (SART) guidelines aimed at reducing, and ultimately eliminating, multiple gestations [40–43]. In 1995, an average of four embryos per cycle were transferred among women < 35 years old undergoing a fresh non-donor cycle. By 2004, the mean number of embryos transferred had been reduced to 2.5 per cycle and SETs were performed in 8.2% of fresh non-donor ART cycles [40]. During the last decade, the percentage of clinics transferring two embryos in women < 35 years old increased from 3.3% in 1996 to 53.6% in 2004 [44]. During this time, the pregnancy rate per cycle increased from 29.7% to 42.5% and the resultant per cycle live birth rate increased from 25.3% to 36.9% [40]. Furthermore, the singleton live birth rate for non-donor, fresh ART cycles increased from 17% in 1996 to 23% in 2004.

Remarkably, the triplet and HOM rates have dramatically declined, while the twin rate has remained largely unchanged [40]. Progress has been made towards reducing the multiple gestation rates, yet there remains the opportunity for continually improved pregnancy outcomes, while further reducing the number of embryos transferred. This was evidenced by a recent study, which found that while the total number of embryos transferred had been reduced, nearly one third of patients undergoing ART in the USA were still receiving more than three embryos per transfer. This is in stark contrast to the experience in Europe where only 6.7% of patient transfers involved more than three embryos [45, 46].

Outcomes in elective single embryo transfer

In order to employ eSET effectively, clinical strategies must maximize per cycle pregnancy rates, while reducing multiple gestations. The essentials to introducing eSET into an ART program include: (1) a high baseline ongoing pregnancy rate among good prognosis patients; (2) an unacceptable multiple pregnancy rate; and (3) a successful cryopreservation program [9]. Elective SET programs should be implemented gradually, in distinct clinical phases, with judicious selection based on patient attributes, embryo quality and professional organization algorithms modified by clinical experience [47]. Physicians should obtain informed consent from couples prior to undergoing eSET and physicians should recognize that personal, financial, societal and regulatory influences might affect the couple's decision to undergo eSET.

When the aforementioned essentials are applied, eSET strategies may result in a similar ongoing pregnancy rate to double embryo transfer (DET) with at least half the twinning rate [48–53]. In total, the application of eSET yielded an ongoing pregnancy rate of approximately 35% (range: 27–61%) and nearly eliminated multiple gestations.

Elective single embryo transfer

In a study of women < 34 years old undergoing their first ART cycle, Gerris *et al.* prospectively randomized 53 women producing ≥ 2 top quality embryos to either eSET or DET. Among those assigned to the eSET, the ongoing pregnancy rate was 38% (10/26), whereas the DET ongoing pregnancy rate was 74% (20/27) [48]. In this study, the corresponding twinning rates were 10% for eSET and 30% for DET.

Meanwhile, Thurin *et al.* performed a prospective randomized multicenter trial at 11 Scandinavian IVF programs to compare the more standard fresh cycle DET to a strategy of eSET with a fresh high-grade embryo, followed by a subsequent transfer of a single frozen-thawed embryo if the fresh cycle was unsuccessful [49]. This study enrolled women < 36 years undergoing their first or second IVF cycle having two "good quality embryos" as defined by the following: < 20% fragmentation; 4–6 cells on culture day 2 or 6–10 cells on culture day 3. Pregnancies resulting in at least one live birth occurred in 43% (142/331) of women undergoing DET compared with 39% (128/330) undergoing the eSET strategy (difference: 4%; 95% CI: −3%–12%). Ultimately, the multiple birth rate in this study was significantly higher among the DET group (DET: 33%, eSET: 1%; $p < 0.001$).

Similarly, van Montfoort *et al.* randomized 308 unselected patients immediately prior to the first embryo transfer to either eSET or DET [50]. In this study, the investigators included a non-randomized comparison arm of subjects undergoing the "standard transfer policy," in which the transfer of a single embryo occurred when patient age was <38 years and when ≥ 1 good embryo was available, otherwise two embryos were transferred. In this study, the ongoing pregnancy rate among those randomized to receive an eSET was significantly lower when compared with those randomized to DET (eSET: 21%, DET: 40%; $p < 0.05$). Notably, the resultant twin gestation rate was eliminated by this practice (DET: 21%, eSET: 0%; $p < 0.05$). When these results were compared with the standard embryo transfer policy of the practice, there was no difference in ongoing pregnancy rates between groups (eSET: 33%, DET: 30%; $p > 0.05$). Likewise, there was a corresponding reduction in the twin pregnancy rate with eSET (eSET: 3%, DET: 22%; $p < 0.05$). The authors concluded that eSET was an effective method of reducing twin pregnancy rates, but that this practice results in approximately a 50% reduction in the ongoing pregnancy rate with a single transfer cycle.

Martikainen *et al.* either randomized women undergoing their first or second ART cycle having ≥ 4 "good quality embryos" to either eSET or DET at four IVF centers. In this study, the investigators found that when frozen-thawed embryo cycles were incorporated into the treatment regimen, there were no differences in the cumulative pregnancy rates between groups (eSET: 47.3%, DET: 58.6%; $p = \mathrm{NS}$) [52]. As in other studies, there was a negligible twinning rate among those undergoing eSET (4%).

Additional cohort studies demonstrating the successful employment of eSET have reported similar results to those abovementioned [54, 55]. At first inspection, eSET seems to be less effective than DET in terms of ongoing pregnancy rates; however, when a heightened selection process is employed, in conjunction with a successful cryopreservation program, these rates can be comparable to DET.

Elective single blastocyst transfers

Improvements in embryo culture have allowed for more than 50% of all zygotes to develop into blastocysts [56]. A distinct advantage of extended culturing has been the longitudinal assessment of embryos beyond genomic activation [57]. This prolonged observation allows a more accurate determination of the embryonic implantation potential and as a result for the selection of the most suitable embryos to transfer [58]. This determination of implantation potential may be the most critical for eSET. Thus, there has been debate regarding whether the blastocyst stage should be favored over early cleavage stage embryos for eSET.

A recent Cochrane review of nine randomized controlled clinical trials comparing blastocyst stage with cleavage stage embryo transfers found significant improvements in the live birth rate by performing blastocyst transfers (Day 2/3: 29.4%, Day 5/6: 36.0%; OR: 1.35; 95% CI: 1.05–1.74) [58]. Interestingly, among good prognosis patients there were no significant differences between groups (OR: 1.50; 95% CI: 0.79–2.84) [53].

By increasing the implantation rates using blastocysts, it has been suggested that fewer embryos need to be transferred to maintain a comparable, satisfactorily high pregnancy rate [59]. Milki et al. demonstrated a 53% ongoing pregnancy rate after a fresh single blastocyst transfer and a cumulative pregnancy rate of 68% when thaw cycles were included [59]. Similarly, Gardner et al. reported an ongoing pregnancy rate of 61% (14/23) among those randomized to receive a single blastocyst and 76% (19/25) among those receiving two blastocysts [53]. A Japanese group reported similar outcomes [60]. Most importantly, this strategy resulted in no cases of twinning among subjects undergoing eSET, while those receiving two blastocysts had a twinning rate of 48%.

Another study comparing single with double blastocyst transfers noted comparable clinical pregnancy and implantation rates (single: 49%, double: 44%), but significantly lower multiple pregnancy rates in the single blastocyst transfer group (single: 3%, double: 42%; $p < 0.01$) [61]. Further evidence supporting the value of performing single blastocyst transfers came from a 2006 study [40, 58]. In this prospective, randomized trial of day 3 versus day 5

transfers in women < 36 years of age, there was a significantly higher delivery rate in patients receiving blastocyst stage day 5 embryos (32%) versus cleavage stage day 3 embryo transfers (22%) (relative risk [RR]: 1.5; 95% CI: 1.0–2.1).

These results suggest that the transfer of a single blastocyst, because of its increased implantation efficiency, does not result in a decrement in implantation and clinical pregnancy rates. More importantly, this strategy virtually eliminates the twinning rate. Resultantly the blastocyst stage may be the optimal timing for eSET. However, many do not perform day 5 blastocyst transfers as a routine because of the reduction in embryo number that occurs with growing embryos to the blastocyst stage, in addition to the poor cryopreservation results with blastocysts [9, 62]. Ultimately, one must conclude that each ART practice must determine its own best approach.

Selection criteria for elective single embryo transfer

Opinions vary as to whether eSET should be accompanied by a strategy of optimized embryo selection. If embryos are too strictly defined, eSET will be applied infrequently and it will have a limited impact on the twinning rate. On the other hand, if only one embryo is transferred without using any selection criteria, the pregnancy rates would likely drop below an acceptable standard. Labeling an embryo as "a top quality, high implantation potential embryo" remains a clinically useful, but an intrinsically oversimplified, representation of graduated implantation potential.

Oocyte and embryo characteristics

Efforts have been made to correlate implantation potential with oocyte and embryo characteristics [49, 52, 63]. Nonetheless, morphological characteristics cannot entirely predict whether a particular embryo will implant, as they do not disclose all the information contained within the embryo. It remains difficult to draw firm conclusions between embryo quality and likelihood of success with eSET for a couple of reasons. First, some studies have used varying descriptions of the stated embryo selection criteria [64–66]. Second, study populations have varied. Some investigations examined unselected populations, while others were limited to subsets of the ART population, typically those with a very good prognosis [9, 51, 66–70]. Therefore, comparisons may be confounded and direct conclusions may be hard to draw.

Preimplantation genetic screening

Originally developed to identify embryonic aneuploidy prior to transfer, preimplantation genetic screening (PGS) has been suggested to improve the eSET outcomes, yet studies examining its use have not yielded convincing results. The limited utility demonstrated thus far has been in the reduction of early pregnancy losses. Munné *et al.* recently reported a significant reduction in pregnancy losses prior to 20 weeks' gestation, particularly among women > 40 years old (PGS: 22.2%, no PGS: 40.6%, $p < 0.001$) [70]. The utility of PGS in eSET remains to be fully determined, as there remain limitations to its use [71, 72]. These limitations include an incomplete assessment of all chromosomes and inherent inaccuracy, in part because of embryo mosaicism (which occurs in up to 50% of embryos), both of which may lead to misdiagnoses [42]. Additionally, embryo biopsy may damage the embryo, impairing its ability to implant and to survive, which may significantly lower live birth rates [42]. However, future technological developments in PGS with embryos or blastocysts may well improve the utility of this procedure.

Selection based on patient age

The patient's age needs to be considered when deciding whether to proceed with eSET or with multiple embryo transfer. Schieve *et al.* demonstrated that among good prognosis patients < 35 years old, transferring three embryos rather than two did not increase pregnancy rates [42]. Among women

≥ 35 years old, the live birth rates were increased if > 2 embryos were transferred. However, multiple birth rates were also increased and varied by age and the number of embryos transferred. With DET, multiple birth rates were 22.7% (age: 20–29), 19.7% (age: 30–34), 11.6% (age: 35–39) and 10.8% (age: 40–44) [73]. When three embryos were transferred, the multiple birth rates increased to 45.7% (age: 20–29), 39.8% (age: 30–34), 29.4% (age: 35–39) and 25% (age: 40–44). For women ≥ 40 years old, the transfer of up to five embryos was associated with slightly higher pregnancy rates. Conversely, in poor prognosis patients (those without supernumerary embryos for cryopreservation), the transfer of two embryos in patients < 35 years of age did increase pregnancy rates. Likewise, the transfer of three to four embryos in the 35- to 39-year-old age group and four to five embryos in the 40- to 44-year-old age group also increased pregnancy rates. For American ART programs, these data confirmed the need to select the number of embryos for transfer based on patient age and embryo quality. While this study did not specifically examine eSET, the aforementioned principles would likely apply.

No single static observation gives all the information contained within an embryo. It may be more reasonable to consider a combination of observations, preferably reflecting varied aspects of implantation potential, to determine those embryos for which eSET should be applied. For example, blastomere asymmetry and multinucleation may reflect aneuploidy, while both correlating with poor pregnancy outcomes. From the prevention of multiple pregnancies point of view, it seems more important to begin implementing eSET rather than wait for any final proof as to which embryo selection technique is "better," because the question will always be: better for whom?

Comparison of the USA to Europe and the World

The approach to multiple births in the USA has received substantial criticism from Europeans, who consider the US twin and triplet rates excessive [73]. Regardless of regional differences, multiple birth remains a complicated issue. Many factors, such as co-morbid conditions and lifestyle factors, affect ART prognosis, which in turn influences treatment decisions [4, 74, 75]. Moreover, in Europe ART often represents a covered benefit; whereas in the USA it often represents an out-of-pocket expense resulting in different approaches to ART [76]. Furthermore, up to 58% of patients undergoing ART preferred having a twin gestation to a singleton gestation [8, 17]. In the USA, for example, there tends to be a cost–benefit approach towards risk; whereas in Europe, many would argue that there is a precautionary principle of "better safe than sorry."

One aspect of multiple pregnancy that has not been adequately addressed includes the value of human life and the value of individuals that result when an additional baby is born. The vast majority of twin multiple pregnancies result in healthy children who produce value not only for parents but also for society. In evaluating SET this value of an additional human life that might not occur because of lower success rates or dropout rates from treatment must be considered. The value is not only subjective to families, but economically quantitative, in the sense of earning power and contribution to society. While it is difficult to specify discrete amounts, legal cases and government actions regarding the value of human life clearly set the benefit in the hundreds of thousands if not millions of dollars per individual, depending on the circumstances. While not arguing for "pregnancy at any price," this beneficial economic contribution to society of healthy (and even some "unhealthy") multiple birth babies clearly mitigates at least some of their cost. Furthermore, if the implementation of SET results in overall lower cumulative pregnancy rates from fresh and cryopreserved embryo transfer, then this will reduce the economic benefit of SET compared to transfer of more than one embryo in appropriately selected patients. United States live birth rates are higher than overall European live birth rates [74]. While the specific reasons for this difference are not clearly understood and are controversial, it is possible that

one of the reasons might be the higher utilization of SET in Europe than in the USA [76, 77].

The number of embryos transferred per cycle and the associated cycle outcomes continue to vary between the USA and Europe [77]. In 2003, 2.9 embryos were transferred per cycle in the USA compared to only 2.2 embryos transferred per cycle in Europe and the proportion of US transfer cycles utilizing one to two embryos increased from 20.4% to 38.6% between 1998 and 2002 [78, 79]. While fewer embryos are utilized, US physicians continue to transfer more embryos than their European counterparts do, where more than 68% of cycles are either eSET or DET [46, 80].

It is clear that decreasing the number of embryos transferred resulted in a dramatic reduction in the overall triplet rate in Europe (3.6% in 1997; 1% in 2003) [46, 80]. During the same time period, the European multiple delivery rate following ART likewise declined from 30% to 23% [80]. However, throughout Europe there has been wide variability in multiple pregnancy rates. The European Society for Human Reproduction and Embryology reported that the United Kingdom had a twin pregnancy rate of 26% and a triplet rate of 3%; whereas, Denmark had a twin rate of 24% and a triplet rate of only 0.4%. Sweden similarly had a triplet rate of only 0.4% [80]. In the USA, the triplet rate was similarly lowered from 4.3% in 2000 to 2.6% in 2004. Problematic, however, was that the triplet rate remained more than twofold higher than in Europe and the twin rate was largely unchanged during this time (2000: 31%, 2004: 30%) [40, 81].

Regulatory mandates and elective SET

Probably the most significant differences between the USA and Europe include the regulatory environment governing ART. The USA is comparatively less regulated than a number of developed countries throughout the world [82]. Assisted reproductive technology practices routinely performed in the USA are prohibited elsewhere, influencing views towards multiple pregnancies, eSET and cryopreservation. Some countries have legislated maximal embryo transfer numbers and considered breaches as felonies [76, 83]. Some countries prohibit embryo cryopreservation for more than a pre-specified number of years, after which time embryos must be discarded by law [82, 84].

Europeans generally tend to accept, support and promote a much stronger regulatory environment with mandatory clinical limitations than their US counterparts [6]. For example, an attempt to refute Europe's most restrictive ART laws in Italy failed, despite evidence that it has negatively affected ART outcomes [69, 76]. The more aggressive drive towards eSET in Europe is a further example for the political discrepancy between American and European authorities advocating for legal mandates in order to further decrease the incidence of ART-conceived multiple pregnancies [85].

Solutions to the problem of multiple births in ART

The compelling problem with moving to eSET is "Can the reduction from a three- to two-embryo transfer (which has largely been accepted and successfully employed) be extrapolated to a two- to one-embryo transfer paradigm?" This is certainly not the case in an indiscriminate and linear way. There are many solutions to the multiple birth problem in ART, including voluntary guidelines or legislative mandates for embryo transfer, increasing physician acceptance of eSET, or increasing patient demand for eSET. Multifetal pregnancy reduction is an acceptable and successful approach to multifetal pregnancy only when strategies to reduce multifetal pregnancy have been implemented but are not successful in individual cases.

Reduce the number of embryos transferred

A major and immediately achievable way to reduce multiple birth rate is to continue to reduce the number of embryos transferred. From a medical perspective, it might also be possible to improve the quality of embryos transferred through enhanced embryo assessment, blastocyst transfers and newer technologies to assess embryos such as complete genomic hybridization and proteomics. Additionally, limiting the number of embryos can be accomplished by reducing patient demand through education, a voluntary change in professional guidelines and/or government regulation.

Legislation may have unintended consequences for numerous reasons. First, patients require individualized treatment to attain an optimal outcome. Second, technology evolves more rapidly than legislation. Third, absolute limits may result in reproductive tourism, or the traveling of patients from one jurisdiction/country/region to another in order to obtain the services desired. Lastly, legislative mandates are discriminatory, involving medicine and politics, and unintentionally criminalize medicine. Thus, it is likely best not to legislate, but rather to leave medical decisions to medical professionals and their patients. The Centers for Disease Control has concurred with this notion, issuing the following guidelines in 2000, "... Efforts are needed ... to limit the number of embryos transferred for patients receiving ART. These approaches ... should follow guidelines issued by organizations such as the American Society for Reproductive Medicine" [86].

Conclusions

Patient autonomy, the consequences of multifetal pregnancies, and issues regarding relative efficacy of cleavage stage embryos and blastocysts remain critical issues with the general application of eSET in clinical practice. Elective SET has trade-offs that may be unacceptable to many couples and their providers [9]. Thus embryo transfer decisions in the context of maintaining high pregnancy and live birth rates remain complex [87]. Cryopreservation success rates, while good, vary from program to program, especially with respect to blastocyst cryopreservation. To effectively incorporate eSET into clinical practice, it remains imperative to improve embryo selection and to perfect blastocyst cryopreservation programs [61, 88].

Furthermore, it remains essential to improve access to care in the USA and to advance our basic and clinical knowledge to increase the eSET rate. It also remains important that we learn to select patients likely to succeed with eSET based on identifiable factors. Lastly, it may be that more regulation will occur if physicians do not meet their professional responsibilities to reduce multiple pregnancies. Numerous regulations already exist around the world regulating the creation of embryos, the number of embryos transferred and embryo cryopreservation.

The practice of ART in the USA and elsewhere has important challenges on the horizon, including continually reducing multiple births. This chapter has highlighted some of the issues surrounding eSET, particularly as it relates to the US experience. In the end, the goal should be to develop future eSET strategies that result in acceptable pregnancy rates, approaching the success observed with multiple embryo transfer, while eliminating the multifetal gestation rate altogether. These efforts should be mindful of the cultural, institutional, political and economic issues affecting eSET in the USA, should be based on scientific and clinical evidence, and should bring maximum benefit to individual patients within acceptable societal moral and ethical standards.

What do we know?
1. Multiple pregnancies are associated with an increased risk of complications for both mother and babies. These complications are associated with significant medical, family and societal financial and psychological costs. As a result, it is imperative that the rate of multiple pregnancies, including twins, be reduced in the USA.
2. Elective SET can reduce the triplet pregnancies to almost zero, and twin pregnancies to approximately 5%. In selected populations, the cumulative live birth rate with eSET and subsequent transfer of cryopreserved embryos can approach that of double embryo transfer. While currently it is possible to identify some patients who are

good candidates for eSET, and those who are poor candidates, the optimal application of eSET in the entire population of patients undergoing IVF is yet to be determined.
3. Further basic science and clinical research efforts must be made to increase our ability to select embryos with both high and low implantation potential so that eSET can be utilized more effectively and more often.

What do we need to know?
1. We need to know how to identify embryos with both high and low implantation rates, and develop standardized systems for identifying these embryos.
2. We need to know which patients should always have eSET, and which can safely have two or more embryos transferred, on their first IVF cycle.
3. We need to know which counseling methods will have the most impact in encouraging patients to undergo eSET.

What do we need to do?
1. We need to begin to implement eSET on good prognosis patients. These include ooctye donation patients and those who meet the American Society for Reproductive Medicine/Society for Assisted Reproductive Technology guidelines for good prognosis patients. This includes the use of eSET for both day 3 embryo and day 5 blastocyst transfers.
2. We need to educate all of our patients about the risks of multiple pregnancy and encourage them to consider the benefits of eSET. We need to educate them that twins are not a desirable outcome from ART.
3. We need to consider ART success in terms of the birth of a healthy singleton baby from both the fresh and all cryopreserved/thaw cycles following a single ovarian stimulation cycle. Reporting of ART success rates should change so that this is emphasized as the desired outcome. Triplets should be reported as a serious complication, and twins as acceptable but much less desirable than a singleton pregnancy.

REFERENCES

1. P. C. Steptoe and R. G. Edwards, Birth after the reimplantation of a human embryo. *Lancet*, **2** (1978), 366.
2. ICMART Committee *World Report of Assisted Reproductive Technology (ART)* Fact Sheet. European Society of Human Reproduction and Embryology 2006. Available from www.eshre.com/emc.osp?pageId=807 (cited 2008 Jul 29).
3. C. J. Hogue, Successful assisted reproductive technology: the beauty of one. *Obstet. Gynecol.*, **100** (2002), 1017–1019.
4. V. C. Wright, J. Chang, G. Jeng, M. Chen, and M. Macaluso, Assisted reproductive technology surveillance – United States, 2004. *MMWR Surveill. Summ.*, **56** (2007), 1–22.
5. J.P. Toner, Progress we can be proud of: U. S. trends in assisted reproduction over the first 20 years. *Fertil. Steril.*, **78** (2002), 943–950.
6. D. D. Braat, J. A. Kremer and W. L. Nelen, Barriers and facilitators for implementation of elective single embryo transfer (eSET) in vitro fertilization (IVF). *Hum. Reprod.*, **20**: Suppl. 1 (2005), i30.
7. M. M. Alper, In vitro fertilization outcomes: why doesn't anyone get it? *Fertil. Steril.*, **81** (2004), 514–516.
8. G. L. Ryan, S. H. Zhang, A. Dokras, C. H. Syrop and B. J. Van Voorhis, The desire of infertile patients for multiple births. *Fertil. Steril.*, **81** (2004), 500–504.
9. J. M. Gerris, Single embryo transfer and IVF/ICSI outcome: a balanced appraisal. *Hum. Reprod. Update*, **11** (2005), 105–121.
10. G. L. Ryan, A. E. Sparks, C. S. Sipe *et al.*, A mandatory single blastocyst transfer policy with educational campaign in a United States IVF program reduces multiple gestation rates without sacrificing pregnancy rates. *Fertil. Steril.*, **88** (2007), 354–360.
11. G. M. Hartshorne and R. J. Lilford, Different perspectives of patients and health care professionals on the potential benefits and risks of blastocyst culture and multiple embryo transfer. *Hum. Reprod.*, **17** (2002), 1023–1030.
12. B. Blondel, M. D. Kogan, G. R. Alexander *et al.*, The impact of the increasing number of multiple births on the rates of preterm birth and low birthweight: an international study. *Am. J. Public Health*, **92** (2002), 1323–1330.
13. J. A. Martin, B. E. Hamilton, P. D. Sutton *et al.*, Births: final data for 2002. *Natl. Vital Stat. Rep.*, **52** (2003), 1–113.
14. B. Stromberg, G. Dahlquist, A. Ericson *et al.*, Neurological sequelae in children born after in-vitro fertilisation: a population-based study. *Lancet*, **359** (2002), 461–465.
15. B. Luke and M. B. Brown, The changing risk of infant mortality by gestation, plurality, and race: 1989–1991 versus 1999–2001. *Pediatrics*, **118** (2006), 2488–2497.
16. B. Luke and L. G. Keith, The contribution of singletons, twins and triplets to low birth weight, infant mortality and handicap in the United States. *J. Reprod. Med.*, **37** (1992), 661–666.
17. A. Hojgaard, L. D. Ottosen, U. Kesmodel and H. J. Ingerslev, Patient attitudes towards twin pregnancies and single embryo transfer – a questionnaire study. *Hum. Reprod.*, **22** (2007), 2673–2678.
18. B. Kallen, Congenital malformations in twins: a population study. *Acta. Genet. Med. Gemellol.* (Roma), **35** (1986), 167–178.
19. P. E. Doyle, V. Beral, B. Botting and C. J. Wale, Congenital malformations in twins in England and Wales. *J. Epidemiol. Community Health*, **45** (1991), 43–48.
20. H. B. Westergaard, A. M. Johansen, K. Erb and A. N. Andersen, Danish National In-Vitro Fertilization Registry 1994 and 1995: a controlled study of births, malformations and cytogenetic findings. *Hum. Reprod.*, **14** (1999), 1896–1902.
21. U. B. Wennerholm, C. Bergh, L. Hamberger *et al.*, Obstetric and perinatal outcome of pregnancies following intracytoplasmic sperm injection. *Hum. Reprod.*, **11** (1996), 1113–1119.
22. A. Ericson and B. Kallen, Congenital malformations in infants born after IVF: a population-based study. *Hum. Reprod.*, **16** (2001), 504–509.
23. J. A. Land, and J. L. Evers, Risks and complications in assisted reproduction techniques: Report of an ESHRE consensus meeting. *Hum. Reprod.*, **18** (2003), 455–457.
24. A. G. Sutcliffe and M. Ludwig, Outcome of assisted reproduction. *Lancet*, **370** (2007), 351–359.
25. H. A. Ghazi, C. Spielberger and B. Kallen, Delivery outcome after infertility–a registry study. *Fertil. Steril.*, **55** (1991), 726–732.
26. J. L. Zhu, O. Basso, C. Obel, C. Bille and J. Olsen, Infertility, infertility treatment, and congenital malformations: Danish national birth cohort. *BMJ*, **333** (2006), 679.
27. Multiple gestation pregnancy. The ESHRE Capri Workshop Group. *Hum. Reprod.*, **15** (2000), 1856–1864.
28. M. van Wely, M. Twisk, B. W. Mol and F. van der Veen, Is twin pregnancy necessarily an adverse outcome of

assisted reproductive technologies? *Hum. Reprod.*, **21** (2006), 2736–2738.

29. M. Garel and B. Blondel, Assessment at 1 year of the psychological consequences of having triplets. *Hum. Reprod.*, **7** (1992), 729–732.

30. M. Garel, C. Salobir and B. Blondel, Psychological consequences of having triplets: a 4-year follow-up study. *Fertil. Steril.*, **67** (1997), 1162–1165.

31. P. Doyle, The outcome of multiple pregnancy. *Hum. Reprod.*, **11**: Suppl. 4 (1996), 110–117.

32. C. Glazebrook, C. Sheard, S. Cox, M. Oates and G. Ndukwe, Parenting stress in first-time mothers of twins and triplets conceived after in vitro fertilization. *Fertil. Steril.*, **81** (2004), 505–511.

33. C. Sheard, S. Cox, M. Oates, G. Ndukwe and C. Glazebrook, Impact of a multiple, IVF birth on postpartum mental health: a composite analysis. *Hum. Reprod.*, **22** (2007), 2058–2065.

34. T. Jain, B. L. Harlow and M. D. Hornstein, Insurance coverage and outcomes of in vitro fertilization. *N. Engl. J. Med.*, **347** (2002), 661–666.

35. G. M. Chambers, M. G. Chapman, N. Grayson, M. Shanahan and E. A. Sullivan, Babies born after ART treatment cost more than non-ART babies: a cost analysis of inpatient birth-admission costs of singleton and multiple gestation pregnancies. *Hum. Reprod.*, **22** (2007), 3108–3115.

36. T. L. Callahan, J. E. Hall, S. L. Ettner *et al.*, The economic impact of multiple-gestation pregnancies and the contribution of assisted-reproduction techniques to their incidence. *N. Engl. J. Med.*, **331** (1994), 244–249.

37. E. D. Levens, Variables affecting the decision for numbers of embryos transferred. *Fertil. Steril.*, **88** (2007), 760–761.

38. E. R. Norwitz, V. Edusa and J. S. Park, Maternal physiology and complications of multiple pregnancy. *Semin. Perinatol.*, **29** (2005), 338–348.

39. C. Bergh, Single embryo transfer: a mini-review. *Hum. Reprod.*, **20** (2005), 323–327.

40. Assisted reproductive technology success rates 2004: national summary and fertility clinic reports. In K. E. Toomey, ed. (Atlanta: U. S. Department of Health and Human Services, Centers for Disease Control and Prevention, 2006). www.cdc.gov/ART/ART2005.

41. Assisted reproductive technology success rates 1995: national summary and fertility clinic reports. In J. S. Marks, ed. (Atlanta: U. S. Department of Health and Human Services, Centers for Disease

Control and Prevention, 1997). www.cdc.gov/ART/ArchivedARTPDFs/95eastern.pdf.

42. L. A. Schieve, H. B. Peterson, S. F. Meikle *et al.*, Live-birth rates and multiple-birth risk using in vitro fertilization. *JAMA*, **282** (1999), 1832–1838.

43. Society for Assisted Reproductive Technology, American Society For Reproductive Medicine Practice Committees. Guidelines on number of embryos transferred. *Fertil. Steril.*, **86** (2006), 551–552.

44. J. E. Stern, M. I. Cedars, T. Jain *et al.*, Assisted reproductive technology practice patterns and the impact of embryo transfer guidelines in the United States. *Fertil. Steril.*, **88** (2007), 275–282.

45. Assisted reproductive technology success rates 2003: national summary and fertility clinic reports. In F. E. Thompson, ed. (Atlanta: U. S. Department of Health and Human Services, Centers for Disease Control and Prevention, 2005). www.cdc.gov/ART/ART2003.

46. A. N. Andersen, V. Goossens, L. Gianaroli *et al.*, Assisted reproductive technology in Europe, 2003. Results generated from European registers by ESHRE. *Hum. Reprod.*, **22** (2007), 1513–1525.

47. D. Adamson and V. Baker, Multiple births from assisted reproductive technologies: a challenge that must be met. *Fertil. Steril.*, **81** (2004), 517–522.

48. J. Gerris, D. De Neubourg, K. Mangelschots *et al.*, Prevention of twin pregnancy after in-vitro fertilization or intracytoplasmic sperm injection based on strict embryo criteria: a prospective randomized clinical trial. *Hum. Reprod.*, **14** (1999), 2581–2587.

49. A. Thurin, J. Hausken, T. Hillensjo *et al.*, Elective single-embryo transfer versus double-embryo transfer in in vitro fertilization. *N. Engl. J. Med.*, **351** (2004), 2392–2402.

50. A. P. van Montfoort, A. A. Fiddelers, J. M. Janssen *et al.*, In unselected patients, elective single embryo transfer prevents all multiples, but results in significantly lower pregnancy rates compared with double embryo transfer: a randomized controlled trial. *Hum. Reprod.*, **21** (2006), 338–343.

51. H. G. Lukassen, D. D. Braat, A. M. Wetzels *et al.*, Two cycles with single embryo transfer versus one cycle with double embryo transfer: a randomized controlled trial. *Hum. Reprod.*, **20** (2005), 702–708.

52. H. Martikainen, A. Tiitinen, C. Tomas *et al.*, One versus two embryo transfer after IVF and ICSI: a randomized study. *Hum. Reprod.*, **16** (2001), 1900–1903.

53. D. K. Gardner, E. Surrey, D. Minjarez *et al.*, Single blastocyst transfer: a prospective randomized trial. *Fertil. Steril.*, **81** (2004), 551–555.

54. G. M. Jones, A. O. Trounson, N. Lolatgis and C. Wood, Factors affecting the success of human blastocyst development and pregnancy following in vitro fertilization and embryo transfer. *Fertil. Steril.*, **70** (1998), 1022–1029.

55. M. C. Scholtes and G. H. Zeilmaker, Blastocyst transfer in day-5 embryo transfer depends primarily on the number of oocytes retrieved and not on age. *Fertil. Steril.*, **69** (1998), 78–83.

56. D. K. Gardner, P. Vella, M. Lane *et al.*, Culture and transfer of human blastocysts increases implantation rates and reduces the need for multiple embryo transfers. *Fertil. Steril.*, **69** (1998), 84–88.

57. R. Z. Karaki, S. S. Samarraie, N. A. Younis, T. M. Lahloub and M. H. Ibrahim, Blastocyst culture and transfer: a step toward improved in vitro fertilization outcome. *Fertil. Steril.*, **77** (2002), 114–118.

58. D. A. Blake, C. M. Farquhar, N. Johnson and M. Proctor, Cleavage stage versus blastocyst stage embryo transfer in assisted conception. *Cochrane Database Syst. Rev.*, **17** (2007), CD002118.

59. A. A. Milki, M. D. Hinckley, L. M. Westphal and B. Behr, Elective single blastocyst transfer. *Fertil. Steril.*, **81** (2004), 1697–1698.

60. N. Yoshioka, A. Egashira, M. Motoisha *et al.*, Single selected blastocyst transfers maintained pregnancy outcome and reduced multiple pregnancies. *Fertil. Steril.*, **82** (2004), S198-S199.

61. E. G. Papanikolaou, M. Camus, E. M. Kolibianakis *et al.*, In vitro fertilization with single blastocyst-stage versus single cleavage-stage embryos. *N. Engl. J. Med.*, **354** (2006), 1139–1146.

62. P. Terriou, C. Sapin, C. Giorgetti *et al.*, Embryo score is a better predictor of pregnancy than the number of transferred embryos or female age. *Fertil. Steril.*, **75** (2001), 525–531.

63. A. Salumets, C. Hyden-Granskog, S. Makinen *et al.*, Early cleavage predicts the viability of human embryos in elective single embryo transfer procedures. *Hum. Reprod.*, **18** (2003), 821–825.

64. J. Gerris, E. Van Royen, D. De Neubourg *et al.*, Impact of single embryo transfer on the overall and twin-pregnancy rates of an IVF/ICSI programme. *Reprod. Biomed. Online*, **2** (2001), 172–177.

65. J. Gerris, D. De Neubourg, K. Mangelschots *et al.*, Elective single day 3 embryo transfer halves the twinning rate without decrease in the ongoing pregnancy rate of an IVF/ICSI programme. *Hum. Reprod.*, **17** (2002), 2626–2631.

66. S. Coskun, J. Hollanders, S. Al-Hassan *et al.*, Day 5 versus day 3 embryo transfer: a controlled randomized trial. *Hum. Reprod.*, **15** (2000), 1947–1952.

67. J. L. Frattarelli, M. P. Leondires, J. L. McKeeby, B. T. Miller and J. H. Segars, Blastocyst transfer decreases multiple pregnancy rates in vitro fertilization cycles: a randomized controlled trial. *Fertil. Steril.*, **79** (2003), 228–230.

68. D. De Neubourg, K. Mangelschots, E. Van Royen *et al.*, Impact of patients' choice for single embryo transfer of a top quality embryo versus double embryo transfer in the first IVF/ICSI cycle. *Hum. Reprod.*, **17** (2002), 2621–2625.

69. L. Rienzi, F. Ubaldi, M. Iacobelli *et al.*, Day 3 embryo transfer with combined evaluation at the pronuclear and cleavage stages compares favourably with day 5 blastocyst transfer. *Hum. Reprod.*, **17** (2002), 1852–1855.

70. S. Munné, J. Fischer, A. Warner *et al.*, Preimplantation genetic diagnosis significantly reduces pregnancy loss in infertile couples: a multicenter study. *Fertil. Steril.*, **85** (2006), 326–332.

71. M. Li, C. M. DeUgarte, M. Surrey *et al.*, Fluorescence in situ hybridization reanalysis of day-6 human blastocysts diagnosed with aneuploidy on day 3. *Fertil. Steril.*, **84** (2005), 1395–1400.

72. C. Staessen, P. Platteau, E. Van Assche *et al.*, Comparison of blastocyst transfer with or without preimplantation genetic diagnosis for aneuploidy screening in couples with advanced maternal age: a prospective randomized controlled trial. *Hum. Reprod.*, **19** (2004), 2849–2858.

73. A. Murdoch, Triplets and embryo transfer policy. *Hum. Reprod.*, **12** (1997), 88–92.

74. G. D. Adamson, J. de Mouzon, P. Lancaster *et al.*, World collaborative report on in vitro fertilization, 2000. *Fertil. Steril.*, **85** (2006), 1586–1622.

75. M. A. Hassan and S. R. Killick, Negative lifestyle is associated with a significant reduction in fecundity. *Fertil. Steril.*, **81** (2004), 384–392.

76. N. Gleicher, A. Weghofer and D. Barad, A formal comparison of the practice of assisted reproductive technologies between Europe and the USA. *Hum. Reprod.*, **21** (2006), 1945–1950.

77. N. Gleicher, A. Weghofer and D. Barad, Update on the comparison of assisted reproduction outcomes

between Europe and the USA: the 2002 data. *Fertil. Steril.*, **87** (2007), 1301–1305.

78. A. N. Andersen, L. Gianaroli, R. Felberbaum, J. de Mouzon and K. G. Nygren, Assisted reproductive technology in Europe, 2002. Results generated from European registers by ESHRE. *Hum. Reprod.*, **21** (2006), 1680–1697.

79. Assisted reproductive technology success rates 2002: national summary and fertility clinic reports. In D. F. Stroup, ed. (Atlanta: U.S. Department of Health and Human Services, Centers for Disease Control and Prevention, 2004). www.cdc.gov/ART/ART02/.

80. K. G. Nygren and A. N. Andersen, Assisted reproductive technology in Europe, 1997. Results generated from European registers by ESHRE. European IVF-Monitoring Programme (EIM), for the European Society of Human Reproduction and Embryology (ESHRE). *Hum. Reprod.*, **16** (2001), 384–391.

81. Assisted reproductive technology success rates 2000: national summary and fertility clinic reports. In J. S. Marks, ed. (Atlanta: U.S. Department of Health and Human Services Centers for Disease Control and Prevention, 2002). www.cdc.gov/ART/ArchivedARTPDFs/ART2000.pdf.

82. Human Fertilisation and Embryology Act. (1990).

83. German Act for the Protection of Embryos. *Official Gazette*, 1 (1990), 2746.

84. L. Hamberger and M. Wikland, Regulations and results concerning assisted reproduction in Sweden. *J. Assist. Reprod. Genet.*, **10** (1993), 243–245.

85. D. Healy, Damaged babies from assisted reproductive technologies: focus on the BESST (birth emphasizing a successful singleton at term) outcome. *Fertil. Steril.*, **81** (2004), 512–513.

86. Centers for Disease Control and Prevention (CDC), Contribution of assisted reproductive technology and ovulation-inducing drugs to triplet and higher-order multiple births–United States, 1980–1997. *MMWR Morb. Mortal Wkly Rep.*, **49** (2000), 535–538.

87. M. D'Alton, Infertility and the desire for multiple births. *Fertil. Steril.*, **81** (2004), 523–525.

88. E. G. Papanikolaou, E. D'Haeseleer, G. Verheyen *et al.*, Live birth rate is significantly higher after blastocyst transfer than after cleavage-stage embryo transfer when at least four embryos are available on day 3 of embryo culture. A randomized prospective study. *Hum. Reprod.*, **20** (2005), 3198–3203.

23

A European perspective on single embryo transfer

André Van Steirteghem

Introduction

After accepting a request to contribute to this monograph on single embryo transfer (SET), a European perspective on SET, I find myself reluctant to write on just a European perspective. The question might be asked as to whether the topic should be limited to a specific area of the world or whether it should be applicable everywhere. In this chapter, I'll discuss a number of recommendations on how to promote the practice of elective SET (eSET).

Elective SET was introduced in the last decade and this monograph covers several aspects of this strategy in the treatment of infertile couples. Assisted reproductive technology (ART) has been around for 30 years since the birth of Louise Brown (25 July 1978) and it seems appropriate not to forget that the reason for ART is to give childless couples an opportunity of having a healthy child [1, 2]. Having children has been for most couples throughout history a strong desire and not being able to fulfil this childwish is a source of grief and suffering. The prevalence of non-voluntary childlessness is quite high; with approximately one out of every ten couples experiencing problems in having children without medical intervention.

Over the last fifty years several major developments contributed to the fact that ART became possible and also more effective. In the 1950s and 1960s major advances were made in reproductive endocrinology as well as in surgical (especially micro-surgical) techniques to correct tubal infertility. At the end of the 1970s and during the 1980s, in vitro fertilization (IVF) and embryo transfer became more and more established to circumvent female-factor and idiopathic infertility [1]. The beginning of the 1990s saw the introduction of intracytoplasmic sperm injection (ICSI), which made it possible to alleviate even severe male-factor infertility [3], and preimplantation genetic diagnosis (PGD) for couples at high risk for a child with a genetic disease [4].

Outcome of ART

The outcome of any infertility treatment has to be evaluated in terms of number of healthy children born, with singleton children being the preferential outcome [5, 6]. Nobody knows exactly how many children have been born after ART but it is fair to estimate a number of at least two million. This is of course very positive but we have to add to this positive statement that around half of this high number of children are not from singleton pregnancies but are mostly from twin gestations and a few from triplet and higher-order pregnancies. This is due to the fact that in IVF/ICSI the number of embryos transferred has been two, three, four or sometimes even more. It has been routine practice to transfer more than one embryo in order to enhance the

Single Embryo Transfer, ed. J. Gerris, G. D. Adamson, P. De Sutter and C. Racowsky. Published by Cambridge University Press.
© Cambridge University Press 2009.

chance of pregnancy, which increases with the number of embryos transferred. A major drawback is, of course, that the number of multiple gestations increases. Reducing the number of embryos to two will all but eliminate triplets but the number of twins remains high. It is clear by now that in order to avoid multiple ART pregnancies there is only one option – that is to transfer a single embryo, in other words to carry out eSET.

Looking back over the history of ART, it is surprising that so much emphasis was put on increasing the pregnancy rate without fully considering that multiple pregnancy is not a desired outcome. Only recently has more emphasis been placed on the way ART results are expressed. All practioners should be convinced that the only proper way to express outcome is to mention the chance a couple has of having a healthy child *per treatment cycle*. Surrogate outcome measures are not what are of interest to a couple seeking treatment for their long-standing infertility. Expressing results per oocyte retrieval, or per embryo transfer as well as reporting positive human chorionic gonadotropin (hCG), the presence of a fetal sac (even with positive heartbeat), or even ongoing pregnancy is not what interests the prospective parents. The primary interest of a couple consulting for infertility is not that they have an "x" percentage implantation chance, but that they want (and have the right) to know their chance of having a healthy child.

Several large-scale studies and reports from especially the last decade have indicated that the major negative outcome from all infertility treatments is multiple gestation [7]. Overall the health of ART children at birth and later in life indicates that there is a slight increase in malformations, from 2% to 3% in naturally conceived children to 3% to 4% in ART children. It is also clear that there is no difference between health of children conceived by conventional IVF or ICSI. Even singleton ART children seem to have more problems than spontaneously conceived children in terms of lower term of gestation and weight at birth [8]. The number of singleton children conceived after eSET is increasing and follow-up of these children will provide evidence of

whether their outcome is similar or different from singleton ART children which were not conceived after eSET (see Chapter 1).

So far studies of older ART children indicate that psychomotor development and health is similar to naturally conceived children. Follow-up studies at birth and later in life need to continue in the future to detect rare diseases such as genomic imprinting defects. The oldest ART children are now at an age that they will be able to have children themselves. Both male and female infertility may have some genetic factors involved and this may be transmitted to the children. Information on outcome as complete and reliable as possible is important in the counseling of prospective parents who need ART [9, 10].

How to put SET into practice

It is obvious that the only way to avoid the iatrogenic epidemic of multiple pregnancies including twins is to transfer a single embryo. This obvious knowledge is and has been there since the beginning of ART but it is only in the last decade that the practice of SET has increased. It started with the initiative of a number of individual centers especially in Northern Europe and in the Low Countries, especially in Belgium and these centers should be recognized as the pioneers of eSET. The adoption of eSET by more and more centers may help to reduce the multiple pregnancy rate in those centers but experience has shown that the overall decrease in twinning in a certain country or region is not assured by such initiatives of individual centres. To illustrate this I want to describe both as a privileged observer and participant what happened in Belgium. Since the mid 1980s there has been a voluntary registration of ART practice and this indicated that overall the delivery rate (slightly less than 20% per started cycle) indicated between 25% and 30% twin deliveries and 2–5% triplet deliveries. This remained constant over the years despite that in the majority of transfers a shift from three to two embryos being replaced occurred. The registration became mandatory in 1999 for all licensed ART centers (18 of them are fully licensed B centers, while a number of them – A centers – can do ART until oocyte retrieval). Notably, two centers in Belgium (Algemeen Ziekenhuis Middelheim and Universitair Ziekenhuis Gent) pioneered the practice of SET and were able to demonstrate that SET was working when a single top quality embryo was transferred, especially in young patients. For these centers, the twinning rate decreased without any real impact on the number of twins being born in Belgium as a whole. Around that time a dialogue was started between the Belgian centers and the health authorities. Before this the B centers all agreed on a common policy to propose. The health authorities were willing to provide a better reimbursement for ART on condition that the twinning rate would be reduced from 25% to 30% to 10% over a 2-year period and that triplets would almost disappear. This reduction in twin and triplet births would reduce the cost of care for prematurely born babies and this money would be available for extra ART funding. A proposal, accepted by all centers, was finally put into a law in mid 2003 and involved the reimbursement of laboratory procedures for six cycles for patients up to the age of 43. Before 2003 the Belgian social security system reimbursed clinical procedures and fertility drugs but not the ART laboratory procedures, which were paid for out-of-pocket by patients. The number of embryos transferred had to be reduced for patients younger than 36 to one in the first two cycles and a maximum of two in the subsequent four cycles; for patients between 36 and less than 40 the number of embryos for transfer was two in the first two cycles and a maximum of three in the subsequent four cycles. There are no restrictions on the number of embryos transferred for patients between 40 and 43 years. One year after the introduction of this practice in Belgium (and after well over 10 000 treatment cycles) the twinning rate had fallen to about 10% (Van Landuyt *et al.* [11] describes the experience of the first year in the author's center). This Belgian approach involved a mandatory, maximum number of embryos to transfer policy. In theory, the same could be achieved if all centers voluntarily adopted this practice, without legal requirements, although I personally doubt that this will work as well. I will illustrate this by another example of the Belgian practice. For patients under 36 there was an exception allowed in the regulation: if no top quality embryo was available two embryos could be transferred in the second cycle. As a clinical embryologist with three decades of experience I think it is fair to say that this "non-availability of at least one good quality embryo" in this young group of patients would be very exceptional. However, this "exceptional" practice of transferring two embryos in young patients occurred in more than half of the second cycles, something I do not attribute to a sudden epidemic of bad quality embryos in this age group! This illustrates that for public health measures to work one can, unfortunately I would say, not include exceptional measures. Although in theory I am in favor of retaining freedom of practice in medicine, rather strict regulation is sometimes needed for measures to be successful.

How to select the embryo for eSET

If SET is to be successful the embryologist should select from the cohort of available embryos the embryo for transfer which has the highest chance of implantation and ultimately leading to the birth of a singleton healthy child. The procedures of in vitro culture are well standardized and culture media are commercially available. Initially a short-time culture of typically 2 days was the standard but since the availability of sequential culture media embryo transfer is currently also done on day 3, day 4, day 5 and day 6 of in vitro culture. Nowadays few centers will transfer oocytes and sperm (gamete intrafallopian transfer – GIFT) or fertilized oocytes (zygote intrafallopian transfer – ZIFT). Morphological criteria are well established to follow fertilization and embryo development: presence of two pronuclei and two polar bodies on day 1 as a sign of normal fertilization, 2- to 4-cell embryos on day 2, 8-cell embryos on day 3, morulae on day 4 and blastocysts on day 5 or 6. Besides the number of blastomeres other morphological criteria include the presence of a single nucleus in each of the blastomeres and the percentage of anucleate cytoplasmic fragments. Different scoring systems are available for developing embryos, morulae and blastocysts (della Ragione *et al.* [12] is one example of scoring of embryos). For SET the clinical embryologist will select the "best" embryo and it has been well documented that the better the morphology of the transferred embryo, the higher the chance of success. Regarding the day of SET a meta-analysis has indicated that transfer at the blastocyst stage resulted in higher chance of birth than transfer on day 3, usually around the 8-cell stage. These studies involved the transfer of fresh embryos and did not include the additional deliveries occurring after transfer of frozen-thawed embryos from the same cycle [13]. The role of cryopreservation in SET practice will be discussed later.

There is agreement that morphological criteria are subjective and are not perfect. For this reason several attempts have been made to improve the selection of embryos. Two of these approaches will be discussed: non-invasive testing of culture media and invasive testing of embryos to select the euploid embryos and discard the embryos with aneuploidy.

The metabolism of a preimplantation embryo can be examined by *analyzing the culture medium* of the developing embryo. Extensive research has been carried out in order to examine whether it would be possible to detect, by analyzing the content of the culture medium, the embryo which has the highest chance of implantation. Advances have been made in understanding the metabolism of different embryos but so far this approach can only be considered as a research tool and is not yet to be considered in clinical practice [14].

Preimplantation genetic diagnosis was developed in the early 1990s and has been introduced into clinical practice. Preimplantation genetic diagnosis *stricto sensu* can be considered as an early form of prenatal diagnosis for couples at high risk of having a child affected by a genetic disease (monogenic or chromosomal disorder). The genetic diagnosis is carried out on a blastomere removed from an 8-cell embryo (blastomere biopsy). Two techniques

are mostly used: polymerase chain reaction (PCR) for monogenic diseases and fluorescent *in situ* hybridisation (FISH) for chromosomal disorders (translocations or inversions or sex determination for X-linked disorders) [4]. When FISH was carried out for 5 to 9 chromosomes it became clear that many human embryos were aneuploid for one or more of the tested chromosomes. Aneuploidy of embryos increased with the age of the female patient. The percentage of aneuploid embryos was always high and varied between 30% and 70% of the embryos. This observation led to the introduction of *preimplantation genetic screening* (PGS) or PGD by aneuploidy screening (PGD-AS). The observation of the high frequency of aneuploid embryos led to the hypothesis that the results of IVF/ICSI may be improved if only euploid embryos are replaced. The question to be answered in a proper study would be: among patients requiring IVF with SET (as part of what we are discussing now) is the chance of having a child increased when PGS is carried out in comparison to the situation when no PGS is carried out? A similar question needs to be answered for all indications where PGS is applied. The value of PGS as a clinical tool is currently a matter of great controversy among the ART community. A number of groups, who were the first to apply PGS, claim that the value of PGS is established by the many observational studies they reported in the literature. So far, only two controlled studies have been carried out for PGS in patients with advanced age [15, 16]. Neither of these two randomized controlled trials (RCTs) indicated that there was an improvement in outcome when PGS was done: in the Brussels' study [15] the delivery rate was similar in both groups, while in the Amsterdam study [16] the chance of having a child was decreased in couples who had PGS. The Mastenbroek study, published in the *New England Journal of Medicine*, was severely criticized by the groups in the USA promoting PGS as valid clinical practice. Without wishing to propagate the controversy surrounding this area, it seems to me that the burden of proof that PGS works must lie with the groups who advocate its routine use. Instead of criticizing the published

RCTs it is up to these groups to carry out rigorous clinical trials where the valid hypothesis of PGS is tested. For the time being it seems appropriate to label PGS as clinical research and not as routine clinical practice.

The results of an RCT of PGS in SET were reported at the 2007 ESHRE Meeting in Lyon by Staessen *et al.* (Abstract O-079) and indicate that single blastocyst transfer in young patients undergoing IVF with or without PGS led to comparably high embryo implantation and ongoing pregnancy rates.

Cryopreservation and SET

The practice of SET has put more emphasis on the performance of cryopreservation. If only one embryo is transferred (especially the case in younger patients) there will usually be several good quality embryos which are not replaced in the fresh cycle and can be frozen for later use. Freezing of supernumerary embryos has been in clinical practice since the mid 1980s. Until recently most cryopreservation methods involved slow freezing and slow thawing procedures with especially propanediol, dimethylsulfoxide (DMSO) or glycerol as the cryoprotectant. Embryos have been cryopreserved at different stages of development (fertilized oocytes, cleaved embryos, morulae and blastocysts). The replacement of frozen and thawed embryos resulted in a moderate number of additional pregnancies and the success of cryoprograms varied widely depending on several factors not least the stage and quality of embryos which were frozen. Recently vitrification has been introduced but, as is the case for PGS, we are still awaiting the outcome of properly designed studies to answer the question whether vitrification really is more successful than conventional freezing procedures [17].

ACKNOWLEDGEMENTS

I am grateful to Andy Williams, managing Editor of *Human Reproduction* for editing the text.

REFERENCES

1. B. C. Fauser and R. G. Edwards, The early days of IVF. *Hum. Reprod. Update*, **11** (2005), 437–438.

2. J. Cohen, A. Trounson, K. Dawson *et al.*, The early days of IVF outside the UK. *Hum. Reprod. Update*, **11** (2005), 439–460.

3. P. Devroey and A. Van Steirteghem, A review of ten years experience of ICSI. *Hum. Reprod. Update*, **10** (2004), 19–28.

4. K. Sermon, A. Van Steirteghem and I. Liebaers, Preimplantation genetic diagnosis. *Lancet*, **363** (2004), 1633–1641.

5. D. H. Barlow, A time for consensus and consistency of reporting in clinical studies and the importance of new basic research. *Hum. Reprod.*, **19** (2004), 1–2.

6. J. K. Min, S. A. Breheny, V. MacLachlan and D. L. Healy, What is the most relevant standard of success in assisted reproduction? The singleton, term gestation, live birth rate per cycle initiated: the BESST endpoint for assisted reproduction. *Hum. Reprod.*, **19** (2004), 3–7.

7. B. C. Fauser, P. Devroey and N. S. Macklon, Multiple birth resulting from ovarian stimulation for subfertility treatment. *Lancet*, **365** (2005), 1807–1816.

8. A. G. Sutcliffe and M. Ludwig, Outcome of assisted reproduction. *Lancet*, **370** (2007), 351–359.

9. F. Belva, S. Henriet, I. Liebaers *et al.*, Medical outcome of 8-year-old singleton ICSI children (born >or = 32 weeks' gestation) and a spontaneously conceived comparison group. *Hum. Reprod.*, **22** (2007), 506–515.

10. L. Leunens, S. Celestin-Westreich, M. Bonduelle, I. Liebaers and I. Ponjaert-Kristoffersen, Follow-up of cognitive and motor development of 10-year-old singleton children born after ICSI compared with spontaneously conceived children. *Hum. Reprod.*, **23** (2008), 105–111.

11. L. Van Landuyt, G. Verheyen, H. Tournaye *et al.*, New Belgian embryo transfer policy leads to sharp decrease in multiple pregnancy rate. *Reprod. Biomed. Online*, **13** (2006), 765–771.

12. T. della Ragione, G. Verheyen, E. Papanikolaou *et al.*, Developmental stage on day-5 and fragmentation rate on day-3 can influence the implantation potential of top-quality blastocysts in IVF cycles with single embryo transfer. *Reprod. Biol. Endocrinol.*, **5** (2007), 2.

13. E. G. Papanikolaou, E. M. Kolibianakis, H. Tournaye *et al.*, Live birth rates after transfer of equal number of blastocysts or cleavage-stage embryos in IVF.

A systematic review and meta-analysis. *Hum. Reprod.*, **23** (2008), 91–99.

14. H. J. Leese, R. G. Sturmey, C. G. Baumann and T. G. McEvoy, Embryo viability and metabolism: obeying the quiet rules. *Hum. Reprod.*, **22** (2007), 3047–3050.

15. C. Staessen, P. Platteau, E. Van Assche *et al.*, Comparison of blastocyst transfer with or without preimplantation genetic diagnosis for aneuploidy screening in couples with advanced maternal age: a prospective randomized controlled trial. *Hum. Reprod.*, **19** (2004), 2849–2858.

16. S. Mastenbroek, M. Twisk, J. van Echten-Arends *et al.*, In vitro fertilization with preimplantation genetic screening. *N. Engl. J. Med.*, **357** (2007), 9–17.

17. K. E. Loutradi, E. M. Kolibianakis, C. A. Venetis *et al.*, Cryopreservation of human embryos by vitrification or slow freezing: a systematic review and meta-analysis. *Fertil. Steril.*, **90**(1) (2008), 186–93. Epub 2007 Nov 5.

Index

Printed in the United States
by Baker & Taylor Publisher Services